AF758194

ANEURYSMS: TYPES, RISKS, FORMATION AND TREATMENT

ANEURYSMS: TYPES, RISKS, FORMATION AND TREATMENT

ALAIN LAURENT
AND
ETHAN MOREL
EDITORS

Nova Biomedical Books
New York

Copyright © 2009 by Nova Science Publishers, Inc.

All rights reserved. No part of this book may be reproduced, stored in a retrieval system or transmitted in any form or by any means: electronic, electrostatic, magnetic, tape, mechanical photocopying, recording or otherwise without the written permission of the Publisher.

For permission to use material from this book please contact us:
Telephone 631-231-7269; Fax 631-231-8175
Web Site: http://www.novapublishers.com

NOTICE TO THE READER

The Publisher has taken reasonable care in the preparation of this book, but makes no expressed or implied warranty of any kind and assumes no responsibility for any errors or omissions. No liability is assumed for incidental or consequential damages in connection with or arising out of information contained in this book. The Publisher shall not be liable for any special, consequential, or exemplary damages resulting, in whole or in part, from the readers' use of, or reliance upon, this material. Any parts of this book based on government reports are so indicated and copyright is claimed for those parts to the extent applicable to compilations of such works.

Independent verification should be sought for any data, advice or recommendations contained in this book. In addition, no responsibility is assumed by the publisher for any injury and/or damage to persons or property arising from any methods, products, instructions, ideas or otherwise contained in this publication.

This publication is designed to provide accurate and authoritative information with regard to the subject matter covered herein. It is sold with the clear understanding that the Publisher is not engaged in rendering legal or any other professional services. If legal or any other expert assistance is required, the services of a competent person should be sought. FROM A DECLARATION OF PARTICIPANTS JOINTLY ADOPTED BY A COMMITTEE OF THE AMERICAN BAR ASSOCIATION AND A COMMITTEE OF PUBLISHERS.

Aneurysms : types, risks, formation, and treatment / [edited by] Alain Laurent and Ethan Morel.
p. ; cm.
Includes bibliographical references and index.
ISBN 978-1-60741-557-2 (hardcover)
1. Aneurysms. I. Laurent, Alain, 1963- II. Morel, Ethan.
[DNLM: 1. Aneurysm. WG 580 A5978 2009]
RC693.A544 2009
616.1'33--dc22

2009029737

Published by Nova Science Publishers, Inc. ✦ New York

Contents

Preface

An aneurysm is a localized dilation of the wall of a blood vessel, usually caused by atherosclerosis and hypertension, or less frequently, by trauma, infection or a congenital weakness in the vessel wall. Aneurysms most commonly occur in arteries at the base of the brain and in the aorta. As the size of the aneurysm increases, there is an increased risk of rupture, which can result in severe hemorrhage and other complications including sudden death. This book describes different types of aneurysms, their causes, diagnosis and how they can be treated.

Chapter 1 - Cerebral aneurysm also known as intracranial aneurysm is a condition in which weakness of the wall of a cerebral artery causes a localized dilatation or ballooning of the blood vessel. Cerebral aneurysm is the most common cause of subarachnoid hemorrhage carrying a mortality rate as high as 50%.

The true incidence of intracranial aneurysm is very difficult to estimate, however, recent autopsy and angiography studies have indicated a prevalence of 2%, and the incidence can be much higher in patients with polycystic kidney disease, fibromuscular dysplasia, connective tissue disorders, arteriovenous malformation of the brain, coarctation of the aorta, hypertension, as well as atherosclerosis. The majority of cerebral aneurysms are the 'berry' type, which usually develops at the bifurcation of the major cerebral vessels of the circle of Willis where it is subjected to maximal hemodynamic stress and thus prone to the development of degenerative changes. Other rare types of aneurysm are mycotic or traumatic in origin.

For patients harboring aneurysms, the risk of rupture appears to be dependent on the size of the aneurysm and its location. Certainly, the risk of bleeding is higher in patients with multiple aneurysms or in those aneurysms that have already ruptured. Subarachnoid hemorrhage from a ruptured aneurysm carries a high mortality, and for those who survive the initial bleed, rebleeding and cerebral infarction are the major causes of death. Therefore, early diagnosis and treatment are essential to reduce the risk of further bleeding. Depending on the circumstances, a procedure to clip or coil the aneurysm may be recommended to prevent future rupture or rebleeding.

Chapter 2 - The diameter of the thoracic and abdominal aorta is central to predicting the risk for incident aortic aneurysms. In this regard, examination of significant risk factors for increasing diameter of the aorta is of scientific and clinical relevance. Accordingly, in this chapter, the authors will be discussing the epidemiology of aortic diameter using the results from two different studies that examined aortic diameter using computed tomography. Results from these studies suggest that age, sex, body mass index, and the presence and extent of calcified atherosclerosis in both the abdominal aorta and iliac arteries are significantly associated with increasing aortic diameter independent of the other cardiovascular disease risk factors. Finally, another data set indicates that the segment-specific variations in aortic diameter can potentially be used as a marker of vascular adaptation. The authors believe the findings described are important in understanding risk for early abdominal aortic dilatation, which may ultimately lead to aneurysmal formation.

Chapter 3 - Abdominal aortic aneurysms (AAAs) are a complex disease with a late age at onset. Causing approximately 15,000 deaths per year, AAAs are among the top twenty leading causes of death in the United States. A main reason for the high mortality rate of AAAs is that most are asymptomatic until rupture. Local inflammation of the aorta, fragmentation of the extracellular matrix and loss of smooth muscle cells are distinct characteristics of AAA formation. Large epidemiological studies have shown that smoking and positive family history are the two most important risk factors for AAAs. Other risk factors include male sex, increasing age, hypertension and high cholesterol. Interestingly, diabetes has a negative association with AAA. A genome-wide approach using DNA linkage analysis has found susceptibility loci for AAAs on chromosomes 19q13 and 4q31 and a genetic association study identified a variant on chromosome 9p21 associated with AAA in addition to other vascular phenotypes. Microarray-based expression profiles have also been generated to determine differentially expressed genes between AAA tissue and non-aneurysmal controls. These genetic and genomic approaches will be critical in determining the pathophysiological mechanisms leading to AAA formation, growth and rupture, and identifying the genetic factors predisposing to AAA later in life.

Chapter 4 - Abdominal aortic aneurysm (AAA) affects approximately 2—4% of the adult population and is the thirteenth leading cause of death in the United States. Patients are mostly asymptomatic but they can present with mild abdominal or back pain, distal embolization of thrombus, compression of ureters and hydronephrosis, pulsatile abdominal mass, as well as rupture, which is characterized by sudden-onset pain, hypotension, syncope, or sudden death. Risk factors for AAA formation and progression include cigarette smoking, hypertension, dyslipidemia, advancing age, male gender, and family history, while protective factors include African race, female gender, and diabetes mellitus. The pathophysiology of thoracic aortic aneurysms (TAA) is cystic medial degeneration, a non-inflammatory process. On the other hand, formation of AAA results from complex interactions between mural inflammation, proteolysis by matrix metalloproteinases, oxidative stress, apoptosis of smooth muscle cells, and neovascularization of the vasa vasorum. Ultrasonography is the method of choice for detection of AAA, while computerized tomography (CT) and magnetic resonance imaging (MRI) are the most frequently used methods for planning therapeutic strategies. Surgical treatment of AAA is generally reserved for larger (> 5 cm), rapidly expanding, or symptomatic aneurysms and consists of open versus endovascular aneurysm repair (EVAR). Although endovascular repair has lower short-term mortality, this does not translate into long-term survival difference. With increased understanding of the pathophysiology of AAA formation, new medications are being investigated for prevention of AAA and their progression, including angiotensin II inhibitors and statins. This review summarizes current knowledge of the incidence, pathophysiology, risk factors, natural history, and treatment of this increasingly more common pathology.

Chapter 5 - Endovascular repair is increasingly popular as a minimally invasive treatment option for patients with abdominal aortic aneurysms. Long-term durability and cost-effectiveness of this technology, however, are still in doubt. Essentially, the mechanical reliability of the exclusion of the aneurysm sac from blood flow and pressure depends on anatomical fit between endograft and aortic-iliac attachment zones and may be challenged over time by continuing aneurysmal degeneration. Failure of endograft seal is associated with the occurrence of endoleaks and graft migration, the need for repeated interventions and a small but continuing risk of re-pressurization of the aneurysm sac potentially leading to aortic rupture.

In this chapter the authors review the mechanical and biological challenges which are currently associated with endovascular abdominal aortic aneurysm repair. The authors discuss promising new approaches and their potential limitations. Clearly, multidisciplinary efforts will be indispensable to facilitate an integrated form of endovascular management including improved patient selection, dedicated stent graft design, pharmacological stabilization of the attachment zones and modulation of the biological background of the disease. Based on current evidence such a strategy has the best prospect of improving long-term durability and cost-effectiveness of endovascular repair and hopefully will eventually translate into optimized safety and quality of life for patients with the disease. Maybe even more importantly, such efforts have the potential to pave future ways for dedicated proteomic and genomic interventions to prevent the genesis of the disease at all in the large population of patients at risk.

Chapter 6 - Atherosclerosis is the most common cause of abdominal aortic aneurysm (AAA). Inflammatory abdominal aneurysm (IAAA), a variant of AAA, is characterized by dense fibrosis and extensive lymphoplasmacytic infiltration of the aortic wall, particularly its adventitia and surrounding connective tissue, and belongs to a spectrum of chronic periaortitis that includes retroperitoneal fibrosis and perianeurysmal retroperitoneal fibrosis. Recent studies disclosed that retroperitoneal fibrosis belongs to the IgG4-related diseases, characterized by numerous infiltrating IgG4-positive plasma cells and fibrosis, and high serum IgG4 concentrations. However, the relationship between IgG4-related diseases and IAAA remains unclarified. Our recent studies comparing IAAA with atherosclerotic AAA and IgG4-related diseases in other organs, showed that IAAA could be classified into 2 types: those aneurysms with IgG4-positive plasma cells (IgG4-related type), and those without (IgG4-unrelated type). All patients with atherosclerotic AAA had only a few IgG4-positive plasma cells. The IgG4-related type was characterized by marked lymphoplasmacytic infiltration with lymph follicle formation and inflammatory extension around nerve fibers, frequent infiltration of eosinophils, and inconspicuous infiltration of neutrophils compared with the IgG4-unrelated type. Obliterative phlebitis, which is found in patients with IgG4-related diseases in other organs, was observed in all cases of IgG4-related IAAA. These histopathological features were identical to those of IgG4-related diseases in other organs such as autoimmune pancreatitis. In addition, serum IgG4 concentrations were significantly higher in IgG4-related IAAA, suggesting it to be one of the IgG4-related diseases. Because some cases of retroperitoneal fibrosis and inflammatory IAAA belong to IgG4-related diseases, such cases are categorized as "IgG4-related chronic periaortitis".

Chapter 7 - The rupture of an arterial aneurysm during pregnancy is a rare event and can potentially be lethal. It is a difficult clinical situation with likely consequences for the maternal and fetal prognosis and it requires immediate and multidisciplinary treatment.

This chapter describes the physiopathology, clinical features, diagnostic methods and therapeutic principles of aneurysmal ruptures of the splenic, renal and ovarian arteries during pregnancy and postpartum.

In previous studies, it has been estimated that 50% of the ruptures of arterial aneurysms in women under 40 are linked to pregnancy [1]. Many elements suggest that pregnancy is involved in the formation and rupture of aneurysms. These mechanisms are still poorly understood, but it seems that the hemodynamic and hormonal modifications caused by the gestation are preponderant factors [2].

In a pregnant women, two-thirds of the ruptures of aneurysms happen during the third trimester and the postpartum period [3,4]. In the abdomen, these ruptures most often take place on the aorta, splenic artery, renal arteries, ovarian arteries [1] and uterine arteries.

Most of the aneurysms are asymptomatic until their rupture [5]. The clinical presentation of the rupture is nonspecific. When it happens during the third trimester of the pregnancy, the rupture of an aneurysm can be a dangerous trap and mislead the obstetrical team to a diagnosis of placental abruption or uterine rupture [2,3,6-8]. Ultrasound examination, CT scan and abdominal arteriography are the main diagnostic means to confirm the presence and the rupture of an aneurysm.

When the rupture happens at the end of the pregnancy and in the presence of signs of hemodynamic instability, resuscitation measures and the realisation of a caesarean section as a matter of urgency, together with an exploratory laparotomy, will have to be carried out without delay. As Pfannenstiel incision does not allow suitably satisfactory access to the sub-mesocolic level, a median longitudinal laparotomy will have to be realised immediately if there is an active hemorrhage causing hemodynamic instability and whose origin remains unexplained after exploring the sub-mesocolic level. The standard reference treatment remains the surgical resection of the aneurysm. Some authors report cases of selective embolisation of the sites of the ruptures, especially for aneurysms of the ovarian arteries [3,9,10]. This therapeutic option seems attractive when the symptomatology occurs during the postpartum period in a stable patient.

Chapter 8 - This review presents the current state and advances in endovascular embolization for the treatment of intracranial aneurysms (IA), including embolic materials, therapeutic and assisting techniques, long-term effectiveness, and limitations.

Over the last decade, endovascular treatment (EVT) of IA has made remarkable progress and has become widely used. EVT by means of detachable coils has been accepted as an alternative to surgical clipping for the treatment of unruptured and ruptured IA. Until recently, EVT was mostly applied in patients with small aneurysms with a small neck. Indeed, these aneurysms have a favorable anatomical configuration that prevents coil protrusion within the parent vessel as well as stable long-term anatomical results. In this particular subgroup of patients, EVT has the same efficacy as surgical clipping and it is associated with lower morbidity and mortality rates. Therefore, EVT is now considered as the first therapeutic option in these patients.

Thanks to the recent development of new endovascular techniques and tools, more and more IA are amenable to EVT. New coils, remodeling balloons, and self-expandable stents allow to treat complex IA including wide-necked aneurysms, fusiform aneurysms, and aneurysms with a branch arising from the neck or the sac. These new techniques have thus enlarged EVT indications but the question remains as to whether these techniques justify EVT as first-intention treatment in all IA. On a technical point of view, most IA are treatable by endovascular approach and EVT is no more limited to small aneurysms with a small neck. It also appears obvious that these techniques require a long learning curve and this may explain contradictory information within the literature about their associated complication rate. On a clinical point of view, EVT as first-line treatment seems a reasonable strategy that is associated with good clinical results. However, these new developments fail to circumvent the major limitation of EVT that remains the anatomical results stability. Among new techniques, intracranial stenting seems the most promising one because stents may induce intra-aneurysmal flow reduction and parent artery healing that might lead to aneurysm thrombosis without even "touching" the sac. For the first time in the history of IA treatment, a causal therapeutic approach – that is focused on the vessel wall defect – seems thus feasible. Therefore, stenting might be the next revolution of IA treatment, 15 years after the advent of detachable coils.

Chapter 9 - Coronary artery aneurysm/ectasia is rare, reported less than 5 % of coronary angiography. That might cause death because of thrombotic occlusion or rupture. The main cause of adult coronary aneurysm is atherosclerosis. Other cause may include Kawasaki disease, inflammatory and infectious arteritis, connective tissue disease, aortic dissection, congenital disease, and diagnostic or interventional coronary angiography. To estimate the etiology of the aneurysm, evaluating plaque component in the aneurysm is essential besides patients' history. Atherosclerotic coronary aneurysm contains yellow plaque by angioscopy and low density eccentric plaque by intravascular ultrasound (IVUS). Coronary artery aneurysms in patients with Kawasaki disease tend to have predominant egg-shell calcification. Recently, Multidetector row computed tomography (MDCT) is an excellent modality for detecting coronary artery disease with high accuracy compared to invasive coronary artery. Many previous reports mentioned that MDCT also can detect coronary anomalous condition. Also, coronary plaque is distinguishable by CT number. The authors developed color-coded analysis based on CT number, Plaque Map for tissue and plaque characterization. Using MDCT with Plaque Map, some kinds of aneurysm may be distinguished by their features, such as calcification and atherosclerotic plaque. The authors present a review of diagnostic imaging of coronary artery aneurysm by MDCT with Plaque Map and invasive plaque imaging, such as IVUS and angioscopy.

Chapter 10 - Coronary aneurysm is uncommon, but occasionally encountered in patients undergoing coronary angiography. Most coronary aneurysms are caused secondarily by atherosclerosis, Kawasaki disease and infectious emboli. Whereas the pathogenesis has not been entirely clarified, an inflammatory process is crucially involved. One of the earliest histopathological changes include granulomatous inflammation within the adventia and outer layers of the affected arteries, and gradual progression to a panarteritis with inflammatory mononuclear cell infiltration. Advential inflammation and subsequent neointimal proliferation promotes the destruction of the elastic lamina and tunica muscularis, leading to formation of aneurysms. At molecular levels, matrix metalloproteinases (MMPs) are up-regulated by chronic inflammation, and promote aneurysm formation through excessive proteolysis of extracellular matrix proteins. Recently, endothelial MMP-9 emerged as a coronary flow-sensitive effector for aneurysm formation. In this section, the authors will summarize the current view of the pathophysiology and management of coronary aneurysms.

Chapter 11 - Each year 15, 000 Americans die due exsanguination following rupture of an abdominal aortic aneurysm (AAA); it is the 13th leading cause of death in the U.S. The prevalence in screening studies is approximately 5% (Scott 1986). Surgical repair in the emergent situation is associated with high mortality rates of about 80%. Elective repair aims at prevention of death from haemorrhage. The UK small aneurysm trial in 1998 and the Aneurysm Detection and Management (ADAM) trial in 2002 have provided evidence that surveillance to an aneurysm diameter of 5.5cm is justified and patients should undergo surgical repair if aneurysms grow beyond this point. Nonetheless once the diagnosis abdominal aortic aneurysm is confirmed patients are at increased risk for cardiovascular death and should therefore be treated like patients with cardiovascular disease (Brady 2001, Norman 2004).

Chapter 12 - This paper considers four factors which could predispose an artery to false aneurysm (pseudoaneurysm) formation when it is cut. It then describes recent findings on the frequency of pseudoaneurysm formation during slaughter in livestock for meat consumption. Pseudoaneurysms can develop when carotid arteries are severed in cattle, calves and water buffalo, but not in sheep or goats. Bilateral carotid artery pseudoaneurysms occur in 7% of cattle slaughtered by shechita and 8% of cattle slaughtered by the halal method, and this can delay the onset of unconsciousness during the slaughter process. It is proposed that the main mechanism causing pseudoaneurysm formation in this situation is retraction of the artery within its connective tissue sheath. Blood leaving the severed end impregnates the sheath which swells as it becomes congested with blood. In some cases the swelling covers and occludes the severed end. This could have a protective effect during unintended injuries, but it creates complications during routine slaughter.

Chapter 13 - The pathogenesis of aortic aneurysms is linked to the presence of inflammatory diseases and smoking. In The Feiring Biopsy Study, the authors found a relatively high occurrence of chronic inflammatory cell infiltrates in deep vascular layers of the ascendant aorta of patients with coronary artery disease. The occurrence and extent of the infiltrates were more pronounced in patients with inflammatory rheumatic diseases (IRD) than non-IRD patients, in current cigarette smokers than non-smokers, and in patients with any history of aortic aneurysms compared to patients without aortic aneurysms. In theory, chronic vascular inflammation may be involved in aneurysm formation and also may contribute to aneurysm instability. Clinicians should be aware of the possibility to detect aortic inflammation using surgical specimens, but also of the pitfalls in the interpretation of the histological criteria of aortitis.

Chapter 14 - An aneurysm is an important complication of thromboembolic phenomena. This disorder is considered problematic and requires good medical management. This disorder can be seen in every country with different patterns. Here, the author will review and summarize the previous reports on aneurysms in Thailand. The epidemiology and clinical characteristics (diagnosis and treatment) as well as prevention will be discussed and conclusions will be reached.

Chapter 15 - Parasitic infestation is a common infectious disease that can be seen around the world. Parasitic infestation can bring several disorders to the host. An interesting complication of parasitic infestation is the formation of an aneurysm. It should be noted that there is a specific group of parasitic infestations that is classified as blood infection. These infections can directly involve the vessel, and an aneurysm can be a complication of these infections. The situation of heartworm infection and Chagas disease will be reviewed and presented.

In: Aneurysms: Types, Risks, Formation and Treatment
Editors: Alain Laurent and Ethan Morel
ISBN: 978-1-60741-557-2
© 2009 Nova Science Publishers, Inc.

Chapter 1

Aneurysms: Risks, Formation and Treatment

Wen-Shan Sung**, *Mei-Jo Sung and Jon Ho Chan
Royal Hobart Hospital and Menzies Research Institute, University of Tasmania, Hobart, Tasmania, Australia 7000

Abstract

Cerebral aneurysm also known as intracranial aneurysm is a condition in which weakness of the wall of a cerebral artery causes a localized dilatation or ballooning of the blood vessel. Cerebral aneurysm is the most common cause of subarachnoid hemorrhage carrying a mortality rate as high as 50%.

The true incidence of intracranial aneurysm is very difficult to estimate, however, recent autopsy and angiography studies have indicated a prevalence of 2%, and the incidence can be much higher in patients with polycystic kidney disease, fibromuscular dysplasia, connective tissue disorders, arteriovenous malformation of the brain, coarctation of the aorta, hypertension, as well as atherosclerosis. The majority of cerebral aneurysms are the 'berry' type, which usually develops at the bifurcation of the major cerebral vessels of the circle of Willis where it is subjected to maximal hemodynamic stress and thus prone to the development of degenerative changes. Other rare types of aneurysm are mycotic or traumatic in origin.

For patients harboring aneurysms, the risk of rupture appears to be dependent on the size of the aneurysm and its location. Certainly, the risk of bleeding is higher in patients with multiple aneurysms or in those aneurysms that have already ruptured. Subarachnoid hemorrhage from a ruptured aneurysm carries a high mortality, and for those who survive the initial bleed, rebleeding and cerebral infarction are the major causes of death. Therefore, early diagnosis and treatment are essential to reduce the risk of further bleeding. Depending on the circumstances, a procedure to clip or coil the aneurysm may be recommended to prevent future rupture or rebleeding.

*Correspondence to: Dr. Wen-Shan Sung; E-mail: wssung@gmail.com

Definition

A cerebral aneurysm (also known as intracranial or intracerebral aneurysm) is a focal outpouching of a cerebral blood vessel, which commonly arises from an arterial branching point, at the base of the brain, at or near the circle of Willis.

Epidemiology

Prevalence of Unruptured Cerebral Aneurysms

The prevalence, which is defined as the number of affected persons present in the population at a specific time divided by the number of persons in the population at that time, of unruptured cerebral aneurysms in a general population varies in the literature from approximately 1-5% (1). An extensive review of the prevalence of unruptured cerebral aneurysms revealed that the rate was dependent largely on the study design. Prevalence figures ranging from 0.4-6.0% are quoted in retrospective autopsy studies (0.4%), prospective autopsy studies (3.6%), retrospective angiography studies (3.7%), and prospective angiography studies (6.0%) respectively (2). The authors concluded that the prevalence of unruptured cerebral aneurysms in a general population without specific risk factors is about 2%; increasing with age (2). Adults with specific risk factors such as autosomal dominant polycystic kidney disease; a familial predisposition; and atherosclerosis have prevalence rates 2-4 times higher than the general population (2).

Incidence of Aneurysmal Subarachnoid Hemorrhage

Cerebral aneurysms can be life-threatening due to their propensity to rupture and are the most common cause of non-traumatic subarachnoid hemorrhage (SAH). SAH due to ruptures of intracranial aneurysms is a devastating event with high rates of morbidity and mortality (3). It accounts for approximately 4-5% of all strokes (4), but is responsible for 25% of all fatalities related to stroke (3). Its global mortality ranges from approximately 30-67% (5). Of those that survive a SAH, only less than 1/3 of patients regain their previous occupation and lifestyle (5). About 12% die before receiving any medical attention, and among those who reach a tertiary hospital, about 1/4 will die from complications of SAH or its treatment within 2 weeks (3, 6). The estimated annual incidence of SAH, which is defined as the estimated number of new cases of SAH that occur in a year, in a population at risk, is around 6-8 per 100 000 people, with females having a greater incidence than males (1.6:1) (7, 8). The incidence may even be higher in the Finnish and Japanese populations, as they are particularly prone to aneurysm development (9-11). Patients who have had an aneurismal SAH are also at increased risk of developing a new aneurysm in the future, and in this group of people, the annual incidence of a ruptured aneurysm is about 6 per 10 000, which is significantly higher than that of the general population (12, 13).

Common Sites

The majority of intracranial aneurysms, about 80%, are located in the anterior circulation, most commonly at the junction of the internal carotid and the posterior communicating arteries (i.e. the so-called posterior communicating artery aneurysm), the anterior communicating artery complex or the trifurcation of the middle cerebral artery in the Sylvain fissure. About 20% of aneurysms arise from the posterior circulation and they are commonly found at the bifurcation of the basilar artery or at the junction of a vertebral artery and the ispilateral posterior inferior cerebellar artery (14).

Pathogenesis of Cerebral Aneurysms

The cause or causes of cerebral aneurysms, how they form, grown and rupture are still yet to be clearly identified. However, there are many types of aneurysms. The most common type of aneurysm resulting in SAH is the saccular aneurysm, which is also known as a 'berry' aneurysm. These are small spherical dilations involving a portion of the arteries, and are often partially or completely filled with thrombus. Fusiform aneurysms are another form of aneurysm and they involve a longer segment of the arteries (15). Microscopically, the aneurysm, in particular the saccular aneurysm, has a defective wall. It has a thin or absent middle muscular layer of the artery (i.e. the tunica media), and also an absent or severely fragmented internal elastic layer (i.e. the internal elastic lamina). These defects, combined with hemodynamic stress, probably lead to the formation of aneurysms (14). Mycotic aneurysms are a rare type of aneurysm that results from the infection of a major artery and thus weakening of the arterial wall. It may originate either from embolization of a septic embolus; as an extension of an adjacent suppurative process; or from direct infection of circulating organisms (15).

Risk Factors

Several factors such as genetics and others are thought to contribute to the formation of aneurysms. Currently there is no definite hereditary basis to the development of intracranial aneurysms, however, there is considerable evidence to support it. The main supporting evidence is the association of cerebral aneurysms with heritable connective-tissue disorders and the familial occurrence of cerebral aneurysm. Cerebral aneurysms have been associated with numerous heritable connective tissue disorders, in particular polycystic kidney disease, Ehlers-Danlos syndrome type IV, Marfan's syndrome and neurofibromatosis type 1 (14, 16, 17). It has been estimated that about 5-40% of patients with autosomal dominant polycystic kidney disease have intracranial aneurysms, and about 10-30% of patients have multiple aneurysms (14). Although most cerebral aneurysms are sporadic (non-familial), familial forms had been described in the literature (14). It has been revealed that about 7-20% of patients with aneurysmal SAH have first or second degree relatives with a diagnosed cerebral aneurysm (6, 18-20).

The incidence of cerebral aneurysm increases with age. The incidence is low in the first two decades of life, however, it increases steadily after the third decade (2). Similarly increasing age has been found to be associated with an increasing risk of rupture, as shown in most of the literature (10, 21-23), however, increasing age may also have a protective effect despite this effect being only demonstrated in patients of extremely old age (23).

Intracranial aneurysms happen more commonly in women than in men. A recent meta-analysis revealed that the prevalence of aneurysms discovered on angiographic studies was 4.6% and 3.5% for women and men respectively (2). In respect to gender and rupture rate, studies have suggested that women may have a higher risk of aneurysm rupture than men, however, the data are inconclusive (2, 24, 25).

Hypertension is another modifiable risk factor that has been hypothesized in the literature as contributing to both the development and rupture of cerebral aneurysms. However, the literature has not clearly demonstrated a link (10, 26-28). In a large study, the prevalence of hypertension in patients with unruptured aneurysms compared to a random sample of hospitalized patients, was 43.2% and 34.4% respectively (25). Furthermore, hypertension was found to be a significant risk factor for future SAH, with a risk ratio of about 1.5 (25).

Natural History of Cerebral Aneurysms

Fortunately, most cerebral aneurysms are small (i.e. less than 10 mm in diameter, averaging 7.5 mm) as the literature suggests that the risk of rupture increases significantly when aneurysms are greater than 10 mm (21). A review revealed that the annual risk of rupture was approximately 1% in the cohort with small aneurysms and 4% in the group with larger ones (2). In the past, the traditional thought was that unruptured intracranial aneurysms pose a high risk of rupture of approximately 1-2% yearly (10, 26, 29, 30). A recent large retrospective study, the International Study of Unruptured Intracranial Aneurysms (ISUIA), challenged this thought and suggested a yearly rate of rupture of 0.05% for aneurysms less than 10 mm in diameter (1). Risk of rupture was about 10 times higher for patients with a history of bleeding aneurysms than those without such a history. Aneurysms larger than 10 mm in diameter and aneurysms of the basilar apex or posterior communicating artery had an even higher rate of rupture. However, this study was not without criticism. The most significant of which was related to the possibility of selection bias i.e. participants were selected in such a way that would create a population with a lower risk of rupture. Despite this criticism, subsequent studies have demonstrated higher risks of rupture for unruptured aneurysms (9, 11).

The rate of rupture may be affected by other factors, with the location of the aneurysm identified as being an important variable in the literature. Aneurysms located at the basilar bifurcation (22, 26), in the anterior (31) and posterior communicating artery locations (22, 26), appear to have a higher likelihood of rupture. Basilar artery aneurysms had a rupture rate of 42% whilst inferior cerebellar artery aneurysms were all less than 7% (26). The anterior communicating artery aneurysms were more than twice as likely to rupture than middle cerebral artery aneurysms and more than 1.5 times as likely as inferior cerebellar artery aneurysms (31). Similarly patients with multiple aneurysms had a higher risk of rupture compared to patients with a solitary aneurysm (2). Other factors such as age, gender and hypertension, as discussed previously, may also predispose patients to aneurysmal bleeding. Cigarette smoking, out of all the risk factors, has been consistently identified in the literature (14, 32). The risk of aneurysm rupture is approximately 3-10 times higher amongst smokers than non-smokers (14). A moderate-to-high level of alcohol consumption has been shown in the literature to be another risk factor for aneurysmal bleeds. This is particularly true in cases of binge drinking (14, 32, 33).

Signs and Symptoms

Most cerebral aneurysms remain asymptomatic until they rupture and cause a subarachnoid hemorrhage. Fortunately, as discussed previously, most aneurysms especially those less than 10 mm do not generally rupture. However, some cerebral aneurysms may become symptomatic because of a mass effect (34). Such aneurysms are often large or giant but not invariably so (35), and are commonly aneurysms of the posterior communicating artery (14). The common signs and symptoms of a mass effect may include any or all of: headache, third cranial nerve palsy or brain stem compression (14). Very rarely, patients with unruptured cerebral aneurysms may manifest with symptoms associated with cerebral ischemia possible due to embolization of an intra-aneurysmal thrombus (35, 36). Most patients with SAH present with an acute onset of severe headache, often being described as the "worst headache of my life" or "thunder-clap" headache. The headache is usually accompanied by nausea or vomiting, and in some cases loss of consciousness. Some patients may have an unusual acute prodromal headache, possibly the result of a minor leakage of blood into the wall of the aneurysm or into the subarachnoid space, preceding the hemorrhage by several days or weeks (37, 38). It is important to recognize these "warning leaks" in the diagnosis of cerebral aneurysms as delaying the diagnosis may lead to a catastrophic SAH. Other signs and symptoms of SAH include global or focal neurologic abnormalities depending on the location and severity of the SAH, meningism and intraocular hemorrhages. Anterior cerebral artery aneurysm rupture may cause transient bilateral lower extremity weakness. Rupture of middle cerebral artery aneurysm is more likely to be associated with hemiparesis, paresthesia, hemianopia, and dysphasia. Third nerve palsy or unilateral retro-orbital pain suggests an aneurysm arising at the junction of the internal carotid and posterior communicating arteries or aneurysms at the origin of the superior cerebellar artery (39).

Diagnosis

As most cerebral aneurysms are asymptomatic, diagnosis of them relies heavily on imaging techniques. Aneurysmal subarachnoid hemorrhage carries a poor prognosis, as discussed previously. The natural history of cerebral aneurysms is not well defined and the benefits of screening in the general population have not been quantified. However, screening has been evaluated as cost-effective in patients at high risk for the development of aneurysms. Patients most commonly screened are those with a family history of intracranial aneurysms and those with autosomal dominant polycystic kidney disease (14). The three main imaging methods are discussed here: computed tomography, magnetic resonance imaging, and cerebral angiography by direct intra-arterial catheterization.

Comupted Tomography

Standard cranial CT without enhancement has generally been the first imaging method for the investigation of patients with suspected SAH. However, standard CT with or without enhancement cannot reliably detect the presence of unruptured cerebral aneurysms, as most CT scanner obtains slices with a thickness of 5-10 mm (40, 41). CT angiography (CTA) on the other hand may detect aneurysms as small as 2-3 mm and are more reliable in delineating the size and morphological features of a cerebral aneurysm (42). CTA provides software-generated 3D images from contrast-enhanced blood vessels. It is shown to have a sensitivity of 97% and a specificity of 87 to 100% (42). Its use has been indicated in patients with partially clipped aneurysms, recent treatment with endovascular techniques, and in conservative follow-ups (43-46). It has also been suggested as a screening tool for high-risk populations (40, 47-49). It is important to note that CTA, like other forms of angiography, carries its own risks. These risks include cerebral infarction, the formation of a hematoma or pseudo-aneurysm at the puncture site, and exacerbation or precipitation of renal failure. The risks are particularly high in elderly patients with severe atherosclerotic disease (14).

Magnetic Resonance Imaging

Magnetic resonance angiography (MRA) is useful in locating aneurysms of 3 to 5 mm (49-53). It is both highly sensitive (69-99%) and specific (100%) (49-53). MRA takes considerably longer to perform compared with CTA and is therefore not suitable for critically ill patients. However, MRA may be useful in detecting changes in the size of aneurysms over time or as a screening tool for patients with previously treated cerebral aneurysms (54). Standard magnetic resonance imaging (MRI) is the best method of detecting the presence of a thrombus within aneurysms that were not seen on standard angiography (4-vessel view) on several instances (55). Furthermore, MRA alone is rarely sufficient for surgical planning (14).

Catheter Angiography

Catheter angiography (CA) can produce higher quality images and is still considered the gold standard in the diagnosis of cerebral aneurysms (56-58). However, it is invasive and is more expensive than either CTA or MRA. Therefore, CA is not recommended as the first approach in the evaluation of suspected unruptured aneurysms. CA has been shown to be associated with a risk of local complications (e.g. groin hematomas, femoral artery injury) of 5%, and neurologic complications of 1% (with permanent impairment in 0.1-0.5% of patients) (13, 59). Similarly to CTA, the risk of complications increase in elderly patients with atherosclerotic vessels (14).

Aneurysmal Hemorrhage

A head CT scan without contrast is the initial diagnostic test of choice for a suspected bleeding aneurysm. It is highly sensitive if done within three days of the hemorrhage and is especially sensitive (i.e. revealing hemorrhages in about 90-95% of cases) if done within 24 hours (60, 61). After this interval, the sensitivity of CT decreases with time. In some cases, despite a normal CT scan, if a strong clinical suspicion of a SAH remains, then a lumber puncture is usually indicated. Even if the cerebrospinal fluid (CSF) is bloodstained, it may still be a result of a traumatic lumber tap as opposed to a true SAH. The "three tube test" (a decrease in the red cell count in the CSF samples from the first to the last tube) is an unreliable method of excluding a SAH (62). Xanthochromia (yellow discoloration of the CSF after centrifugation) of the supernatant, however, is diagnostic of SAH (62). It is formed by the sufficient lysis of red blood cells circulating in the CSF over an appropriate period of time. A lumber puncture done too soon after the SAH may therefore fail to show xanthochromia. Xanthochromia is best detected using spectrophotometry, and will be shown in all patients with SAH of 12 hour to 2 weeks old (62). MRI is not sensitive in detecting acute hemorrhage, however, may be useful in detecting subacute or chronic SAH, long after the findings of CT scan have become normal (63).

Management of Unruptured Aneurysms

The overall risk of SAH from an unruptured aneurysm is reported to be 1-2% per year, with the median time between discovery of an aneurysm and subsequent rupture being estimated to be 9.6 years (22, 24, 27, 64). The clinical risk of bleeding from an unruptured aneurysm is different from an aneurysm that has already ruptured, therefore, the management of unruptured aneurysms would also be different in the setting of aneurysmal SAH. At the moment there is still debate with regards to the optimal treatment of unruptured aneurysms. Therefore, each individual patient must be carefully evaluated weighing up the risk of rupture versus the risk of treatment by either surgical clipping and/or endovascular coiling. The risk of rupture must outweigh the risk of any treatment modality for treatment to be instituted.

In each individual, the annual risk of rupture depends on patient factors as well as aneurysm characteristics. In view of the patient factors, there is an increased risk of aneurysmal SAH if the patients has: (i) family history of aneurysms, (ii) history of previous SAH from a separate aneurysm, (iii) advanced age, (iv) female sex, (v) cigarette smoking, (vi) hypertension, and (vii) binge alcohol drinking (2, 22, 32, 65). Several characteristics of aneurysms have been shown to be associated with an increased risk of rupture: (i) large aneurysm size, (ii) location within the posterior circulation, (iii) morphological appearance, especially the presence of a daughter sac or a large aneurysm angle, (iv) symptomatic aneurysm, (v) aneurysms associated with arteriovenous malformations, and (vi) enlarging aneurysms on follow-up imaging (10, 22, 27, 66, 67). Of all the factors mentioned above, aneurysm size is the most important predictor of future rupture. In a large, retrospective study of unruptured intracranial aneurysms conducted in multiple centers internationally, the annual risk of rupture of aneurysms that were less than 10 mm in diameter at diagnosis was less than 0.05% per year (22). In contrast, the rupture rate of aneurysms that were 10 mm or more in diameter was approximately 1% per year (22).

The surgical outcome after repair of unruptured aneurysms has been described in several study series, and most of them demonstrated a mortality ranging from 0-1% and a morbidity ranging from 2-7.3% (68, 69). Once again, aneurysm size is the most important factor with regards to the likely surgical outcome and possibility of complications with an operative morbidity of 2.3% for aneurysms smaller than 5 mm, 6.8% for aneurysms between 6-15 mm, and 14% for aneurysms larger than 16 mm (70). The association between increased aneurysm size and a poorer surgical outcome may be explained by a poorer technical result requiring multiple clips, a wider aneurysm neck, and calcification within the aneurysm neck. Also the morbidity can vary with the location of the aneurysm. A meta-analysis of 2460 patients found that the repair of unruptured non-giant posterior circulation aneurysms has an almost 10-fold increase in surgical risk when compared with similar-sized lesions in the anterior circulation (71). Of all the posterior circulation aneurysms, a basilar bifurcation aneurysm is associated with the greatest surgical risk (70, 71). Similarly, within the anterior circulation an aneurysm of the anterior communicating artery and the bifurcation of the internal carotid artery appears to have the greatest risk (70, 71). Furthermore, patient-related factors such as advanced age, history of cerebrovascular disease, diabetes, and other concurrent medical conditions may also increase the surgical risks associated with unruptured aneurysms.

The management goal of unruptured aneurysms is to prevent future rupture and subsequent aneurysmal SAH. In general, surgical clipping appears be a preferable method to occlude aneurysms as the current literature suggests that endovascular coiling plays a limited role in the setting of unruptured aneurysms, as complete aneurysm occlusion can only be achieved in half of patients, and thus aneurysm recurrence rate is high (72). However, endovascular therapy has the potential advantage in elderly patients with multiple co-morbid medical conditions, or in patients where there may be surgical difficulty due to the location of the aneurysms. Furthermore, it has become clear that not everyone with an unruptured aneurysm should be actively treated, as there are times when any form of treatment may provide more harm than benefit. Therefore, the most important question to be asked is: *Who should be treated?* A thorough understanding of the natural history, surgical risk, life expectancy, as well as alternative treatments for an unruptured aneurysm is required to make an informed decision. Based on the available evidence and research, we believe that patients with unruptured aneurysms with the following characteristics should be treated (54, 73): previous SAH due to another aneurysm, symptomatic aneurysm, family history of aneurysm or SAH, aneurysm larger than 10 mm, or aneurysm measuring 6-9 mm in young and middle-aged patients. Patients with aneurysms smaller than 6 mm should undergo periodic follow-up with angiography and be treated if the lesion enlarges or change configuration. Treating preventable risk factors such as hypertension, cigarette smoking, and alcohol binge drink is also important to minimize the chance of aneurysm rupture (32, 33, 65).

Management of Ruptured Aneurysms

Patients suffering from a ruptured intracranial aneurysm have a mortality rate of approximately 45% and among those surviving the initial hemorrhage treated without surgery, rebleeding is the major cause of subsequent death and severe disability (5, 74, 75). Therefore, aneurysm obliteration to prevent rebleeding is essential to the successful management of SAH. The management of patients following the rupture of an aneurysm is invariably more complicated, and can be broadly divided into three stages: immediate, short-term, and long-term management.

Immediate Management

The aim of initial management is to assess the severity of SAH and to stabilize the patient's clinical condition. The initial emergency care after rupture would include: assessment of airway patency, breathing, and circulatory function. A complete neurological assessment including conscious level, cranial nerves and sensory, motor function will help to determine if urgent surgical interventions such as extraventricular drainage device insertion, or evacuation of intracranial hematoma are required. Patients should be admitted to an intensive care unit with vigilant care and monitoring. Typical admitting orders are listed below (39, 76):

- Bed rest with bed head elevation of 30° until aneurysm obliteration,
- Placement within a darkened room, restriction of visitation, and avoidance of unnecessary sensory stimulation,
- Vital signs and neurological assessment hourly,
- Nil by mouth in preparation for early surgery; if not then oral clear fluids only,
- Strict fluid intake and output, and daily monitoring of body weight,
- Venous thromboembolism prevention with intermittent pneumatic compression stockings,
- Indwelling Foley catheter insertion if patient is bedridden or unable to void,
- Intravenous normal saline with 20 mmol KCl/L at 125-150 ml/hour to gently expand the intravenous volume and to elevate blood pressure (systemic BP 120-150 mmHg) which can minimize the effect of vasospasm and cerebral salt wasting,
- Intubation and ventilation in patients who are obtunded or unable to protect their airway,
- Pulmonary artery catheter insertion in poor grade patients (Hunt and Hess grade > 3), and in patients with severe cardiopulmonary disease, or hemodynamic instability,
- Cardiac rhythm monitoring as arrhythmias may occur following SAH,
- Intraventricular catheter for intracranial pressure monitoring and drainage in the settings of acute hydrocephalus, the presence of significant intraventricular blood, or poor clinical grading; drain for pressure of >20mmHg until aneurysm obliteration and then for pressure >5-10 mmHg,
- Phenytoin for seizure prophylaxis along with mild sedation if required,

- Pain relief with analgesics such as fentanyl, morphine, or codeine,
- Histamine-2 blockers or proton pump inhibitors to reduce the risk of stress induced gastric ulcers,
- Stool softeners in patients who tolerate oral intake,
- Calcium channel blockers should be initiated within 4 days of SAH for vasospasm neuroprotection, and the duration of treatment is ~21 days or until the patient is discharged home in good neurological condition.

Short-Term Management

After initial stabilization, the next stage of management would be deciding the appropriate treatment of the ruptured aneurysm for the individual patient. There are two important questions to consider: (i) *When should the surgery be performed?* and (ii) *Should this patient undergo surgical or endovascular aneurysm occlusion?*

The timing of aneurysm obliteration is critical in obtaining an optimal result following SAH. Controversy exists between "early surgery" (defined as less than 2-4 days post SAH) and "late surgery" (usually more than 10-14 days post SAH). In the past, many neurosurgeons believed that a better operative result could be achieved if the surgery is delayed because (i) brain edema is often severe immediately after SAH, therefore, requiring more brain retraction during the surgery, (ii) the presence of solid clots that have not had time to lyse can hamper the surgery, and (iii) the risk of intra-operative aneurysm rupture is higher with early surgery (76). However, it is now increasingly recognized that early surgery is associated with an improved outcome as it virtually eliminates the risk of rebleeding and also facilitates the preventative treatment of vasospasm by allowing early introduction of hypertensive hypervolemic therapy without danger of aneurysm rupture (77). Although there is a general trend towards a better outcome with early surgery than with late surgery, delaying surgery may still be preferable for complex lesions such as giant aneurysms or in patients with medical comorbidity and advanced age (73, 76, 78). Recent advances in endovascular therapy have allowed this technique to become a viable alternative approach for the early treatment of ruptured aneurysms. The potential advantage of endovascular therapy is that it is less physically stressful as brain retraction and vessel dissection are not required. Consequently, it may be the preferred treatment choice in some poor-grade patients where extensive cerebral edema is seen on CT, or when intracranial pressure is uncontrollable, or in the situation where technical difficulty is anticipated due to the location of the aneurysm (73). Endovascular aneurysm occlusion may even be considered as a primary treatment in elderly patients for whom long-term coil stability may be less relevant (79). It is also important to note that several factors may limit the success of the endovascular procedure. It appears that only about 50% of ruptured aneurysms can be completely occluded using endovascular techniques (72, 80). Large aneurysm size, a wide aneurysm neck, and aneurysm morphology with dome-to-neck ratio less than 2 account for the majority of incomplete aneurysm occlusions, thereby increasing the risk of aneurysm recurrence and rebleed (81-83).

In general, treatment should be instituted as soon as possible after the cerebral angiogram. Surgical clip ligation remains the conventional therapy for many ruptured aneurysms. The endovascular approach can be considered as a complement to surgical techniques in the settings of medical contraindication, anticipated surgical difficulty, and in some instances, the primary treatment for selected aneurysms. The decision as to whether an aneurysm should be clipped or coiled is best made jointly by neurovascular surgeons and interventional neuroradiologists. The careful study of imaging is essential to determine the aneurysm size and configuration as well as the relationship between the aneurysm and surrounding structures, as this can be closely associated with the success and risk of either endovascular or surgical treatment. Finally, in situations where both early surgery and endovascular therapy are contraindicated, most neurosurgeons would agree to delay surgery to a later date when a clinical improvement has been observed.

Long-Term Management and Complication Prevention

Aggressive care and monitoring should be established soon after securing the aneurysm. In the postoperative period, several problems may arise as a result of SAH, and the goal of the "long-term" management is to treat and to prevent the potential complications. Here we have described 4 commonly encountered complications associated with SAH: (i) vasospasm, (ii) hydrocephalus, (iii) hyponatremia and hypovolemia, and (iv) cardiovascular abnormalities.

Vasospasm of the cerebral arteries is the major cause of preventable death and disability in patients surviving SAH, and it may even exceed the direct effects of aneurysmal rupture or rebleeding. The overall incidence of angiographic vasospasm after SAH is roughly 50%, one half of this group would become symptomatic, and one half of these symptomatic patients would die of ischemic infarction (84, 85). The onset of vasospasm generally begins 2-3 days after the initial hemorrhage, peaking in incidence during day 6-8, and rarely delayed beyond 14 days (84, 86). Once angiographic vasospasm has been demonstrated, it usually resolves slowly over the next 3-4 weeks (87). The exact pathogenesis of vasospasm is poorly understood, but it is certainly related to vasoconstrictor substances in the CSF as a result of hemorrhage (88). There appears to be a direct correlation between the amount and location of subarachnoid blood seen on the CT scan and the risk and distribution of vasospasm (89). Several other factors such as poor neurological condition on admission, cigarette smoking, history of preexisting hypertension, and advanced age can also predispose to vasospasm (87, 90, 91). In view of the treatment of vasospasm, early surgery can provide the neurosurgeon the opportunity to reduce subarachnoid clots, which may be useful in reducing the risk of vasospasm. Furthermore, it eliminates the risk of rebleeding by excluding aneurysms from the circulation, and also facilitates the treatment of vasospasm by permitting the safe use of hyperdynamic therapy (also known as the 'triple H therapy': hypertension, hypervolemia, and hemodilution) to overcome hypoperfusion (92). In addition, recent studies have shown promising results with the prophylactic use of calcium channel blockers (e.g. nimodipine and nifedipine), and nowadays they have been frequently used in SAH to prevent vasospasm, although there is still some doubt as to whether their effects are due to their action on cerebral blood vessels or due to a "brain protection" effect (93).

Hydrocephalus after SAH has been observed in approximately 20% of patients, and 3% of those without ventricular dilatation on initial CT may develop hydrocephalus within 1 week (94). Acute hydrocephalus is more likely to occur with increasing age, preexisting or postoperative hypertension, intraventricular hemorrhage, diffuse SAH, focal thick SAH, posterior circulation aneurysms, and poor clinical grading on admission (95). Among these predisposing factors, intraventricular hemorrhage and a larger volume of subarachnoid clots have been shown to be the most important predictors of acute hydrocephalus (96). The pathogenesis of ventricular dilatation is related to CSF flow blockade through the Sylvian aqueduct, fourth ventricle outlet, or subarachnoid space, or to the interference of CSF reabsorption at the arachnoid granulations. Insertion of a ventricular drain is usually indicated in patients with a depressed level of consciousness or increased ICP (94). There is probably an increased risk of aneurysmal rebleeding in patients undergoing ventriculostomy shortly after SAH because ventricular drainage may increase the transmural pressure gradient across the aneurysmal wall leading to subsequent rupture (94, 97). Therefore, recommendations exist that when a ventriculostomy is performed, ICP should be kept within the range of 15-25 mmHg to avoid rapid pressure reduction (98). If a drain is not placed preoperatively, it is usually inserted at the time of surgery to achieve optimal brain relaxation, then the catheter is left in place postoperatively to monitor ICP, to drain CSF as necessary, and to administer fibrinolytic agents if indicated (99). Instances where the catheter cannot be removed within 7 day of insertion due to uncontrolled ICP or when chronic hydrocephalus has developed, permanent diversion of CSF with a ventriculoperitoneal shunt is required (100).

Hyponatremia and hypovolemia frequently ensure following a SAH as a result of natriuresis and diuresis. It had been formerly postulated that hyponatremia in SAH patients was a result of the syndrome of inappropriate secretion of antidiuretic hormone (SIADH) as this condition had been reported in association with other neurological conditions and ADH has been identified in SAH-related hyponatremia (101). However, the ADH increment in the post SAH period is usually transient, lasting only about 4 days whereas hyponatremia usually develops on average 7 days after SAH (102). Furthermore, up to 50% of patients suffering SAH may become volume depleted with the administration of maintenance fluids, which is not consistent with SIADH (103). Therefore the negative sodium and fluid balance has now been attributed to a condition called "cerebral salt wasting" in which there is a urinary loss of sodium as a result of intracranial disease producing hyponatremia and a decrease in extracellular fluid volume. The actual mechanism whereby the kidney fails to retain sodium in cerebral salt wasting in unknown, and may be either a result of a yet to be identified natriuretic factor or a direct neural control mechanism (104, 105). Factors that may increase the risk of hyponatremia after SAH include: history of diabetes, congested heart failure, cirrhosis, adrenal insufficiency, or the use of specific drugs such as non-steroidal anti-inflammatories, narcotics, and thiazide diuretics (76). It is important to note that patients with aneurysmal SAH can have cerebral salt wasting with hyponatremia that mimics SIADH. In this setting, fluid restriction may be hazardous since dehydration increases blood viscosity which exacerbates vasospasm induced ischemia (106). The principle of fluid and sodium management is to make an accurate diagnosis and the key differentiating feature between SIADH and salt wasting is volume status. The goal of treatment is to replace water and sodium deficit with normal saline and supplemental oral salt, or hypertonic saline in order to maintain at least normovolemia and normal serum sodium. Extra caution must be taken in correcting hyponatremia as rapid inordinate sodium replacement carries the risk of central pontine myelinolysis (107).

Almost all patients with SAH develop some type of cardiovascular abnormality. The most common are electrocardiogram (ECG) changes and cardiac arrhythmia. The possible mechanism for its occurrence may be due to the cerebral vasospasm induced hypothalamic ischemia leading to an increased sympathetic tone with a resultant catecholamine surge producing subendocardial ischemia or coronary artery spasm (108, 109). Occasionally, SAH may produce a condition called "stunned myocardium" which appears compatible with a myocardial infarction on ECG, yet enzymes are negative and it is reversible in most cases before progressing on to an actual acute myocardial infarction (109). Patients with SAH should have continuous cardiac monitoring as well as frequent monitoring of electrolytes, particularly potassium. Hypokalemia should be avoided because it may aggravate arrhythmia and has been associated with prolonged QT interval, ventricular fibrillation, and torsades de pointes (110). Although, a double-blinded, randomized trial has demonstrated less cardiac related death and a better outcome with adrenergic blockade, this treatment has not been widely used, probably because it is at odds with other reports demonstrating that antihypertensive treatment worsens outcomes post SAH (111).

Conclusion

Patients with ruptured aneurysms, the appropriate selection of surgical or endovascular occlusion requires a collaborative approach between neurosurgeons and neuroradiologists and an understanding of the anatomical and physiological characteristics of both techniques. The selection of one treatment over another often requires consideration of patient- and aneurysm-specific factors. Complete aneurysm occlusion effectively prevents rebleeding, but outcome optimization also requires ongoing vigilant care and monitoring to facilitate the early detection of complications and the institution of appropriate treatment for them. It is hoped that optimal neurosurgical and medical care will improve the outcome of patients suffering aneurysmal SAH.

References

[1] Wiebers, DO; Whisnant, JP; Huston, J; 3rd, Meissner, I; Brown, RD; Jr., Piepgras, DG; et al. Unruptured intracranial aneurysms: natural history, clinical outcome, and risks of surgical and endovascular treatment. *Lancet*, 2003, Jul., 12, 362(9378), 103-10.

[2] Rinkel, GJ; Djibuti, M; Algra, A; Van Gijn, J. Prevalence and risk of rupture of intracranial aneurysms: a systematic review. *Stroke*, 1998 Jan., 29(1), 251-6.

[3] Ferro, JM; Canhao, P; Peralta, R. Update on subarachnoid haemorrhage. *J Neurol*, 2008 Apr., 255(4), 465-79.

[4] Ingall, TI; Wiebers, DO. Natural history of subarachnoid hemorrhage. In: Whisnant JP, editor. Stroke: Populations, Cohorts, and Clinical Trials. *Boston*: Butterworth-Heinemann Ltd., 1993, p. 174-86.
[5] Hop, JW; Rinkel, GJ; Algra, A; Van Gijn, J. Case-fatality rates and functional outcome after subarachnoid hemorrhage: a systematic review. *Stroke*, 1997, Mar., 28(3), 660-4.
[6] Schievink, WI; Wijdicks, EF; Parisi, JE; Piepgras, DG; Whisnant, JP. Sudden death from aneurysmal subarachnoid hemorrhage. *Neurology*, 1995 May, 45(5), 871-4.
[7] Linn, FH; Rinkel, GJ; Algra, A; Van Gijn, J. Incidence of subarachnoid hemorrhage: role of region, year, and rate of computed tomography: a meta-analysis. *Stroke*, 1996 Apr., 27(4), 625-9.
[8] Epidemiology of aneurysmal subarachnoid hemorrhage in Australia and New Zealand: incidence and case fatality from the Australasian Cooperative Research on Subarachnoid Hemorrhage Study (ACROSS). *Stroke*, 2000 Aug., 31(8), 1843-50.
[9] Tsutsumi, K; Ueki, K; Morita, A; Kirino, T. Risk of rupture from incidental cerebral aneurysms. *J Neurosurg*, 2000 Oct., 93(4), 550-3.
[10] Juvela, S; Porras, M; Heiskanen, O. Natural history of unruptured intracranial aneurysms: a long-term follow-up study. *J Neurosurg*, 1993 Aug., 79(2), 174-82.
[11] Juvela, S; Porras, M; Poussa, K. Natural history of unruptured intracranial aneurysms: probability of and risk factors for aneurysm rupture. *J Neurosurg*, 2000 Sep., 93(3), 379-87.
[12] Miller, CA; Hill, SA; Hunt, WE. "De novo" aneurysms. A clinical review. *Surg Neurol*, 1985 Aug., 24(2), 173-80.
[13] Rinne, JK; Hernesniemi, JA. De novo aneurysms: special multiple intracranial aneurysms. *Neurosurgery*, 1993 Dec., 33(6), 981-5.
[14] Schievink, WI. Intracranial aneurysms. *N Engl J Med.*, 1997 Jan., 2, 336(1), 28-40.
[15] Schoen, FJ. Blood vessels. In: Kumar V, Abbas AK, Fausto N, editors. Robbins and Cotran Pathologic Basis of Disease. 7th ed. Philadephia: *Saunders*, 2005, p. 511-54.
[16] Schievink, WI; Michels, VV; Piepgras, DG. Neurovascular manifestations of heritable connective tissue disorders. *A review. Stroke*, 1994, Apr., 25(4), 889-903.
[17] Schievink, WI; Schaid, DJ; Rogers, HM; Piepgras, DG; Michels, VV. On the inheritance of intracranial aneurysms. *Stroke*, 1994 Oct., 25(10), 2028-37.
[18] Norrgard, O; Angquist, KA; Fodstad, H; Forsell, A; Lindberg, M. Intracranial aneurysms and heredity. *Neurosurgery*, 1987 Feb., 20(2), 236-9.
[19] Ronkainen, A; Hernesniemi, J; Ryynanen, M. Familial subarachnoid hemorrhage in east Finland, 1977-1990. *Neurosurgery,* 1993 Nov., 33(5), 787-96; discussion 96-97.
[20] De Braekeleer, M; Perusse, L; Cantin, L; Bouchard, JM; Mathieu, J. A study of inbreeding and kinship in intracranial aneurysms in the Saguenay Lac-Saint-Jean region (Quebec, Canada). *Ann Hum Genet*, 1996 Mar., 60(Pt 2), 99-104.
[21] Wiebers, DO; Whisnant, JP; Sundt, TM; Jr., O'Fallon, WM. The significance of unruptured intracranial saccular aneurysms. *J Neurosurg*, 1987 Jan., 66(1), 23-9.
[22] Unruptured intracranial aneurysms--risk of rupture and risks of surgical intervention. International Study of Unruptured Intracranial Aneurysms Investigators. *N Engl J Med.*, 1998 Dec 10, 339(24), 1725-33.

[23] Weir, B. Aneurysms Affecting the Nervous System. Baltimore: *Williams & Wilkins*, 1987.

[24] Juvela, S. Natural history of unruptured intracranial aneurysms: risks for aneurysm formation, growth, and rupture. *Acta Neurochir Suppl.*, 2002, 82, 27-30.

[25] Taylor, CL; Yuan, Z; Selman, WR; Ratcheson, RA; Rimm, AA. Cerebral arterial aneurysm formation and rupture in 20,767 elderly patients: hypertension and other risk factors. *J Neurosurg*, 1995 Nov., 83(5), 812-9.

[26] Wiebers, DO; Whisnant, JP; O'Fallon, WM. The natural history of unruptured intracranial aneurysms. *N Engl J Med.*, 1981 Mar 19, 304(12), 696-8.

[27] Asari, S; Ohmoto, T. Natural history and risk factors of unruptured cerebral aneurysms. *Clin Neurol Neurosurg*, 1993 Sep., 95(3), 205-14.

[28] Brown, RD; Jr., Huston, J; Hornung, R; Foroud, T; Kallmes, DF; Kleindorfer, D; et al. Screening for brain aneurysm in the Familial Intracranial Aneurysm study: frequency and predictors of lesion detection. *J Neurosurg*, 2008 Jun., 108(6), 1132-8.

[29] Mount, LA; Brisman, R. Treatment of multiple aneurysms--symptomatic and asymptomatic. *Clin Neurosurg*, 1974, 21, 166-70.

[30] Winn, HR; Almaani, WS; Berga, SL; Jane, JA; Richardson, AE. The long-term outcome in patients with multiple aneurysms. Incidence of late hemorrhage and implications for treatment of incidental aneurysms. *J Neurosurg*, 1983 Oct., 59(4), 642-51.

[31] Inagawa, T; Hada, H; Katoh, Y. Unruptured intracranial aneurysms in elderly patients. *Surg Neurol*, 1992 Nov., 38(5), 364-70.

[32] Juvela, S; Hillbom, M; Numminen, H; Koskinen, P. Cigarette smoking and alcohol consumption as risk factors for aneurysmal subarachnoid hemorrhage. *Stroke*, 1993 May, 24(5), 639-46.

[33] Longstreth, WT; Jr., Nelson, LM; Koepsell, TD; Van Belle, G. Cigarette smoking, alcohol use, and subarachnoid hemorrhage. *Stroke*, 1992 Sep., 23(9), 1242-9.

[34] Connolly, ES; Solomon, RA. Management of unruptured aneurysms. In: Le Roux PD, Winn HR, Newell DW, editors. Management of cerebral aneurysms. Philadelphia: *Saunders,* 2004, p. 271-85.

[35] Raps, EC; Rogers, JD; Galetta, SL; Solomon, RA; Lennihan, L; Klebanoff, LM; et al. The clinical spectrum of unruptured intracranial aneurysms. *Arch Neurol*, 1993, Mar., 50(3), 265-8.

[36] Przelomski, MM; Fisher, M; Davidson, RI; Jones, HR; Marcus, EM. Unruptured intracranial aneurysm and transient focal cerebral ischemia: a follow-up study. *Neurology*, 1986 Apr., 36(4), 584-7.

[37] Leblanc, R. The minor leak preceding subarachnoid hemorrhage. *J Neurosurg*, 1987, Jan., 66(1), 35-9.

[38] Ostergaard, JR. Headache as a warning symptom of impending aneurysmal subarachnoid haemorrhage. *Cephalalgia*, 1991, Feb., 11(1), 53-5.

[39] MacDonald, RL; Weir, B. Perioperative management of subarachnouid hemorrhage. In: Winn HR, editor. Youmans Neurological Surgery. 5th ed. Philadelphia: *W. B. Saunders*, 2004, p. 1813-37.

[40] Hsiang, JN; Liang, EY; Lam, JM; Zhu, XL; Poon, WS. The role of computed tomographic angiography in the diagnosis of intracranial aneurysms and emergent aneurysm clipping. *Neurosurgery*, 1996 Mar., 38(3), 481-7 discussion 7.

[41] Findlay, JM. Current management of aneurysmal subarachnoid hemorrhage guidelines from the Canadian Neurosurgical Society. *Can J Neurol Sci.*, 1997 May, 24(2), 161-70.

[42] Hope, JK; Wilson, JL; Thomson, FJ. Three-dimensional CT angiography in the detection and characterization of intracranial berry aneurysms. *AJNR Am J Neuroradiol*, 1996 Mar, 17(3), 439-45.

[43] Dorsch, NW; Young, N; Kingston, RJ; Compton, JS. Early experience with spiral CT in the diagnosis of intracranial aneurysms. *Neurosurgery*, 1995 Jan., 36(1), 230-6, discussion 6-8.

[44] Vieco, PT; Shuman, WP; Alsofrom, GF; Gross, CE. Detection of circle of Willis aneurysms in patients with acute subarachnoid hemorrhage: a comparison of CT angiography and digital subtraction angiography. *AJR Am J Roentgenol.* 1995 Aug., 165(2), 425-30.

[45] Zeman, RK; Silverman, PM; Vieco, PT; Costello, P. CT angiography. *AJR Am J Roentgenol*, 1995 Nov., 165(5), 1079-88.

[46] Vieco, PT; Morin, EE; 3rd, Gross CE; CT angiography in the examination of patients with aneurysm clips. *AJNR Am J Neuroradiol*, 1996 Mar., 17(3), 455-7.

[47] Harbaugh, RE; Schlusselberg, DS; Jeffery, R; Hayden, S; Cromwell, LD; Pluta, D. Three-dimensional computerized tomography angiography in the diagnosis of cerebrovascular disease. *J Neurosurg*, 1992 Mar., 76(3), 408-14.

[48] Tampieri, D; Leblanc, R; Oleszek, J; Pokrupa, R; Melancon, D. Three-dimensional computed tomographic angiography of cerebral aneurysms. *Neurosurgery*, 1995 Apr., 36(4), 749-54, discussion 54-5.

[49] Raaymakers, TW; Rinkel, GJ; Ramos, LM. Initial and follow-up screening for aneurysms in families with familial subarachnoid hemorrhage. *Neurology*, 1998 Oct., 51(4), 1125-30.

[50] Ross, JS; Masaryk, TJ; Modic, MT; Ruggieri, PM; Haacke, EM; Selman, WR. Intracranial aneurysms: evaluation by MR angiography. *AJR Am J Roentgenol*, 1990 Jul., 155(1), 159-65.

[51] Ronkainen, A; Puranen, MI; Hernesniemi, JA; Vanninen, RL; Partanen, PL; Saari, JT, et al. Intracranial aneurysms: MR angiographic screening in 400 asymptomatic individuals with increased familial risk. *Radiology*, 1995 Apr., 195(1), 35-40.

[52] Korogi, Y; Takahashi, M; Mabuchi, N; Nakagawa, T; Fujiwara, S; Horikawa, Y; et al. Intracranial aneurysms: diagnostic accuracy of MR angiography with evaluation of maximum intensity projection and source images. *Radiology*, 1996 Apr., 199(1), 199-207.

[53] Maeder, PP; Meuli, RA; De Tribolet, N. Three-dimensional volume rendering for magnetic resonance angiography in the screening and preoperative workup of intracranial aneurysms. *J Neurosurg*, 1996 Dec., 85(6), 1050-5.

[54] Bederson, JB; Awad, IA; Wiebers, DO; Piepgras, D; Haley, EC; Jr., Brott, T; et al. Recommendations for the management of patients with unruptured intracranial

aneurysms: A Statement for healthcare professionals from the Stroke Council of the American Heart Association. *Stroke*, 2000 Nov., 31(11), 2742-50.

[55] Curnes, JT; Shogry, ME; Clark, DC; Elsner, HJ. MR angiographic demonstration of an intracranial aneurysm not seen on conventional angiography. *AJNR Am J Neuroradiol*, 1993 Jul-Aug., 14(4), 971-3.

[56] Pryor, JC; Setton, A; Nelson, PK; Berenstein, A. Complications of diagnostic cerebral angiography and tips on avoidance. *Neuroimaging Clin N Am*, 1996 Aug., 6(3), 751-8.

[57] Setton, A; Davis, AJ; Bose, A; Nelson, PK; Berenstein, A. Angiography of cerebral aneurysms. *Neuroimaging Clin N Am.*, 1996 Aug., 6(3), 705-38.

[58] Tu, RK; Cohen, WA; Maravilla, KR; Bush, WH; Patel NH; Eskridge J; et al. Digital subtraction rotational angiography for aneurysms of the intracranial anterior circulation: injection method and optimization. *AJNR Am J Neuroradiol*, 1996 Jun-Jul, 17(6), 1127-36.

[59] Ronkainen, A; Miettinen, H; Karkola, K; Papinaho, S; Vanninen, R; Puranen, M; et al. Risk of harboring an unruptured intracranial aneurysm. *Stroke*, 1998 Feb., 29(2), 359-62.

[60] Van Gijn, J; Van Dongen, KJ. The time course of aneurysmal haemorrhage on computed tomograms. *Neuroradiology*, 1982, 3(3), 153-6.

[61] Kassell, NF, Torner, JC; Haley, EC; Jr.; Jane, JA; Adams, HP; Kongable, GL. The International Cooperative Study on the Timing of Aneurysm Surgery. Part 1: Overall management results. *J Neurosurg*, 1990 Jul., 73(1): 8-36.

[62] Vermeulen, M; Hasan, D; Blijenberg, BG; Hijdra, A; Van Gijn, J. Xanthochromia after subarachnoid haemorrhage needs no revisitation. *J Neurol Neurosurg Psychiatry*, 1989 Jul., 52(7), 826-8.

[63] Ogawa, T; Inugami, A; Fujita, H; Hatazawa, J; Shimosegawa, E; Noguchi, K; et al. MR diagnosis of subacute and chronic subarachnoid hemorrhage: comparison with CT. *AJR Am J Roentgenol*, 1995 Nov., 165(5), 1257-62.

[64] Yasui, N; Suzuki, A; Nishimura, H; Suzuki, K; Abe T. Long-term follow-up study of unruptured intracranial aneurysms. *Neurosurgery*, 1997 Jun., 40(6), 1155-9, discussion 9-60.

[65] Bonita, R. Cigarette smoking, hypertension and the risk of subarachnoid hemorrhage: a population-based case-control study. *Stroke*, 1986 Sep-Oct., 17(5), 831-5.

[66] Brown, RD; Jr.; Wiebers, DO; Forbes, GS. Unruptured intracranial aneurysms and arteriovenous malformations: frequency of intracranial hemorrhage and relationship of lesions. *J Neurosurg*, 1990 Dec., 73(6), 859-63.

[67] Dhar, S; Tremmel, M; Mocco, J; Kim, M; Yamamoto, J; Siddiqui, AH; et al. Morphology parameters for intracranial aneurysm rupture risk assessment. *Neurosurgery*, 2008 Aug., 63(2), 185-96; discussion 96-7.

[68] King, JT; Jr., Berlin, JA, Flamm, ES. Morbidity and mortality from elective surgery for asymptomatic, unruptured, intracranial aneurysms: a meta-analysis. *J Neurosurg*, 1994 Dec., 81(6), 837-42.

[69] Piepgras, DG. Management of incidental intracranial aneurysms. *Clin Neurosurg*, 1989, 35, 511-8.

[70] Wirth, FP; Laws, ER; Jr., Piepgras, D; Scott, RM. Surgical treatment of incidental intracranial aneurysms. *Neurosurgery*, 1983 May, 12(5), 507-11.
[71] Raaymakers, TW; Rinkel GJ; Limburg, M; Algra, A. Mortality and morbidity of surgery for unruptured intracranial aneurysms: a meta-analysis. *Stroke*, 1998 Aug., 29(8), 1531-8.
[72] Thornton, J; Debrun, GM; Aletich, VA; Bashir, Q; Charbel, FT; Ausman, J. Follow-up angiography of intracranial aneurysms treated with endovascular placement of Guglielmi detachable coils. *Neurosurgery*, 2002 Feb., 50(2), 239-49; discussion 49-50.
[73] Le Roux, PD; Winn, HR. Surgical Decision Making for the Treatment of Cerebral Aneurysms. In: Winn HR, editor. Youmans Neurological Surgery. 5th ed. Philadelphia: *W. B. Saunders,* 2004, p. 1793-812.
[74] Kassell, NF; Torner, JC. Aneurysmal rebleeding: a preliminary report from the Cooperative Aneurysm Study. *Neurosurgery*, 1983 Nov., 13(5), 479-81.
[75] Rosenorn, J; Eskesen, V; Schmidt, K; Ronde, F. The risk of rebleeding from ruptured intracranial aneurysms. *J Neurosurg*, 1987 Sep., 67(3), 329-32.
[76] Greenberg, MS; Arredondo, N; Duckworth, EAM; Nichols, TA; Youssef, AS. SAH, and aneurysms. In: Greenberg MS; editor. Handbook of Neurosurgery. New York: *Thieme*, 2006, p. 781-834.
[77] Haley, EC; Jr., Kassell, NF; Torner, JC. The International Cooperative Study on the Timing of Aneurysm Surgery. The North American experience. *Stroke*, 1992 Feb., 23(2), 205-14.
[78] Kassell, NF; Torner, JC; Jane, JA; Haley, EC; Jr., Adams, HP. The International Cooperative Study on the Timing of Aneurysm Surgery. Part 2: Surgical results. *J Neurosurg*, 1990 Jul., 73(1), 37-47.
[79] Molyneux, A; Kerr, R; Stratton, I; Sandercock, P; Clarke, M; Shrimpton, J; et al. International Subarachnoid Aneurysm Trial (ISAT) of neurosurgical clipping versus endovascular coiling in 2143 patients with ruptured intracranial aneurysms: a randomised trial. *Lancet*, 2002 Oct 26, 360(9342), 1267-74.
[80] Vinuela, F; Duckwiler, G; Mawad, M. Guglielmi detachable coil embolization of acute intracranial aneurysm: perioperative anatomical and clinical outcome in 403 patients. *J Neurosurg*, 1997 Mar., 86(3), 475-82.
[81] Raymond, J; Roy, D. Safety and efficacy of endovascular treatment of acutely ruptured aneurysms. *Neurosurgery*, 1997 Dec., 41(6)., 1235-45; discussion 45-6.
[82] Debrun, GM; Aletich, VA; Kehrli, P; Misra, M; Ausman, JI; Charbel, F. Selection of cerebral aneurysms for treatment using Guglielmi detachable coils: the preliminary University of Illinois at Chicago experience. *Neurosurgery*, 1998 Dec., 43(6), 1281-95; discussion 96-7.
[83] Brilstra, EH; Rinkel, GJ; Van der Graaf, Y; Van Rooij, WJ; Algra, A. Treatment of intracranial aneurysms by embolization with coils: a systematic review. *Stroke*, 1999 Feb., 30(2), 470-6.
[84] Dorsch, NW; King, MT. A review of cerebral vasospasm in aneurysmal subarachnoid haemorrhage Part I: Incidence and effects. *J Clin Neurosci*, 1994 Jan., 1(1), 19-26.
[85] Heros, RC; Zervas, NT; Varsos, V. Cerebral vasospasm after subarachnoid hemorrhage: an update. *Ann Neurol*, 1983 Dec., 14(6), 599-608.

[86] Weir, B; Grace, M; Hansen, J; Rothberg, C. Time course of vasospasm in man. *J Neurosurg*, 1978 Feb., 48(2), 173-8.
[87] Findlay, JM. Cerebral Vasospasm. In: Winn HR; editor. Youmans Neurological Surgery. 5th ed. Philadelphia: *W. B. Saunders,* 2004, p. 1839-67.
[88] Cook, DA; Vollrath, B. Free radicals and intracellular events associated with cerebrovascular spasm. *Cardiovasc Res.*, 1995 Oct., 30(4), 493-500.
[89] Kistler, JP; Crowell, RM; Davis, KR; Heros, R; Ojemann, RG; Zervas, T; et al. The relation of cerebral vasospasm to the extent and location of subarachnoid blood visualized by CT scan: a prospective study. *Neurology*, 1983 Apr., 33(4), 424-36.
[90] Rabb, CH; Tang, G; Chin, LS; Giannotta, SL. A statistical analysis of factors related to symptomatic cerebral vasospasm. *Acta Neurochir (Wien)*, 1994, 127(1-2), 27-31.
[91] Lasner, TM; Weil, RJ; Riina, HA; King, JT; Jr., Zager, EL; Raps, EC; et al. Cigarette smoking-induced increase in the risk of symptomatic vasospasm after aneurysmal subarachnoid hemorrhage. *J Neurosurg*, 1997 Sep., 87(3), 381-4.
[92] Origitano, TC; Wascher, TM; Reichman, OH; Anderson, DE. Sustained increased cerebral blood flow with prophylactic hypertensive hypervolemic hemodilution ("triple-H" therapy) after subarachnoid hemorrhage. *Neurosurgery*, 1990 Nov., 27(5), 729-39, discussion 39-40.
[93] Barker, FG; 2nd, Ogilvy, CS. Efficacy of prophylactic nimodipine for delayed ischemic deficit after subarachnoid hemorrhage: a metaanalysis. *J Neurosurg*, 1996 Mar., 84(3), 405-14.
[94] Hasan, D; Vermeulen, M; Wijdicks, EF; Hijdra, A; Van Gijn, J. Management problems in acute hydrocephalus after subarachnoid hemorrhage. *Stroke*, 1989 Jun., 20(6), 747-53.
[95] Graff-Radford, NR; Torner, J; Adams, HP; Jr., Kassell, NF. Factors associated with hydrocephalus after subarachnoid hemorrhage. A report of the Cooperative Aneurysm Study. *Arch Neurol*, 1989 Jul., 46(7), 744-52.
[96] Hasan, D; Tanghe, HL. Distribution of cisternal blood in patients with acute hydrocephalus after subarachnoid hemorrhage. *Ann Neurol*, 1992 Apr., 31(4), 374-8.
[97] Kusske, JA; Turner, PT; Ojemann, GA; Harris, AB. Ventriculostomy for the treatment of acute hydrocephalus following subarachnoid hemorrhage. *J Neurosurg*, 1973 May, 38(5), 591-5.
[98] Voldby, B; Enevoldsen, EM. Intracranial pressure changes following aneurysm rupture. Part 3: Rccurrent hemorrhage. *J Neurosurg*, 1982 Jun., 56(6), 784-9.
[99] Paine, JT; Batjer, HH; Samson, D. Intraoperative ventricular puncture. *Neurosurgery*, 1988 Jun., 22(6 Pt 1), 1107-9.
[100] Vale, FL; Bradley, EL; Fisher, WS; 3rd. The relationship of subarachnoid hemorrhage and the need for postoperative shunting. *J Neurosurg*, 1997 Mar, 86(3), 462-6.
[101] Wise, BL. Syndrome of inappropriate antidiuretic hormone secretion after spontaneous subarachnoid hemorrhage: a reversible cause of clinical deterioration. *Neurosurgery*, 1978 Nov-Dcc, 3(3), 412-4.
[102] Shimoda, M; Yamada, S; Yamamoto, I; Tsugane, R; Sato, O. Atrial natriuretic polypeptide in patients with subarachnoid haemorrhage due to aneurysmal rupture. Correlation to hyponatremia. *Acta Neurochir (Wien)*, 1989, 97(1-2), 53-61.

[103] Wijdicks, EF; Vermeulen, M; ten Haaf, JA; Hijdra, A; Bakker, WH; Van Gijn, J. Volume depletion and natriuresis in patients with a ruptured intracranial aneurysm. *Ann Neurol*, 1985 Aug., 18(2), 211-6.

[104] Wijdicks, EF; Ropper, AH; Hunnicutt, EJ; Richardson, GS; Nathanson, JA. Atrial natriuretic factor and salt wasting after aneurysmal subarachnoid hemorrhage. *Stroke*, 1991 Dec., 22(12), 1519-24.

[105] Diringer, M; Ladenson, PW; Stern, BJ; Schleimer, J; Hanley, DF. Plasma atrial natriuretic factor and subarachnoid hemorrhage. *Stroke*, 1988 Sep., 19(9), 1119-24.

[106] Wijdicks, EF; Vermeulen, M; Hijdra, A; Van Gijn, J. Hyponatremia and cerebral infarction in patients with ruptured intracranial aneurysms: is fluid restriction harmful? *Ann Neurol*, 1985 Feb., 17(2), 137-40.

[107] Ayus, JC; Krothapalli, RK; Arieff, AI. Changing concepts in treatment of severe symptomatic hyponatremia. Rapid correction and possible relation to central pontine myelinolysis. *Am J Med.*, 1985 Jun., 78(6 Pt 1), 897-902.

[108] Marion, DW; Segal, R; Thompson, ME. Subarachnoid hemorrhage and the heart. *Neurosurgery*, 1986 Jan., 18(1), 101-6.

[109] Yuki, K; Kodama, Y; Onda, J; Emoto, K; Morimoto, T; Uozumi, T. Coronary vasospasm following subarachnoid hemorrhage as a cause of stunned myocardium. Case report. *J Neurosurg*, 1991 Aug., 75(2), 308-11.

[110] Estanol Vidal, B; Badui Dergal, E; Cesarman, E; Marin San Martin, O; Loyo M; Vargas Lugo B; et al. Cardiac arrhythmias associated with subarachnoid hemorrhage: prospective study. *Neurosurgery,* 1979 Dec., 5(6), 675-80.

[111] Walter, P; Neil-Dwyer, G; Cruickshank, JM. Beneficial effects of adrenergic blockade in patients with subarachnoid haemorrhage. *Br Med J* (Clin Res Ed), 1982 Jun 5, 284(6330), 1661-4.

In: Aneurysms: Types, Risks, Formation and Treatment
Editors: Alain Laurent and Ethan Morel
ISBN: 978-1-60741-557-2
© 2009 Nova Science Publishers, Inc.

Chapter 2

The Epidemiology of Aortic Diameter

Nicole E. Jensky[1], *Lakshmi Venkitachalam*[2] *and Matthew A. Allison*[3]

[1]Dept. of Family and Preventive Medicine, Univ. of California San Diego.
[2]Cardiovascular Inst., Univ. of Pittsburgh, PA.
[3]Associate Professor, Dept. of Family and Preventive Medicine, Univ., of California San Diego

Abstract

The diameter of the thoracic and abdominal aorta is central to predicting the risk for incident aortic aneurysms. In this regard, examination of significant risk factors for increasing diameter of the aorta is of scientific and clinical relevance. Accordingly, in this chapter, we will be discussing the epidemiology of aortic diameter using the results from two different studies that examined aortic diameter using computed tomography. Results from these studies suggest that age, sex, body mass index, and the presence and extent of calcified atherosclerosis in both the abdominal aorta and iliac arteries are significantly associated with increasing aortic diameter independent of the other cardiovascular disease risk factors. Finally, another data set indicates that the segment-specific variations in aortic diameter can potentially be used as a marker of vascular adaptation. We believe the findings described are important in understanding risk for early abdominal aortic dilatation, which may ultimately lead to aneurysmal formation.

Introduction

An aortic aneurysm is a weakened and bulging area in the aorta that can develop anywhere along the aorta, but most commonly occurs in the abdomen. The basic defect is destruction of the elastic fibers in the media, which permits the remaining fibrous tissue to stretch, leading to an increase in aortic diameter and wall tension. Aneurysms are typically asymptomatic until rupture. Therefore, methods for screening and detection of those at risk for developing an aneurysm is of public health importance.

The major concern of aneurysmal disease is rupture, which is associated with mortality rates of 50–75% [1]. In the United States, AAA is the 15th leading cause of death [2] and can cause approximately 13,000 deaths a year. The aging population as well as increased screening in high-risk populations has led some to suggest that the incidence of AAAs is increasing. Accordingly, routine ultrasound surveillance screening for AAA has been recommended for males over the age of 65 and selected high-risk females [1]. Surgery is currently the only therapy for individuals with AAA, but intervention is costly and associated with morbidity and mortality.

There is controversy as to whether the predominant etiology of AAA is arteriosclerosis (the process leading to muscular thickening of the arterial wall) or atherosclerosis (deposition of lipid into and accompanied by inflammation of the intima-media complex) [3, 4]. Some data indicate that coronary heart disease (CHD) risk factors are differentially associated with AAA [5]. Individuals with AAA and without severe intimal atherosclerosis have excessive arterial dilation and reduced distensibility [6]. The associations between aortic diameter and calcium due to atherosclerosis in the aorta are mixed with some showing negative associations [7] while others show the opposite [8, 9].

The diameter of the abdominal aorta is central to the diagnosis of AAA. Abdominal aortic aneurysm is commonly defined as a diameter > 3.0 cm; however autopsy studies have indicated that AAA's of smaller diameter can potentially rupture and larger ones may not rupture. Other definitions such as ≥ 4 cm and an infrarenal to suprarenal diameter ratio of 1.2 to 1.5 have also been used [10, 11]. The importance of diameter in predicting subsequent aneurysm growth has also been clearly indentified in studies of small AAAs [10, 12-16].

Traditional Risk Factors for Aortic Diameter

From February 2001 to June 2001, 504 ambulatory patients presented for preventive medicine services at The LifeScore Clinic, a private, university affiliated disease prevention center in La Jolla, California. Most patients were asymptomatic and free of clinical cardiovascular disease. This is a clinical population where subjects were either self-referred or referred on the recommendation of their personal physician as an adjunct to their preventive healthcare. All study data was collected at the same patient visit.

The age range of these study subjects was between 25 and 87 years of age and 41% were women, while nearly 68% of the subjects were classified as overweight or obese. None of the participants had a history of myocardial infarction or stroke, five had undergone coronary artery bypass grafting, and 10 had a history of percutaneous transluminal angioplasty of the coronary arteries.

During the study participant's visit, they completed a detailed health history questionnaire that collected information on history of hypertension, diabetes, cholesterol, smoking, family history of coronary heart disease, medications, diet, exercise, and prior surgeries. Casual (not necessarily fasting) serum total, high-density (HDL) and low-density lipoprotein (LDL) cholesterol, and blood glucose measurements were obtained, as well as body mass index (BMI) and body fat measurements. Hypertension was defined as a systolic (SBP) >140 mm Hg or diastolic blood pressure (DBP) >90 mm Hg, or self-report of physician-diagnosed hypertension and current use of an antihypertensive medication. Smoking status was defined as current, former, or never. Diabetes was defined by current use of physician-prescribed anti-glycemic medications or a glucose level >200 mg/dL. Individuals with a total to HDL cholesterol ratio >5 or who reported the use of a medication to treat high cholesterol were classified as dyslipidemic.

Subjects were evaluated by electron beam computed tomography (EBCT) for the extent of atherosclerosis in five different vascular beds: the carotid, coronary, thoracic, aorta, abdominal aortal, and iliac vessels. Images for each vascular bed were obtained using 100-ms scan time and proceeding caudally from the base of the skull to the symphysis pubis. Each bed was obtained by a distinct scan of the segment in question using the following slice thicknesses: 3 mm for the coronary bed, 5 mm for the thorax, and 6 mm through the neck, abdomen, and pelvis. Cardiac CT imaging was electrocardiographically triggered at 40% or 65% of the R-R interval, depending on the subject's heart rate. Imaging of the heart, thorax, and abdomen was conducted during separate breath-holds at half-maximal inspiration.

Atherosclerotic calcium was defined as a plaque area ≥1 mm^2 with a density of ≥130 Hounsfield units (HU). Quantitative calcium scores were determined by Agatston et al [17]. In brief, the calcium score per lesion was calculated by multiplying the area of three contiguous pixels by the corresponding density number using the following scale for density (1 = 130 to 199 HU, 2 = 200 to 299 HU, 3 = 300 to 399 HU, and 4 = ≥400 HU). The total calcium score was then determined by summing the lesion scores from all of the slices for that segment. Agatston calcium scores for vascular beds other than the coronaries were adjusted for slice thickness using the following formula: adjusted score = original score × slice thickness/3.0. Volume averaging was avoided by scoring each homogeneous slice thickness segment separately.

The current study of aortic diameter was a retrospective analysis of the images obtained using the following technique. In brief, computer software equipped to view CT images and conduct the appropriate measurements for aortic diameter was used to measure the diameters of the abdominal aorta at (1) the first slice inferior to the superior mesenteric artery (SMA), (2) the first slice superior to the aortic bifurcation, and (3) at the midpoint between the SMA and the aortic bifurcation. At these locations, an adjustable-size electronic caliper in the shape of a circle was used to measure the diameter (d) by fitting the caliper around the circumference (C) of the adventitia of the aorta. The computer then calculated the diameter from the circumference measurement using the equation, $C = \pi d$. Each location was measured three times, and the average of these measurements was used in the analysis. For those images where the image quality was questionable, the principal investigator adjudicated the image, and a consensus was made on the measurement. The average percentage difference in measurements at each of these three sites was 4.1%, 4.0%, and 4.0%, and the intra-class correlation was 0.93. A single reader who was unaware of the subject characteristics conducted the measurements for aortic diameter.

Analysis of covariance was used to calculate the adjusted mean value or prevalence of the subject characteristics by quartile of aortic diameter. The mean age and sex adjusted risk factor values by quartile of aortic diameter at each of the three sites studied are presented in

Table 1. As shown, there were trends for increasing age, BMI, body fat percentage and SBP by quartile of aortic diameter. Age and sex adjusted prevalence of calcium in the coronaries, abdominal aorta, and iliac arteries increased from the first to fourth quartile at the SMA and midpoint locations. At the former, the overall trends for the presence of calcium in both the abdominal aorta and iliac arteries were borderline significant, whereas, for the midpoint location, the prevalence trends for calcium in the coronary and iliac arteries were statistically significant.

Table 1. Distribution of characteristics by aortic diameter quartile

	Superior mesenteric artery					*Aortic midpoint*					*Aortic bifurcation*				
Characteristic	*Q1*	*Q2*	*Q3*	*Q4*	P[a]	*Q1*	*Q2*	*Q3*	*Q4*	P[a]	*Q1*	*Q2*	*Q3*	*Q4*	P[a]
Sample size	124	129	126	125	...	131	125	126	121	...	128	125	126	125	...
Age, years[b]	53.8	56.6	57.9	62.8	<.01	55.2	56.6	58.2	61.3	<.01	55.0	57.5	58.6	60.1	<.01
Female sex[c]	83.1	49.6	21.4	10.4	<.01	85.5	54.4	17.5	5.0	<.01	84.4	52.0	21.4	6.4	<.01
BMI, kg/m[2b]	24.9	26.6	27.8	28.6	<.01	24.7	26.3	27.8	29.1	<.01	25.4	26.7	27.8	28.3	<.01
Total BF%[b]	28.1	28.8	30.9	31.6	<.01	28.8	29.0	29.8	31.6	<.01	29.1	29.7	29.4	31.1	.05
Ever smoker[b]	46.4	46.6	49.2	49.0	.69	39.5	48.2	57.2	46.2	.51	49.4	46.1	53.7	42.2	.58
TC/HDL ratio[b]	3.9	4.0	4.1	4.4	.08	4.0	3.9	4.2	4.4	.08	4.1	4.0	4.1	4.2	.81
Dyslipidemia[b]	29.8	33.6	32.3	31.1	.94	32.6	27.5	32.5	34.6	.72	36.8	32.1	29.0	29.3	.25
SBP[b]	122	127	130	131	<.01	125	127	129	131	.02	124	129	128	130	.05
DBP[b]	76	79	80	82	<.01	78	78	80	81	.07	77	79	80	81	.05
Hypertension[b]	26.0	33.4	48.3	44.7	<.01	35.3	36.2	38.0	43.1	.38	31.8	40.8	34.9	45.2	.20
Diabetes mellitus[b]	1.0	4.1	3.5	2.4	.74	0.6	1.8	2.1	1.9	.28	5.6	3.8	0.5	1.2	.06
Family history CHD[b]	28.4	27.1	22.0	21.7	.26	19.3	29.7	28.7	21.7	.88	18.6	29.1	28.0	23.6	.52
Calcium[c]															
Carotid (>0)	32.3	33.8	32.9	41.1	.21	34.3	28.6	36.2	41.0	.22	31.7	35.6	36.9	36.8	.43
Coronary (>0)	61.3	61.3	62.2	67.5	.34	55.3	62.8	66.2	68.9	.05	58.4	65.3	61.9	68.3	.21
Thoracic aortic (>0)	50.5	47.8	44.8	45.7	.42	52.6	44.7	46.9	43.7	.23	51.9	47.2	47.8	41.5	.13
Abdominal aortic (>0)	56.4	57.0	63.8	66.4	.07	59.5	56.2	59.9	67.7	.18	62.9	62.3	56.8	61.9	.71
Renal aortic (>0)	22.7	19.7	18.4	24.6	.74	25.6	22.8	16.2	20.4	.32	26.2	21.7	20	17.6	.14
Iliac aortic (>0)	53.6	61.3	58.8	67.5	.07	50.7	58.4	67.3	65.6	.02	58.6	60.1	58.3	65.2	.38
Total vascular (>0)	79.8	83.5	88.0	84.8	.29	79.9	85.6	86.1	85.1	.40	79.2	87.9	82.9	87.5	.23

BF%, Body fat percentage; *BMI*, body mass index; *DBP*, diastolic blood pressure; *CHD*, coronary heart disease; HDL, high-density lipoprotein; *TC*, total cholesterol.

[a] *P*-value for trend.

[b] Age and sex-adjusted means.

[c] Age and sex-adjusted percentages.

From the lowest to highest quartile of aortic diameter at each of the three sites, the median calcium scores increased in the coronaries, abdominal aorta, and iliac arteries (Figure 1). Similarly, the age- and sex-adjusted prevalence of calcium in the coronaries, abdominal aorta, and iliac arteries increased from the first to fourth quartile at the SMA and midpoint locations (Table 1). At the former, the overall trends for the presence of calcium in both the abdominal aorta and iliac arteries were of borderline significance ($P = .07$ for both), whereas for the midpoint location, the prevalence trends for calcium in the coronary and iliac arteries were statistically significant ($P = .05$ and $.02$, respectively).

Multivariable linear regression was used to determine the simultaneous significance of the associations between the cardiovascular disease risk factors, as well as the presence and extent of vascular calcium in distinct vascular beds, and aortic diameter (Table 2). These data indicate that the diameter of the abdominal aorta just inferior to the SMA, just superior to the aortic bifurcation, and at the midpoint between these two sites that were significantly associated with age, male sex, BMI, (Table 2). Additionally, there was a significant association between total body fat and aortic diameter at all three locations, but this was not independent of BMI. Of note, diabetes was significantly and inversely associated with increments in the diameter of the abdominal aorta just superior to the aortic bifurcation but not at the SMA or the midpoint.

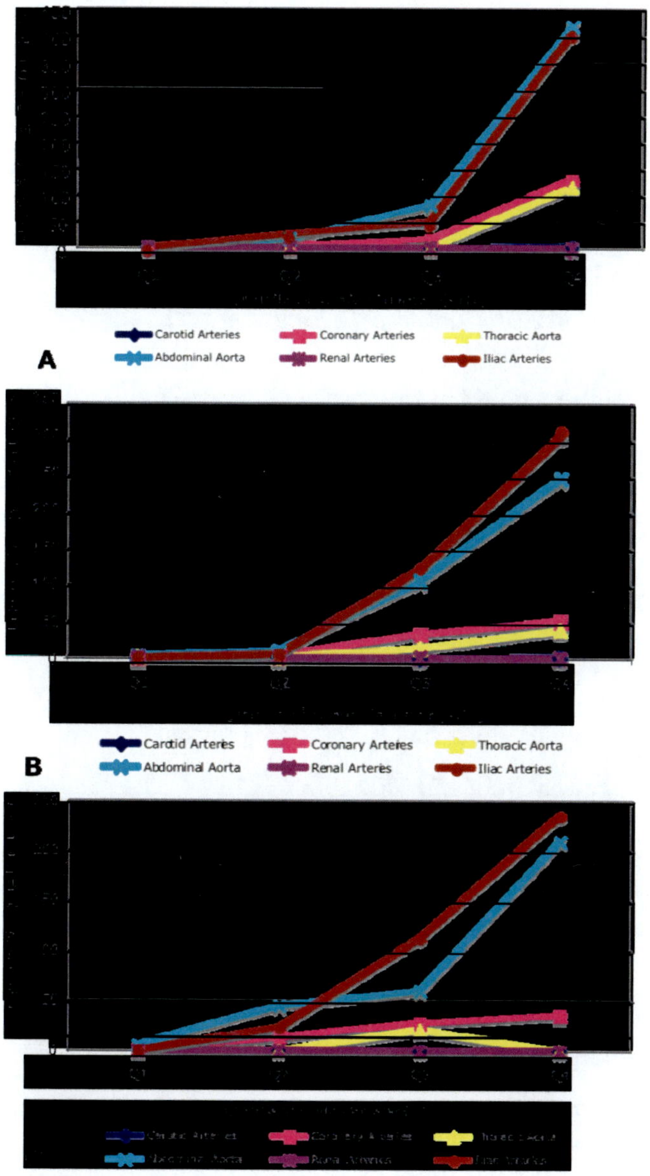

Figure 1. Vascular bed median calcium scores are shown by quartile of the aortic diameter

Figure 2 shows the results of multivariable linear regression analysis where the calcium score for each vascular bed was separately added to a model containing all of the cardiovascular disease risk factors listed above. On average, a 1-unit increment in calcium score in the abdominal aorta and iliac arteries was associated with 0.13-mm ($P < .01$) and 0.09-mm ($P = .02$) increases, respectively, in aortic diameter at the SMA. The results were similar for the midpoint and aortic bifurcation. The total amount of calcium in the vascular beds studies was also associated with increasing aortic diameter at the SMA and midpoint, but not at the bifurcation.

Table 2. Multivariable linear regression for associations between traditional CVD risk factors and aortic diameter

	SMA		Midpoint		Bifurcation	
Variable[a]	β^b	P	β	P	β	P-value
Age ([illegible])	[illegible]	< .01	[illegible]	< .01	[illegible]	< .01
Sex (male vs female)	[illegible]	< .01	[illegible]	< .01	[illegible]	< .01
Body mass index ([illegible])	[illegible]	< .01	[illegible]	< .01	[illegible]	< .01
Diabetes (yes vs no)	[illegible]	[illegible]	[illegible]	[illegible]	[illegible]	[illegible]
Hypertension (yes vs no)	[illegible]	[illegible]	[illegible]	[illegible]	[illegible]	[illegible]
[illegible] (yes vs no)	[illegible]	[illegible]	[illegible]	[illegible]	[illegible]	[illegible]
Smoking (yes vs no)	[illegible]	[illegible]	[illegible]	[illegible]	[illegible]	[illegible]

[illegible]
[a] [illegible]
[b] Linear regression coefficient.

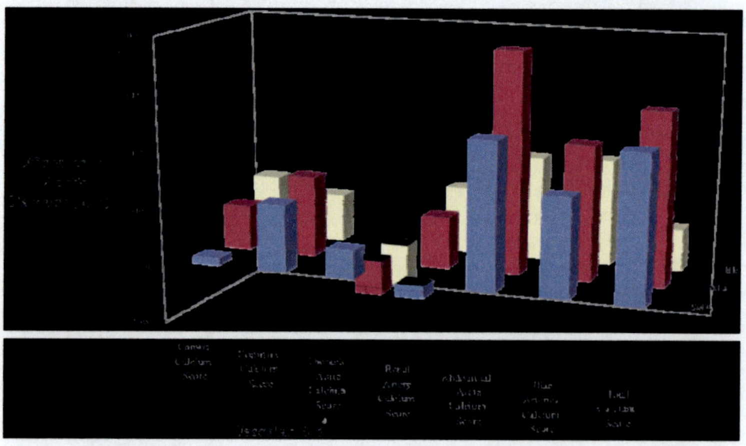

Figure 2. Linear Regression analyses shows differences in aortic diameter per 1-unit increases in calcium scores in various vascular beds

In this cross-sectional study of ambulatory patients who underwent whole-body CT scanning as part of their routine health maintenance, increments in the diameter of the abdominal aorta just inferior to the SMA, just superior to the aortic bifurcation, and at the midpoint between these two sites, were significantly associated with age, male sex, BMI, and calcified atherosclerosis in the abdominal aorta and iliac arteries, even after adjustment for the other traditional cardiovascular disease risk factors. There was also a significant association between the total body fat and aortic diameter at all three locations, but this was not independent of BMI. In total, these results expand the literature on the cardiovascular epidemiology of abdominal aortic diameter by demonstrating significant positive associations with calcified atherosclerosis. Of note, similar to findings from a previous study [18] diabetes was significantly and inversely associated with increments in the diameter of the abdominal aorta just superior to the aortic bifurcation but not at the SMA or the midpoint. However, owing to the small number of 14 patients with diabetes in this study, these results should be viewed with caution.

Our results confirm the significant associations between abdominal aortic diameter and age, sex, and the measures of body morphology described above. However, our study also found a significant inverse association between abdominal aortic diameter and diabetes mellitus. Importantly, this finding was only for the abdominal aorta just proximal to the aortic bifurcation and is in accordance with previous epidemiologic studies that have demonstrated a significant inverse association between diabetes and AAA [18]. The reason for this "protective" effect of diabetes on AAA—and now aortic diameter—is currently unknown.

Overall, these data indicate that age, sex, BMI and the presence and extent of calcified atherosclerosis in both the abdominal aorta and iliac arteries are significantly associated with increasing aortic diameter independent of other cardiovascular disease risk factors except in diabetic subjects, where an inverse association exists with the diameter at the aortic bifurcation.

Segment-Specific Association of Risk Factors with Aortic Diameter in Women

A recent ancillary project [19] (as an abstract), from the Study of Women's Health Across the Nation (SWAN) Heart study [20], described the segment-specific association of aortic diameter with cardiovascular risk factors in a bi-racial cohort of 544 women (37% African-American, mean age: 50 years, mean BMI: 29 kg/sq.m). Aortic diameter was measured at the following segments - aortic root (AR), ascending (AA), descending (DA), thoracic (TA) and abdominal aorta (AbA) - using previously recorded electron beam computed tomography scans. The segments were identified using the following landmarks - aortic root (AR, segment immediately cranial to the origin of the left coronary artery), ascending aorta (AA, segments following after the transverse aortic arch up to the pulmonary artery bifurcation), descending aorta (DA, after the origin of the left subclavian artery and before the apex of the heart), thoracic aorta (TA, immediately cranial to the diaphragmatic hiatus), and abdominal aorta (AbA, after the origin of both renal arteries and before the iliac bifurcation). Measurements were to be taken at eye level to avoid parallax error. Additionally, only those images with no branches, calcification or obvious aneurysmal dilatation and with ≤ 2 mm difference between AP and transverse values were to be selected, in order to avoid oblique slices. The average of measures obtained at both the antero-posterior (AP) and transverse planes was recoded for each segment.

Regression analysis, using mixed linear models that accounted for within-person correlations, revealed interesting results. Age and weight showed positive associations, but of varying magnitude, with aortic diameter in the five segments. Change in diameter (millimeters) associated with a unit increase in age, by segment, was as follows: AR: 0.10, AA: 0.18, DA: 0.20, TA: 0.21, and AbA: 0.10 (P interaction with segment: 0.001). Similarly, a 10-kg increase in weight was associated with 0.05 mm increase in the aortic root and descending segments, 0.06 mm in the ascending aorta and 0.04 mm increase in the thoracic and abdominal diameters (P interaction: 0.04). Other risk factors that showed segment-specific variation in their relationship with aortic diameter, after adjusting for age and weight, were: systolic and diastolic blood pressures, blood glucose, insulin, visceral adipose tissue, lipoprotein A1, and factor VII. Interestingly, increase in blood glucose was associated with significant increase in descending aortic diameter, but a negative, albeit non-significant, association with abdominal aortic diameter. African-Americans, compared to Caucasians, had larger diameters in every segment ($p < 0.05$ for all but aortic root and abdominal aorta), which persisted after adjustment for age, weight, site and degree of education.

Pathology of the aorta, like its physiology, is heterogeneous in that the thoracic aorta is relatively spared from hemodynamically significant plaque formation and aneurismal dilatation while the infra-renal aorta is prone to both [21]. This heterogeneity maybe attributed to differential vascular response to disease process or perhaps, a varying relationship with predisposing risk factors. The above reported findings in a large sample of women demonstrate novel segment-specific impact of risk factors on aortic morphology and provide support to the latter hypothesis. Segment-specific variation in aortic diameter, as a marker of vascular adaptation, deserves further exploration in larger cohorts.

Use of Computed Tomography (CT) to Measure Aortic Diameters

Choice of imaging modality is of central importance when measuring aortic diameters with ultrasonography (US) and CT being commonly used for this purpose. Early studies predominantly in the setting of aneurysms, have shown that reader variability differs by the measurement planes (transverse and antero-posterior) in normal and aneurysmal aortas [22] that differences $\geq$ 5 mm between duplicate reads were not uncommon [23] , and inter-reader variability was higher than that of intra-reader, irrespective of the modality used. It must be noted that reader reproducibility in the studies discussed above were good and ranged form 0.8-0.9. Even so, concerns regarding the use of CT including those related to use of 2-D images to characterize the 3-D aorta exist. Comparisons of 3-D reconstruction of CT images with aortography [24] and conventional CT [25], have shown that 2-D minor axis measurements correlate well with 3-D measures and this may be adequate in the absence of severe tortuosities or angulations. Studies evaluating CT have also yielded equivocal results (Table 3). Nevertheless, some limitations of EBCT in measuring aortic diameters must be acknowledged and include the inability to measure at the aortic arch and differentiate between the layers of the arterial wall. Patient characteristics like waist circumference or BMI that affect soft tissue attenuation [26-28], generate scatter or image noise, affecting scan quality. Recently, the field of vascular imaging has witnessed rapid technological advancements that include magnetic resonance imaging, multi-detector CT and improved Doppler ultrasound techniques, which may overcome some of these limitations. Thus, future studies, incorporating these advancements, are needed to gain more insight into vascular adaptation and remodeling.

Table 3. Studies comparing imaging modalities for measuring aortic diameter

Study (Author, year, place)	Study Sample, Modalities compared	Summary
Lederle 1995, Multicenter study.[23]	Patients with AAA who are not at high surgical risk (N=258, 50-79 years). CT, Ultrasound	Mean difference (SD), mm: -2.7 (4.9), P<0.001 It is possible to achieve high degree of precision using CT. In most cases, Ultrasound measurements of AAA diameter were smaller than that by CT
Jaakkola 1996, Kuopio, Finland. [23, 32]	Patients (N=33) underwent imaging for aneurysms or other reasons. CT, Ultrasound	Mean difference (SD), mm: Normal Aorta: AP: 2.4 (1.9), Transverse: 2.1 (1.5) AAA: AP: 2.0 (1.6), Transverse: 3.1 (3.5) Marked interobserver variability in measuring AAA diameters for both Ultrasound and CT. For normal aortas, Ultrasound was more repeatable for normal aortas.
Wanhainen 2002, Sweden.[33]	Patients (N=61, 65-75 years) screened for AAA. CT, Ultrasound	Mean difference (SD), mm: Normal aorta: AP: 2.8 (2.9), Transverse: 3.8 (3.9) AAA: AP: -0.7 (4.1), Transverse: 0.4 (5.4) Ultrasound gives larger diameters in AP and transverse planes in non-aneurysmal aorta; no significant difference in mean diameters was seen in AAAs
Sprouse II 2003, Norfolk, Virginia.[34]	Patients with AAA (N=334) enrolled in multicenter endograft trial. CT, Ultrasound	Mean difference (SD), mm: Ultrasound-CT: 9.4 (6.9) Maximal AAA diameter by CT was consistently larger than Ultrasound, with lesser discrepancy in smaller AAAs. Limits of agreement exceeded clinically acceptable limits set at -5 to 5 mm.
Dillavou 2003, Pittsburgh, PA.[25]	Patients (N=31) referred for AAA repair. Spiral CT -2D vs 3D scans; AD measured at neck, AAA sac, left and right iliacs	Intraobserver difference 3D: 0.21 to 0.29 2D Minor axis: 0.04 to 0.15 2D Major axis: 0.20 to 0.92 Interobserver difference 3D: 0.34 to 1.17 2D Minor axis: 0.33 to 0.41 2D Major axis: 0.98 to 1.61 2D vs 3D Minor axis: 0.20 to 1.28 Major axis: 0.95 to 1.65 Minor axis measurements using 2D CT have high correlation with 3D measurements in all areas of the aorta.

Table 3. Studies comparing imaging modalities for measuring aortic diameter

Study (Author, year, place)	Study Sample, Modalities compared	Summary
Elkouri 2004, Rochester, MN.[35]	Follow-up of 107 patients following endovascular repair of AAA. CT and Ultrasound	Mean difference (SD), mm: AP: 2.9 Transverse: 1.8 Excellent correlation (0.9) but significant disagreement between the two measures
Sprouse II 2004, Norfolk, Virginia.[36]	Patients (N=38) with asymptomatic aneurysm > 40 mm Ultrasound compared to axial and orthogonal CT images	Mean difference (SD), mm: Axial - Ultrasound: 4.1, $p<0.05$ Orthogonal - Ultrasound: 0.8 (1.8) Axial - Orthogonal: 3.3, $p<0.05$ Ultrasound measurements are not affected by angulations of the aorta and agree with orthogonal measurements, better than axial measurements. Axial CT values are unreliable when angulations exceeds 25 degrees
Parker 2004, USA.[24]	Consecutive AAA patients (N=20, mean age: 73.2 years) being considered for endovascular repair. Conventional CT, 3D-CT and aortography (AG). Diameter was measured at 4 levels and length measured at 6 levels.	Mean difference (SD), mm: AG-3DCT: ranged from -17 (15) to -0.17 (3.6) CT-3DCT: ranged from -4.8 (13) to 1.0(6) 3DCT measurements of aortoilliac diameter do not correlate well with aortography. Acceptable correlation for both diameters and length seen with conventional CT. CT alone may be adequate in patients without significant aortoiliac tortuosities or angulations
de Gracia 2006, Madrid Spain.[37]	Candidates for endovascular repair of infrarenal aneurysm (N=35). Dual-slice Helical CT and digital subtraction aortography (DSA)	Difference in proximal neck diameter: 1.74 , $p<0.001$ Expected values for proximal neck diameter by DSA can be estimated from CTA, given the high correlation between the 2 methods

Conclusion

The strongest risk factor for the rupture of an AAA is maximal aortic diameter [29, 30]. The results from the studies provided above indicate that age, sex, BMI, and the presence and extent of calcified atherosclerosis in both abdominal aorta and iliac arteries are significantly associated with increasing aortic diameter independent of the other cardiovascular disease risk factors [31]. Additionally, segment-specific variations in aortic diameter can potentially be used as a marker of vascular adaptation. We believe these findings are important in understanding risk for early abdominal aortic dilation, which may ultimately lead to aneurysm formation. Novel biomarkers, including genetic markers, may provide insight into the links between atherosclerosis and aneurysmal formation. Future studies are required to elucidate these findings.

References

[1] Schermerhorn, M; Zwolak, R; Velazquez, O; Makaroun, M; Fairman, R; Cronenwett, J. Ultrasound screening for abdominal aortic aneurysm in medicare beneficiaries. *Ann Vasc Surg,* 2008, 22(1), 16-24.

[2] Gillum, RF. Epidemiology of aortic aneurysm in the United States. *J Clin Epidemiol,* 1995, 48(11), 1289-1298.

[3] Sinha, S; Frishman, WH. Matrix metalloproteinases and abdominal aortic aneurysms: a potential therapeutic target. *J Clin Pharmacol,* 1998, 38(12), 1077-1088.

[4] Xu, C; Zarins, CK; Glagov, S. Aneurysmal and occlusive atherosclerosis of the human abdominal aorta. *J Vasc Surg.,* 2001, 33(1), 91-96.

[5] Wanhainen, A; Bergqvist, D; Boman, K; Nilsson, TK; Rutegard, J; Bjorck, M. Risk factors associated with abdominal aortic aneurysm: a population-based study with historical and current data. *J Vasc Surg.,* 2005, 41(3), 390-396.

[6] Makita, S; Ohira, A; Tachieda, R; Itoh, S; Moriai, Y; Niinuma, H; Nakamura, M; Hiramori, K. Dilation and reduced distensibility of carotid artery in patients with abdominal aortic aneurysms. *Am Heart J.,* 2000, 140(2), 297-302.

[7] Matsushita, M; Nishikimi, N; Sakurai, T; Nimura, Y. Infrarenal aortic dilatation less than 4 cm is not unusual in patients with aortoiliac occlusive disease. *Int Angiol.,* 2002, 21(3), 222-227.

[8] Paivansalo, MJ; Merikanto, J; Jerkkola, T; Savolainen, MJ; Rantala, AO; Kauma, H; Lilja, M; Reunanen, YA; Kesaniemi, A; Suramo, I. Effect of hypertension and risk factors on diameters of abdominal aorta and common iliac and femoral arteries in middle-aged hypertensive and control subjects: a cross-sectional systematic study with duplex ultrasound. *Atherosclerosis,* 2000, 153(1), 99-106.

[9] Reynolds, HR; Tunick, PA; Kort, S; Rosenzweig, BP; Freedberg, RS; Katz, ES; Applebaum, RM; Portnay, EL; Adelman, MA; Attubato, MJ; Kronzon, I. Abdominal aortic aneurysms and thoracic aortic atheromas. *J Am Soc Echocardiogr,* 2001, 14(11), 1127-1131.

[10] Lederle, FA; Johnson, GR; Wilson, SE; Chute, EP; Littooy, FN; Bandyk, D; Krupski, WC; Barone, GW; Acher, CW; Ballard, DJ. Prevalence and associations of abdominal aortic aneurysm detected through screening. Aneurysm Detection and Management (ADAM) Veterans Affairs Cooperative Study Group. *Ann Intern Med.,* 1997, 126(6), 441-449.

[11] Alcorn, HG; Wolfson, SK; Jr., Sutton-Tyrrell, K; Kuller, LH; O'Leary, D. Risk factors for abdominal aortic aneurysms in older adults enrolled in The Cardiovascular Health Study. *Arterioscler Thromb Vasc Biol.,* 1996, 16(8), 963-970.

[12] Lederle, FA; Wilson, SE; Johnson, GR; Reinke, DB; Littooy, FN; Acher, CW; Ballard, DJ; Messina, LM; Gordon, IL; Chute, EP; Krupski, WC; Busuttil, SJ; Barone, GW; Sparks, S; Graham, LM; Rapp, JH; Makaroun, MS; Moneta, GL; Cambria, RA; Makhoul, RG; Eton, D, Ansel, HJ, Freischlag, JA, Bandyk, D. Immediate repair compared with surveillance of small abdominal aortic aneurysms. *N Engl J Med.,* 2002, 346(19), 1437-1444.

[13] Lederle, FA; Johnson, GR; Wilson, SE; Ballard, DJ; Jordan, WD; Jr.; Blebea, J; Littooy, FN; Freischlag, JA; Bandyk, D; Rapp, JH; Salam, AA. Rupture rate of large abdominal aortic aneurysms in patients refusing or unfit for elective repair. *JAMA.,* 2002, 287(22), 2968-2972.

[14] Brady, AR; Thompson, SG; Fowkes, FG; Greenhalgh, RM; Powell, JT. Abdominal aortic aneurysm expansion: risk factors and time intervals for surveillance. *Circulation.,* 2004, 110(1), 16-21.

[15] Norman, P; Le, M; Pearce, C; Jamrozik, K. Infrarenal aortic diameter predicts all-cause mortality. *Arterioscler Thromb Vasc Biol.,* 2004, 24(7), 1278-1282.

[16] Brown, LC; Powell, JT. Risk factors for aneurysm rupture in patients kept under ultrasound surveillance. UK Small Aneurysm Trial Participants. *Ann Surg.,* 1999, 230(3), 289-296; discussion 296-287.

[17] Agatston, AS; Janowitz, WR; Hildner, FJ; Zusmer, NR; Viamonte, M; Jr., Detrano, R. Quantification of coronary artery calcium using ultrafast computed tomography. *J Am Coll Cardiol.,* 1990, 15(4), 827-832.

[18] Golledge, J; Muller, J; Daugherty, A; Norman, P. Abdominal aortic aneurysm: pathogenesis and implications for management. *Arterioscler Thromb Vasc Biol.,* 2006, 26(12), 2605-2613.

[19] Venkitachalam, L. Elevated Pulse Wave Velocity Increases the Odds of Coronary Calcification in Overweight Postmenopausal Women. American Journal of Hypertension. *American Journal of Hypertension,* 2007, 20, 469-475.

[20] Sowers, M. Design; survey sampling and recruitment methods of SWAN: a multi-center, multi-ethnic, community-based cohort study of women and menopausal transition, 2000.

[21] Zarins, CK. Atherosclerotic enlargement of the human abdominal aorta. *Atherosclerosis,* 2001, 155, 157-164.

[22] Jaakkola, P. Interobserver variability in measuring the dimensions of the abdominal aorta: comparison of ultrasound and computed tomography. *Eur J Vasc Endovasc. Surg,* 1996, 12, 230-237.

[23] Lederle, FA; Wilson, SE; Johnson, GR; Reinke, DB; Littooy, FN; Acher, CW; Messina, LM; Ballard, DJ; Ansel, HJ. Variability in measurement of abdominal aortic aneurysms. Abdominal Aortic Aneurysm Detection and Management Veterans Administration Cooperative Study Group. *J Vasc Surg,* 1995, 21(6), 945-952.

[24] Parker, MV; O'Donnell, SD; Chang, AS; Johnson, CA; Gillespie, DL; Goff, JM; Rasmussen, TE; Rich, NM. What imaging studies are necessary for abdominal aortic

endograft sizing? A prospective blinded study using conventional computed tomography, aortography, and three-dimensional computed tomography. *Journal of Vascular Surgery,* 2005, 41(2), 199.

[25] Dillavou, E. Two-Dimensional Versus Three-Dimensional CT Scan for Aortic Measurement. . *Journal of Endovascular Therapy.* 2003, 10, 531-538.

[26] McCullough, EC; Morin, RL. CT-number variability in thoracic geometry. *American Journal of Roentgenology,* 1983, 141(1), 135.

[27] Raggi, P. Calcium Scoring of the Coronary Artery by Electron Beam CT: How to Apply an Individual Attenuation Threshold. . *Am. J. Roentgenol,* 2002, 178, 497-502.

[28] Edmundowicz, D. Technical vs Statistical Adjustment of Calcium Scores to Account for the Confounding Influence of Weight. . *Circulation,* 2005, 111, 184-296.

[29] Nevitt, MP; Ballard, DJ; Hallett, JW. Jr. Prognosis of abdominal aortic aneurysms. A population-based study. *N Engl J Med.,* 1989, 321(15), 1009-1014.

[30] Glimaker, H; Holmberg, L; Elvin, A; Nybacka, O; Almgren, B; Bjorck, CG; Eriksson, I. Natural history of patients with abdominal aortic aneurysm. *Eur J Vasc Surg.,* 1991, 5(2), 125-130.

[31] Allison, MA; Kwan, K; DiTomasso, D; Wright, CM; Criqui, MH. The epidemiology of abdominal aortic diameter. *J Vasc Surg.,* 2008, 48(1), 121-127.

[32] Jaakkola, P; Hippelainen, M; Farin, P; Rytkonen, H; Kainulainen, S; Partanen, K. Interobserver variability in measuring the dimensions of the abdominal aorta: comparison of ultrasound and computed tomography. *Eur J Vasc Endovasc. Surg.,* 1996, 12(2), 230.

[33] Wanhainen, A. Measuring the Abdominal Aorta with Ultrasonography and Computed Tomography - Difference and Variability. . *European Journal of Vascular and Endovascular Surgery.* . 2002, 24, 428-434.

[34] Sprouse, II; Meier, III; LeSar, CJ; DeMasi, RJ; Sood, J; Parent, FN; Marcinzyck, MJ; Gayle, RG. Comparison of abdominal aortic aneurysm diameter measurements obtained with ultrasound and computed tomography: is there a difference? *Journal of Vascular Surgery,* 2003, 38(3), 466.

[35] Stephane, E. Computed Tomography and Ultrasound in Follow-up of Patients after Endovascular Repair of Abdominal Aortic Aneurysm. *Annals of Vascular Surgery,* 2004, V18, 271-279.

[36] Sprouse, II; Meier, III; Parent, FN; DeMasi, RJ; Glickman, MH; Barber, GA. Is Ultrasound More Accurate than Axial Computed Tomography for Determination of Maximal Abdominal Aortic Aneurysm Diameter? *European Journal of Vascular and Endovascular Surgery,* 2004, 28(1), 28.

[37] Milagros. Correlation between the Measurement of Transverse Diameter in the Proximal Neck on Computed Tomography and on Aortography before Endovascular Treatment of Infrarenal Aortic Aneurysm. *Annals of Vascular Surgery,* 2006, 20, 488-495.

In: Aneurysms: Types, Risks, Formation and Treatment ISBN: 978-1-60741-557-2
Editors: Alain Laurent and Ethan Morel © 2009 Nova Science Publishers, Inc.

Chapter 3

Abdominal Aortic Aneurysms – A Complex Genetic Disease

Jennifer Nischan, Guy M. Lenk, Amy M. Boddy, John H. Lillvis, Gerard Tromp and Helena Kuivaniemi*

Center for Molecular Medicine and Genetics, Wayne State University School of Medicine, 3305 Gordon H. Scott Hall of Basic Medical Sciences, 540 East Canfield Avenue,Detroit, Michigan 48201,U.S.A.

Abstract

Abdominal aortic aneurysms (AAAs) are a complex disease with a late age at onset. Causing approximately 15,000 deaths per year, AAAs are among the top twenty leading causes of death in the United States. A main reason for the high mortality rate of AAAs is that most are asymptomatic until rupture. Local inflammation of the aorta, fragmentation of the extracellular matrix and loss of smooth muscle cells are distinct characteristics of AAA formation. Large epidemiological studies have shown that smoking and positive family history are the two most important risk factors for AAAs. Other risk factors include male sex, increasing age, hypertension and high cholesterol. Interestingly, diabetes has a negative association with AAA. A genome-wide approach using DNA linkage analysis has found susceptibility loci for AAAs on chromosomes 19q13 and 4q31 and a genetic association study identified a variant on chromosome 9p21 associated with AAA in addition to other vascular phenotypes. Microarray-based expression profiles have also been generated to determine differentially expressed genes between AAA tissue and non-aneurysmal controls. These genetic and genomic approaches will be critical in determining the pathophysiological mechanisms leading to AAA formation, growth and rupture, and identifying the genetic factors predisposing to AAA later in life.

* Corresponding author: Tel.: (570) 271-5593, FAX: (570) 271-6701, e-mail: shkuivaniemi@geisinger.edu

1. Introduction

1.1. Definition and Historical Perspective

Abdominal aortic aneurysm (AAA) is a balloon-like dilatation that occurs in the infrarenal segment of the aorta below the renal arteries (Figures 1 and 2) [1, 2]. If left untreated, the aortic wall continues to weaken and becomes unable to withstand the forces of the luminal blood pressure resulting in progressive dilatation and eventual rupture [2, 3].

The first definitive record of an aneurysm dates back to approximately 800-600 BC India in the ancient writings of surgeon Sushruta. It is here that he refers to swollen, pulsating vessels in various parts of the body, which he believed to be caused by exertion in tired and weakened persons [4]. It would not be until the 16th century AD, however, that aneurysms of the aorta were documented. In 1555, European physician Vesalius was the first to diagnose an AAA in a patient suffering from severe and constant pain after a fall from a horse. Following the patient's death two years later, Vesalius was able to confirm the diagnosis when an autopsy revealed that the patient's aorta had expanded to the size of a palm [4, 5].

Perhaps the most well known person to have had an AAA is Albert Einstein. In 1948, after several years of abdominal pain associated with occasional vomiting, Einstein consulted thoracic surgeon Rudolph Nissen who, through exploratory surgery, located a large AAA and wrapped it with cellophane. Amazingly, this treatment lasted from 1949 to 1955 after which Einstein's abdominal pain returned. At this time Einstein rejected the recommended surgical intervention dying six days later on April 18, 1955 of a ruptured AAA [6, 7].

Today, AAAs are responsible for over 15,000 deaths per year in the United States and are among the top twenty leading causes of death in industrialized Western countries [8, 9]. Up to 10% of people over the age of 65 harbor an AAA making it a significant problem in the aging population [10]. Typically, AAA diagnosis is given with an aortic diameter of 3.0 cm or larger, or a ratio of infrarenal to suprarenal diameter of at least 1.2 [10, 11].

1.2. Risk Factors for AAA

AAAs are a complex disorder with both genetic and environmental components. Non-modifiable risk factors for the development of AAA include increasing age and male sex, with males being ten times more likely than women to have AAAs greater than 4.0 cm (Figure 3) [10-12]. Additionally, family history is a significant risk factor [10, 11, 13-17]. Former and current smoking have consistently been identified as the most significant risk factors for AAAs, with current smokers showing a faster rate of AAA expansion [10, 11, 18]. Interestingly, African Americans and diabetics are at lower risk for AAAs and one study has even shown that AAA expansion is slower in patients with diabetes (Figure 3) [11, 18].

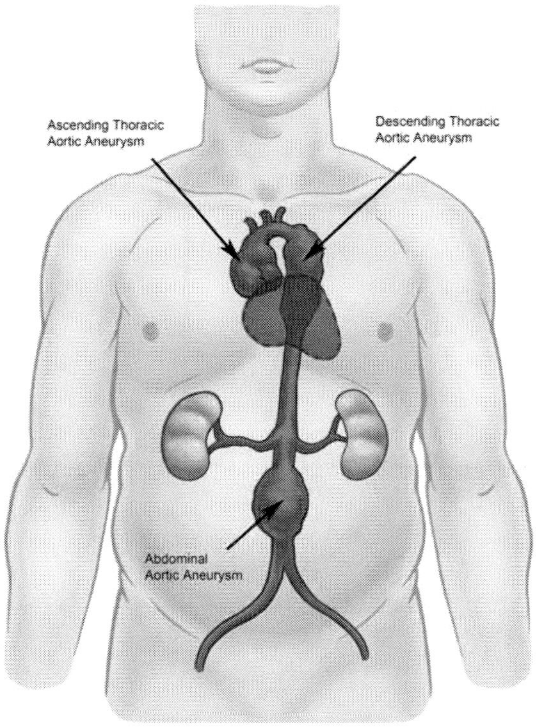

Figure 1. Sites of the most common locations of aneurysms in the aorta. Along the length of the aorta, significant heterogeneity occurs in the distribution of aneurysmal disease. About 50% of TAADs are located in the ascending aorta, 10% in the arch and 40% in the descending thoracic aorta. Only about 25% of patients with TAAD have a concomitant AAA, and multi-segmental disease is found in only bout 10% of cases. AAAs occur in the infrarenal part of the aorta below the renal arteries and their prevalence is at least three times higher than that of TAAD. Illustration by Marc Nischan.

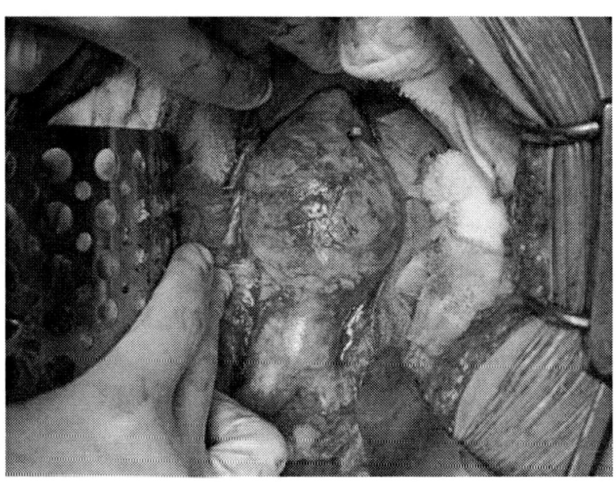

Figure 2. Unruptured human AAA. A 74 year-old Japanese male patient with an AAA of 5.5 cm in diameter is about to undergo an open repair operation. Picture compliments of Yoshiki Kyo, MD, from the Department of Cardiovascular Surgery, Higashihirosima Medical Center, Hiroshima, Japan.

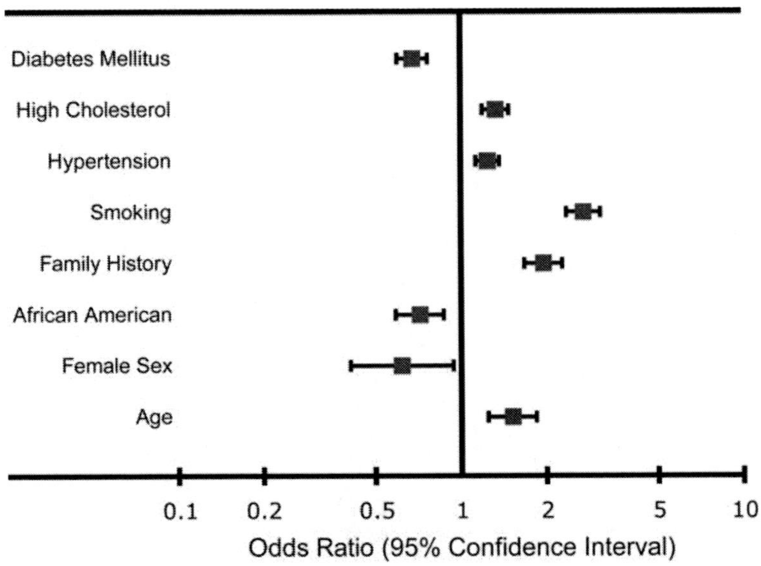

Figure 3. Risk factors for AAAs. Data gathered on 2,217 cases and 66,638 control individuals and reported by Lederle et al. 1997 [36] were used to create a plot of the most significant positive and negative risk factors for AAAs [OR (fixed 95% CI)].

1.3. Detection of AAAs

The original method of AAA detection was abdominal palpation in which the physician feels for a pulsatile mass in the patient's abdomen indicating abnormal widening of the aorta. This method is moderately sensitive but cannot be relied upon to exclude AAA [19]. Today more accurate tools exist for the detection and monitoring of AAAs. Procedures such as abdominal ultrasonography and computed tomography (CT) have close to 100% sensitivity and specificity in detecting AAAs [19, 20]. Ultrasonography is a practical detection method as it is quick, inexpensive and non-invasive [20, 21]. Although more expensive, CT has advantages over ultrasonography in that it is more precise and better able to determine the shape and extent of an AAA [21, 22].

In the late nineties, researchers began using population-based studies to determine the benefits of ultrasound screening for AAAs in people greater than 65 years of age. A review of these randomized, controlled trials for the U.S. Preventive Services Task Force found that screening was associated with a significant reduction in AAA-related mortality for men 65 to 75 years of age [1]. Additionally, results from the Cardiovascular Health Study showed that a one-time screening can not only identify those at risk for AAA, but those at increased risk for future cardiovascular events and total mortality, as these are associated with infrarenal aortic diameters greater than 2.0 cm [23]. Today, the American College of Cardiology and American Heart Association (ACC/AHA) Practice Guidelines for the management of patients with AAA recommend ultrasound screening for men 60 years of age or older who are siblings or offspring of patients with AAA and men aged 65 to 75 years of age who have a history of smoking [24].

1.4. Treatment of AAAs

Presently, the only option available for AAA patients is open or endovascular repair. These types of procedures are only recommended, however, when patients have AAAs larger than 5.5 cm in diameter. This is the result of two large randomized trials looking at elective open repair versus surveillance of AAAs 4.0 to 5.4 cm in diameter. Both studies found that long-term survival is not increased with elective open surgery of small aneurysms when compared to surveillance [25-27].

These procedures also carry some risk of operative mortality. Open repair of AAAs is a major surgical procedure in which an abdominal aortic graft is placed around the aneurysm (Figure 4) [4]. The 30-day operative mortality associated with this procedure can be as high as 6% [28]. Endovascular repair is less invasive and was developed in order to reduce the risks involved with open surgery. This type of repair involves the positioning of an endovascular stent-graft using guidewires inserted through both the ipsilateral common femoral and the lateral iliac arteries, followed by balloon inflation along the stent-graft [29].

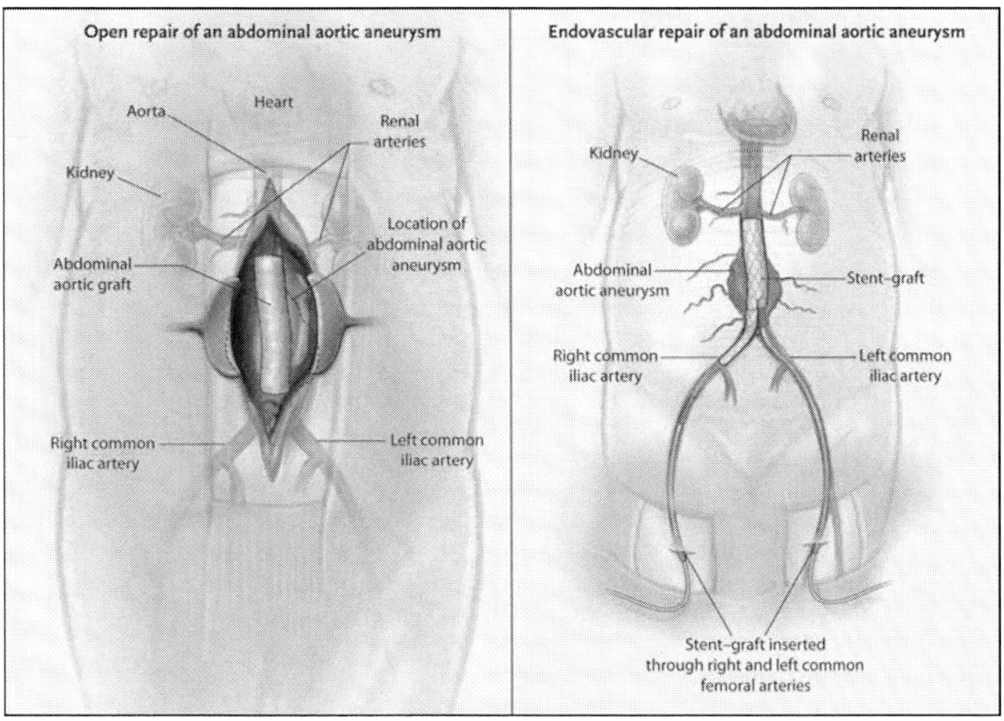

Figure 4. Open repair and endovascular repair of an AAA. In endovascular repair, a stent-graft inserted through the right groin is placed just below the renal arteries, and the left limb of the bifurcated device is inserted through the left groin to overlap with the main body of the stent-graft. Reproduced with permission from an article by Schermerhorn and colleagues [30]. Figure Copyright © *[2008] Massachusetts Medical Society. All rights reserved.*

Although endovascular repair has shown reduced operative mortality along with fewer complications than open surgery, the long-term survival benefit compared to open repair has yet to be established [30-32]. A randomized trial comparing two-year outcomes in patients after open or endovascular repair found a lower post-operative mortality for patients undergoing endovascular repair but found no difference in the overall survival rate between the two groups at two years [33]. Additionally, the need for reintervention is higher after endovascular repair than open repair [30, 31]. A dilemma arises with those patients, many of whom are elderly, who have AAAs greater than 5.5 cm in diameter but are unfit for such a major surgery as open repair. A study examining the use of endovascular aneurysm repair in this patient population found a considerably higher post-operative mortality and a need for continued reinterventions in the surgery population [34]. The long-term durability of endovascular repair has not yet been determined and the ideal AAA patient profile is still being defined [29].

Although there are currently no approved drug therapies shown to reduce the rate of expansion or decrease the incidence of rupture in humans with AAA, the ACC/AHA guidelines recommend adequate blood pressure control and the use of beta-adrenergic blocking agents to lower adverse cardiac events in patients with existing coronary artery disease (CAD) undergoing surgical repair of AAA. The use of beta-adrenergic blocking agents is also recommended based on evidence that they reduce the rate of expansion in a mouse model that develops spontaneous aneurysms [24].

2. Pathophysiologies of AAA

2.1. Are AAAs Distinct from Aortic Occlusive Disease?

AAA development occurs over several years with gradual weakening and slow dilatation of the aortic wall. Unfortunately, most aneurysms are identified only after they have either grown quite large or ruptured, making it difficult to identify the precise mechanisms underlying the initial formation of an aneurysm. Rather, our primary perspective on aneurysms comes from late-stage disease and animal models (see section 4). Typically, these late-stage aneurysms show extensive degradation of the aortic wall and a lumen filled with atherosclerotic plaque and thrombus. Conventionally, this finding has resulted in AAA formation and development being attributed to atherosclerotic disease; atherosclerotic aneurysm is still a commonly used term in textbooks to describe AAA [35]. Since most aneurysms are associated with severe atherosclerotic changes and many AAA patients exhibit risk factors for atherosclerotic disease, particularly smoking (Figure 3), it is quite likely that atherosclerosis plays a role in aneurysm development. Several pieces of evidence, however, suggest that in addition to atherosclerotic changes, there are aneurysm-specific disease mechanisms.

As noted previously, epidemiological evidence suggests that aneurysms are a distinct disease process. First, aneurysms display familial clustering and characteristics of a multifactorial genetic disorder (discussed at length in section 3). Additionally, there is divergence in risk factors between AAA and aortoiliac occlusive disease (AOD). Most notable is the negative association with type II diabetes, a known risk factor of atherosclerotic disease (Figure 3) [36]. Additionally, unlike AAA, AOD has an approximately equal number of affected males and females.

Histological examination of AAA further supports the hypothesis that there are disease-specific mechanisms. Findings characteristic of AAA are inflammation in the entire aortic wall, especially adventitia, loss of smooth muscle cells (SMCs), and disruption of elastic fibers in the tunica media (Figure 5) [37, 38]. In contrast, AOD is primarily an intimal disease, with some invasion deeper into the vessel wall. AAA can also be differentiated from other forms of aortic aneurysms; thoracic aortic aneurysms and dissections (TAAD) show a characteristic pattern known as cystic medial necrosis [37]. Based upon the findings in AAA, several mechanisms have been proposed to be important in AAA formation, including breakdown of extracellular matrix (ECM) by proteinases, infiltration of immune cells to the site of the aneurysm and apoptosis of SMCs (Figure 5).

2.2. Structure of Aorta: Regional Variation

AAA formation may in part be explained by the specific structure of the abdominal aorta. Aneurysms tend to occur in a limited number of blood vessels and do not occur at all sites associated with occlusive atherosclerotic disease, indicating that local vessel biology may be important in aneurysm development [38]. Furthermore, the abdominal aorta may be distinct even from other vessels that develop aneurysms; AAA clusters into different families than intracranial aneurysms (IA) and TAAD, suggesting that the abdominal aorta has characteristics that differentiate it from other arteries, including other regions of the aorta.

The organization of the abdominal aorta is that of a typical artery; it is divided into an intima, media and adventitia. As an elastic artery, the media is the primary component and contains elastic lamellae consisting of alternating layers of SMCs and elastin fibers. The abdominal aorta is distinguished from the thoracic aorta, however, by the number of lamellae. Although the number of lamellae is typically proportionate to the hemodynamic stress on an artery, the abdominal aorta has fewer than would be predicted, perhaps indicating a greater susceptibility to medial damage [38]. The nutrient and gas exchange to the media of the abdominal aorta is also unique, with a relative lack of microvasculature [38]. Unlike the thoracic aorta, which has an extensive network of *vasa vasorum* in the adventitia and outer media, exchange in the media of the abdominal aorta is mainly by diffusion. This exchange is sufficient for up to approximately 29 lamellae, as would be present near the bifurcation, but may result in a relative hypoxia higher in abdominal aorta [38]. Embryological differences between the regions of the aorta may help to explain such differences. Topouzis and Majesky [39] have shown that the SMC lineages of the thoracic and abdominal aorta differ, with origins in neuroectoderm and mesenchyme, respectively. Although similar, these two lineages showed an important difference in response to transforming growth factor beta (TGF-β; *TGFB1*) signaling, which has been implicated in the Marfan syndrome and TAAD [40], perhaps indicating a difference in media formation. [Note that the HUGO Gene Nomenclature Committee (HGNC) [41] symbols for genes and gene products, and their equivalent for other species will be used throughout.]

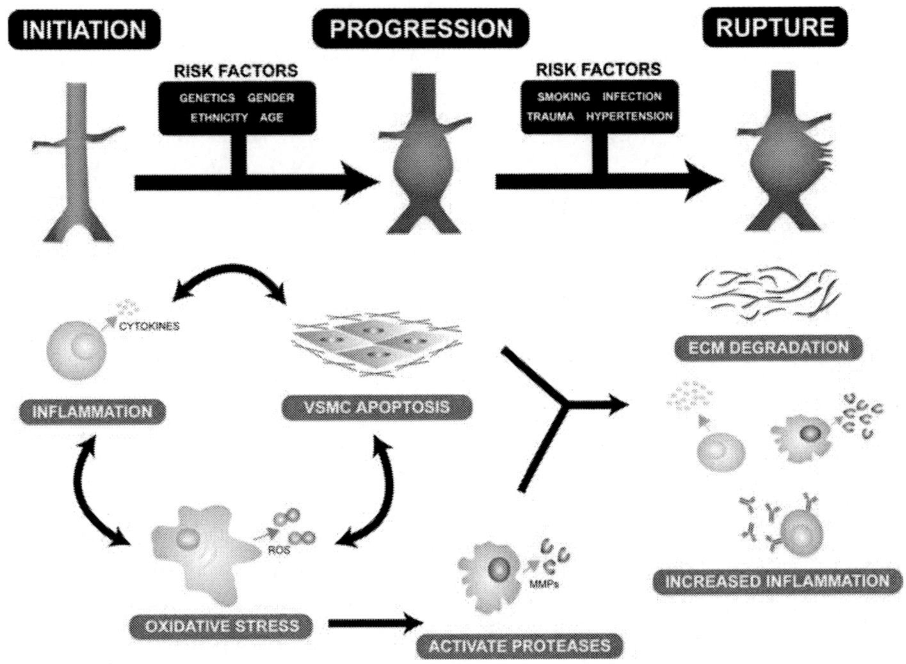

Figure 5. Processes involved in, and risk factors associated with AAA pathogenesis. Risk factors contributing to, and biological processes observed in AAA formation, growth and rupture are summarized. How AAAs form, grow and rupture is not fully understood, but it is clear that AAA is a complex disease with both genetic and environmental risk factors. Many of the same risk factors and processes are involved in initiation and progression as well as rupture. Genes participating in these processes have been studied as candidate genes for AAA. VSMC, vascular smooth muscle cell; ECM, extracellular matrix; ROS, reactive oxygen species; MMPs, matrix metalloproteinases. Reproduced with permission from Boddy et al. 2008 [230].

2.3. ECM Degradation and Increased MMP Expression in AAA

During formation of AAAs, one of the most distinctive and consistent characteristics is the destruction of the elastic lamellae. Elastin is the most abundant protein in the abdominal aorta, accounting for 30% of the aorta by weight [38]. The elastin structure of a blood vessel is formed during development and elastin production does not continue in adulthood. Under normal conditions elastin is quite stable, making the breakdown of elastin in aneurysms particularly striking. The primary structural role of elastin is load bearing; it provides distensibility in response to hemodynamic stress, therefore helping the vessel to maintain its shape. In contrast, collagen, the other major ECM component, provides tensile strength and stiffness to the aorta. A set of experiments by Dobrin and colleagues demonstrated these biophysical effects of elastin and collagen loss in an artery [42]. Under perfusion at physiological pressures, arteries treated with elastase exhibited dilatation and stiffening, whereas collagenase-treated arteries did not dilate but ruptured. Arteries treated with both enzymes dilated rapidly and then ruptured. Given that the elastin of a structurally sound aorta maintains vessel shape even in hypertensive conditions, elastin degradation appears to play a key role in aneurysm growth. Collagen loss in aneurysms, which is typically not detected as early in aneurysm growth, appears to have a more important role in aneurysm rupture. This is supported by the evidence that mutations in the gene for type III procollagen (*COL3A1*) lead to the type IV form of the Ehlers-Danlos syndrome (EDS), the hallmark of which is a rupture of hollow organs such as the aorta, uterus or bowel [43].

Several enzymes have been studied in AAA for their potential role in ECM degradation. Most of this work has focused on the matrix metalloproteinases, or MMPs, and their inhibitors, the tissue inhibitors of metalloproteinases (TIMPs), although other families of enzymes, such as the cathepsins, serine elastases and plasmin, have been studied. The MMPs are a family of related enzymes that break down ECM components including elastin and collagen, although each MMP targets a different repertoire of ligands [44-46]. MMPs have the necessary function of degrading damaged ECM so that new matrix can be regenerated, but can also quickly cause tissue damage if unregulated. Therefore, MMPs are regulated by several mechanisms: by transcription in response to cytokines and growth factors, by secretion in inactive zymogen form, and by inhibition by TIMPs [44]. TIMPs are secreted proteins that bind to activated MMPs. MMPs and TIMPs are often secreted together so as to prevent excess MMP activity. Immunohistochemical analysis of AAA tissue shows that the MMP to TIMP ratio is increased, suggesting that the balance between the two types of proteins influences aneurysm development [47, 48].

MMP2 and MMP9, also known as gelatinase A and B, are two MMPs which specifically cleave gelatin, types IV and V collagen, and fibronectin [46]. More importantly, MMP2 and MMP9 are able to efficiently cleave elastin. Multiple studies examining *MMP2* and *MMP9* transcript and activity have found them to be increased in AAA tissue [49-53]. There is some variability in findings, and of the two, *MMP9* appears to be present more consistently. Additionally, it appears to have a more significant increase in expression in AAA when compared to AOD [50]. Immunohistochemical analysis reveals most MMP9 expression in an aneurysm deriving from infiltrating macrophages, although evidence exists for SMC production of MMP9 [52, 54, 55]. Wilson and colleagues also found that MMP9 levels were increased near the site of aneurysm rupture [56]. Several studies found increased levels of MMP9 in the blood of AAA patients [57, 58], which decreased following surgical repair; these levels do not, however, have a strong predictive value for identifying AAAs.

In contrast to MMP9, MMP2 may have a more generalized role in vascular inflammation. MMP2 is overexpressed in aneurysms, particularly in small ones. It is produced by both resident SMCs and macrophages, and can be found in normal aorta as well as AOD tissue [52]. Increased MMP2 production and activation may therefore be a tissue reaction to inflammation, as evidenced by the observation that SMC MMP2 production increases in the presence of inflammatory cells [52]. Goodall and colleagues also reported that MMP2 levels were increased in remote vasculature of AAA patients, suggesting that the increase is part of a systemic response [59].

Although their primary function is in ECM breakdown, MMP2 and MMP9 may also have roles in ECM signaling. Johnson and colleagues showed that deficiency of both proteins led to decreased SMC invasion *in vitro* [60]. Additionally, it was found that MMP9 may function in the interaction between SMCs and ECM proteins since *Mmp9* knockout mice ($Mmp9^{-/-}$), but not $Mmp2^{-/-}$ mice, had an impaired ability of SMCs to reorganize collagen [60]. Goodall and colleagues [61] confirmed that MMP2 might increase SMC migration by showing that SMCs from AAA patients have higher levels of MMP2 and increased invasiveness *in vitro*.

In addition to MMP2 and MMP9, several other MMPs have been implicated in AAA. MMP12, also known as metalloelastase, has been studied because of its ability to degrade elastin. Comparison of AAA and control tissue has shown that MMP12 is increased in AAA tissue, particularly in macrophages and in association with elastin fibers [62, 63]. MMP8, which is a collagenase, is found at the site of aneurysm rupture, consistent with the hypothesis that collagen breakdown is a necessary condition for AAA rupture. Two MMPs involved in activation of other MMPs, namely MMP3 and MMP14, are also present in AAA tissue. MMP3 is a known activator of MMP9 and is significantly increased in AAA over AOD [64, 65]. In contrast, MMP14, which is also increased in AAA tissue, is known to activate MMP2 and colocalizes with it in AAA tissue [63, 66]. Finally, there are more recently discovered MMPs that have yet to be evaluated in AAA tissue.

2.4. Other Proteases and AAA

Other families of proteases have been studied in AAA. For instance, plasmin (*PLG*), a known activator of MMP3, has been found in AAA tissue [38, 64]. Of particular interest are cathepsins, a family of cysteine proteases that also have the ability to degrade elastin fibers. Immunohistochemistry has identified cathepsins S, K and L in the atheroma and intima of AAA tissue [67, 68]. Similar to MMPs, the cathepsins were found in macrophages and SMCs exposed to inflammatory stimuli, such as interferon gamma (*IFNG*) and interleukin-1 beta (*IL1B*) [67, 68]. Also as with MMPs, cathepsins might have a role in angiogenesis, as inhibition of cathepsin S reduced endothelial cell invasion in culture.

2.5. AAAs are an Immunological Disease

Another prominent histological feature of AAA is infiltration of immune cells into the aortic wall (Figure 5). Inflammation has long been recognized in a subset of aneurysms known as inflammatory aneurysms, but there is growing evidence that AAA is an immune-mediated disease [69]. This observation was first published in a study by Koch and colleagues [70] demonstrating that AAA and inflammatory aneurysms displayed an immune phenotype distinct from AOD. Subsequent studies have identified virtually every leukocyte type in the aneurysmal wall, as well as characterized the cytokine and chemokine makeup. Animal models (see section 4) and whole genome microarray analysis also suggest that the immune system has a critical role in aneurysm formation and growth [71]. By analysis with Kyoto Encyclopedia of Genes and Genomes (KEGG) pathways, Lenk and colleagues [71] found that several immune-related pathways, including Natural Killer (NK) Cell Mediated Cytotoxicity, Leukocyte Transendothelial Migration, T Cell Receptor Signaling, and Antigen Processing and Presentation, are significantly increased in AAA tissue as compared to control aorta. Furthermore, of the top 100 differentially expressed genes, 24 belonged to a Gene Ontology (GO) category with immune-function (Figure 6).

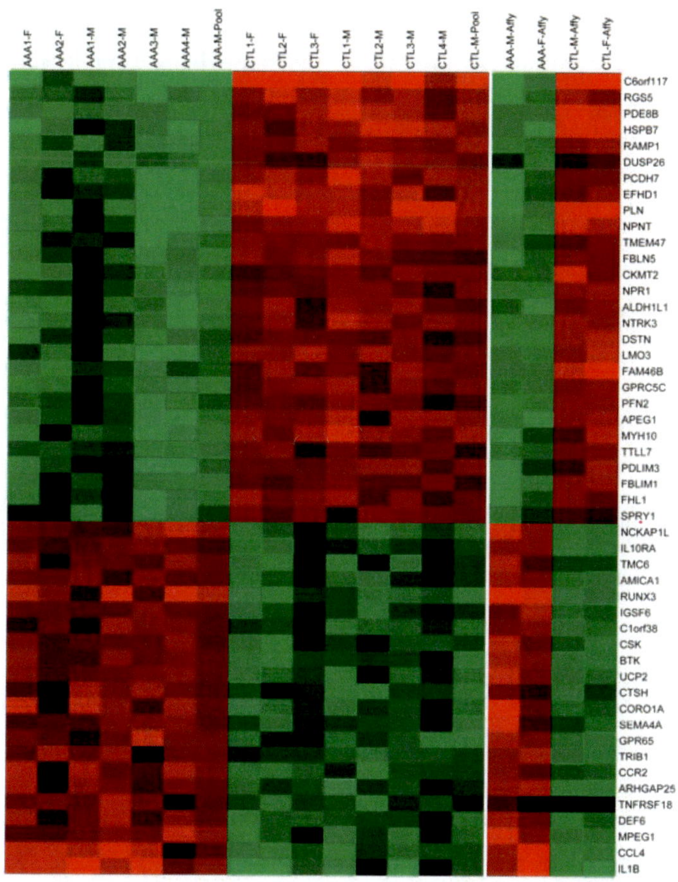

Figure 6. Whole-genome expression profile for AAA tissue. The 50 most significantly different genes between AAA and control tissue are shown as determined by the Illumina microarray platform in ascending order (the most differentially expressed genes are located on the top and bottom, with decreasing difference towards the center). To show consistency of the results between the two platforms (Affymetrix and Illumina), data from both Illumina (15 left columns) and Affymetrix (4 right columns) platforms are presented. Sample IDs are on top of each column (AAA1-F=female aneurysm patient; CTL1-F=female control; etc.). The "Pool" samples were age, sex, and ethnicity matched pools of RNA. All four samples run on Affymetrix arrays were pooled samples. Data were log2-transformed, and gene-centered for each individual platform. Gene IDs shown on the right represent official IDs found at http://www.genenames.org/. For details, see Lenk et al. 2007 [71]. Reproduced with permission from Lillvis et al. 2009 [231].

2.5.1. Inside-out versus outside-in

Histological comparison of AAA and AOD shows that the inflammatory components of these two diseases differ. The pathological appearance of the intimal layer is similar in both diseases, with atherosclerotic plaques containing macrophage-derived foam cells interspersed with T-cells and a small number of dendritic cells as well as macrophages and T-cells infiltrating into the first layers of the underlying media. AAA tissue also shows an additional transmural component, with significant adventitial inflammation infiltrating into the outer media [70]. Conventionally, it has been proposed that inflammation from the atheroma infiltrates into the aortic wall in an "inside-out" manner. This is supported by the presence of neovascularization at the interface of atherosclerotic plaque and the media of the aorta where *vasa vasorum* are scarce [38]. This neovascularization could plausibly provide a route for infiltration of the media and adventitia leading to aneurysm formation.

Growing evidence also points to an "outside-in" component of AAA inflammation [44, 72]. This hypothesis states that vascular injury may cause inflammatory cells to accumulate in the adventitia that then work their way towards the lumen. An example of this process is restenosis following balloon angioplasty where early inflammation occurs in the adventitia and then progresses inwards [72]. Following injury, neovascularization occurs in the outer layers of the vessel, subsequently allowing greater recruitment of immune cells into the adventitia. This may be particularly applicable to AAA development, as the abdominal aorta has fewer *vasa vasorum* and may therefore be more prone to an angiogenic response to injury and greater immune infiltration. Similar to injury from balloon angioplasty, a recently reported porcine model of AAA requires balloon injury of the aorta as well as luminal treatment with elastase to induce aneurysm formation [73]. This indicates that adventitial injury may be necessary in addition to atherosclerosis for AAA formation.

2.5.2. Immune cells in AAA

Several cell types have been identified in AAA tissue, including macrophages, T-cells, B-cells, dendritic cells, mast cells, NK cells, and natural killer T (NKT) cells. Macrophages are perhaps the best studied of these cell types as they are known producers of MMPs and cathepsins. Macrophages are primarily found in the intima, but can also be detected in the adventitia. Surprisingly, however, macrophages represent only a small percentage (~2%) of leukocytes by flow cytometry, although this may be an artifact of cell isolation from tissue [74, 75]. In addition to their direct involvement in ECM breakdown, macrophages also produce several pro-inflammatory cytokines and chemokines including *IL1B*, *TNF*, *CCL2* and *IL8*, which all show increased production in aneurysmal tissue [71]. Finally, macrophages produce other substances such as prostaglandins, which have roles in *IL1B* production and modulating effects on SMCs, and syndecan-1, a proteoglycan which functions in tissue repair [38, 76, 77].

Likely as important to our understanding of AAA are lymphocytes, which comprise a majority of the leukocytes in the aneurysmal wall. Most of these are T-cells (~50 – 70%) which can be found in both the adventitia and intima, but there is also a large proportion of B-cells found in the adventitia (~20 – 40%) [74, 75]. NK and NKT cells are also present in smaller numbers (7%), but may have an important role in aneurysm development (see below) [74, 75]. Histological examination of the adventitia shows that the lymphocytic infiltration is arranged into lymphoid follicle-like structures. Bobryshev and colleagues [78] identified these structures as hypertrophied vascular-associated lymphoid tissue (VALT), which may play a similar role in antigen presentation as mucosa-associated lymphoid tissue (MALT) in the gut and lungs.

Flow cytometry of aneurysm lymphocytes has greatly helped to characterize the B- and T-cell populations [74, 79]. An extensive study by Ocana and colleagues compared expression of ~50 cell surface markers on lymphocytes obtained from AAA tissue and peripheral blood of aneurysm patients [74]. Aneurysmal T-cells showed a similar CD4/CD8 distribution to peripheral blood T-cells, with approximately twice as many $CD4^+$ cells. Significantly more aneurysmal T-cells than blood T-cells expressed an activated phenotype, as measured by CD69 and HLA-DR expression. Additionally, significantly more aneurysmal T-cells showed $CD45RO^+$ $CD45RA^-$ memory phenotype. Findings in B-cells were similar with increased expression of activation markers CD69 and CD80 and memory marker CD27. Also interesting was an increased number of IgA expressing B-cells, which is unusual considering that IgA is the primary immunoglobulin type in mucosal surfaces.

Since $CD4^+$ T-lymphocytes are the primary immune cell in aneurysms, a logical question is what type of T-cell response this represents. Evidence exists supporting both Th1 and Th2 responses in aneurysmal tissue, such as the activation of both macrophages and B-cells, and several studies have addressed this problem. Galle and colleagues [79] used quantitative RT-PCR to study expression of Th1 and Th2 cytokines, *IFNG* and *IL4*, and found increased *IFNG* expression in aneurysmal compared to control tissue but no increase in *IL4*, suggesting a Th1 response. Additionally, expression of the Th1 transcription factor T-bet (*TBX21*) was increased whereas the Th2 transcription factor *GATA3* was not. In contrast, Schönbeck and colleagues [80] found significant amounts of Th2 cytokines IL4 and IL10 by immunohistochemistry and western blotting but no evidence of a Th1 response. To explain these conflicting results, Shimizu and colleagues [81] proposed a model that involved a Th1 response early in atherogenesis and a shift to a Th2 response later in aneurysm development. One complication, however, is that some studies do not distinguish between the intimal and adventitial infiltrates, and cytokine production might vary from layer to layer.

Several studies have found evidence for both immune responses simultaneously. Lindeman and colleagues [82] used several protein and mRNA detection methods and found Th1 cytokines *IL2*, *IFNG*, *IL1A*, and *IL1B* as well as Th2 cytokine *IL13* were significantly increased in AAA over AOD. Another study by Forester and colleagues [75] examined T-cells *ex vivo* and found that they produced primarily Th1 cytokines but also IL5, suggesting a Th0 phenotype that could differentiate into either Th1 or Th2. Array-based analyses add further evidence to this hypothesis. A cytokine protein array study by Middleton and colleagues [83] comparing AAA versus controls found evidence of increased expression of Th1 cytokines TNF, LTA, and CCL2 and increased Th2 cytokine IL10, a result that was fairly consistent with the microarray expression profile by Lenk and colleagues [71]. Since IL10 can also be produced by some Th1 cells, this would suggest a Th1 predominant response. Neither study, however, found a statistically significant increase in levels of Th1 cytokines IFNG, IL2, or CSF2.

Since it is not clear whether the T-cells in aneurysms represent a Th1 or Th2 response, determining their precise role is difficult. It is evident from the increased production of CCL2 and numerous macrophages that there is a likely role for T-cells driving macrophage recruitment into the aneurysm. Conversely, the presence of activated B-cells in follicle-like structures suggests a role for chronic antigen-driven inflammation. This is supported by the fact that dendritic cells, known for their role in antigen processing, can be found localized with T-cells and B-cells in the adventitia [78, 84]. Evidence for antigen processing has even led to the suggestion that aneurysms are a chronic autoimmune disorder in which an aortic antigen drives inflammation [85, 86]. This is supported by the finding that the aneurysmal T-cell receptor (TCR) repertoire is clonal by CDR3 length analysis in $\gamma\delta$ T-cells, although another study found that TCR V beta expression was polyclonal by RT-PCR [87, 88]. Unfortunately, the search for autoantigens has not been particularly successful. One proposed candidate was *Chlamydia pneumoniae*, but this association has not been consistently reproduced [38, 89]. Another putative antigen is a microfibrillar protein associated with collagen, but this hypothesis has not been fully elucidated [90].

Another cell type that may have a small yet important role in aneurysm development is the mast cell. Although mast cells are typically associated with IgE mediated immunity and allergies, they produce several substances, such as histamine and heparin that could contribute to inflammation in AAA. Furthermore, knockout of mast cells prevented formation of aneurysms in two different animal models [91]. A study by Tsuruda and colleagues [92] examined the antifibrotic effect of one mast-cell derived substance, adrenomedullin, and found it to decrease collagen production by fibroblasts *in vitro*.

2.6. Smooth Muscle Cell Apoptosis

A third characteristic feature of aneurysms is loss of SMCs (Figure 5). Terminal transferase dUTP nick end-labeling (TUNEL) of the aortic wall revealed SMCs undergoing cell death, but the precise cause is not fully known [93].

One possibility is that SMC apoptosis is mediated by cytotoxic lymphocytes. Although not a majority, $CD8^+$ T-cells represent a significant proportion of lymphocytes in the aortic wall [74, 75]. Also low in numbers by flow cytometry, NK and NKT cells have been detected by immunostaining in aneurysm tissue [94], as well as apoptotic mediators perforin and Fas [95]. When isolated from AAA plaques, NKT and $CD4^+$ T-cells induced differential effects in vascular SMCs, with the T-cells enhancing proliferation and NKT cells increasing apoptosis [96]. Additionally, peripheral blood NK cells are significantly increased in AAA patients compared to controls.

An important role for cytotoxic lymphocytes is further supported by microarray analysis. Of the immune-related KEGG pathways, "Natural Killer Cell Mediated Cytotoxicity" was statistically the most enriched pathway in AAA tissue compared to non-aneurysmal aorta tissue [71]. Despite the name, this pathway is not specific to NK cells, but may also indicate an increase in NKT cells or cytotoxic lymphocytes.

Other mechanisms of SMC death in aneurysms have also been proposed. One logical explanation, given the age at onset of AAA, is that SMC senescence is responsible [38]. Another theory is that macrophage-derived osteoprotegrin (OPG) can cause SMC apoptosis. OPG can act as a decoy receptor for TRAIL, a TNF-related apoptosis-inducing ligand, and has been shown to slow down SMC proliferation *in vitro* [97]. Alternatively, macrophage-derived prostaglandin E_2 may have similar effects [38].

2.7. Oxidative Stress

Oxidative stress is another mechanism that could be involved in all the above-mentioned aspects of aneurysm development (Figure 5). Reactive oxygen species (ROS) and reactive nitrogen species (RNS) have been implicated in the pathology of several conditions, such as Alzheimer's disease and atherosclerosis [98, 99]. Consistent with the concept of oxidative stress in AAA, it has been shown that levels of enzymes responsible for eliminating ROS, superoxide dismutase, glutathione peroxidase, and glutathione reductase, are decreased in AAA tissue [100]. Simultaneously, there is an increase in inducible nitric oxide synthase.

Production of ROS and RNS in aneurysms is likely from several sources. NADPH and myeloperoxidase activity in infiltrating immune cells, particularly macrophages, can produce large amounts of O_2^- and hypochlorous acid (HOCl), which in turn oxidize LDL and cause tissue damage [100]. Additionally, SMCs can increase ROS production through NADPH oxidase in response to stimulation by angiotensin or TNF [101]. SMCs can also produce ROS in response to pulsatile forces [100].

ROS and RNS could have several effects on aneurysm formation [100] (Figure 5). First, they could induce cytokine production that then leads to immune cell infiltration. Alternatively, they can lead to activation of NFKB, an inflammatory transcription factor implicated in AAA. ROS can also have an effect on the ECM through activation of *MMP2* and *MMP9*. Finally, ROS could possibly lead to SMC apoptosis, although this is debatable as ROS have been shown to increase SMC proliferation.

3. AAA is a Complex Genetic Disease

Whereas simple Mendelian disease is characterized by easily recognizable modes of inheritance and a strong correlation between the presence of a disease gene and the disease phenotype, a complex disease is characterized by a weak correlation and poorly recognizable modes of inheritance. Frequently multiple genes contribute to the disease, either independently or through gene-gene interaction. In addition, environmental or non-genetic risk factors often contribute to the disease and further weaken the gene-phenotype correlation. The most common genetic model for complex disease is the multifactorial model in which at least one environmental factor and one gene contribute to the disease process. Analysis of complex genetic disease therefore involves characterization of both environmental and genetic risk factors.

3.1. Risk Factors for AAA

3.1.1. Smoking

Smoking is consistently identified as the most significant risk factor for AAA development (Figure 3) [10, 36]. Aneurysms occur eight times (95% CI: 3.3 – 17.8%) more frequently in one to two pack a day smokers than in non-smokers [102, 103]. Although smoking cessation reduces the risk of AAA, ex-smokers are still three times (OR = 3.0, 95% CI: 1.4 – 6.4%) more likely to develop AAA than non-smokers [103, 104]. Additionally, a large cohort study including 1,743 patients used ultrasonography screening to monitor AAA expansion over a mean follow-up of 1.9 years and found that current smokers had a 15 – 20% greater increase in AAA expansion (approximately 0.4 mm/y greater) [18].

3.1.2. Male sex

The prevalence of AAA in men is six times higher than women [105, 106] with males ten times more likely to have AAAs greater than 4.0 cm [10-12]. Based on large epidemiological studies, female sex is a protective factor with an OR = 0.22 (95% CI: 0.07 – 0.68) (Figure 3) [36]. The average age of female AAA patients is six years older than male patients [107] and interview and ultrasonography screening studies found that younger female patients were more likely to have a family history of AAA [108].

The higher prevalence in the male sex has resulted in a bias of ultrasonography screening being targeted towards males only [109, 110]. Some have even suggested that screening women is not economically viable [106]. However, women typically have a higher rupture rate than men [111] and a worse outcome in open repair surgery for AAA [112]. Additionally, the mortality rate for ruptured AAA is significantly worse in women than men, 90% compared to 76% ($p < 0.0001$), respectively [107]. Furthermore, AAAs in females grow faster than in males [113]. Given that the aortic diameter is typically larger in males than in females [114], it has been suggested the threshold for surgery should be lowered for women from 5.5 cm to 5.2 cm [113].

Differences between male and female susceptibility to AAA might be a result from the hormonal component estrogen, since the risk of AAA typically increases in women after menopause [115]. Estrogen has been shown to play a protective role in other cardiovascular diseases [116], such as CAD. Women with irregular menstrual cycles were at a significantly increased risk of developing CAD (RR = 1.8, CI = 1.1 – 2.9) [117]. Interestingly, in animal models, male and female rodents also show a difference in susceptibility to AAA formation (see Section 4.2). Mechanistically these animal studies point to a more important role for androgens in worsening the outcome rather than estrogens having a protective effect. Since human observational studies are unable to determine mechanism, this suggests that the protective role of estrogen has been overestimated (see Section 4.2).

3.1.3. Age

Age is one of the leading risk factors for the development of AAA (Figure 3; OR = 1.52, 95% CI: 1.45 – 1.60), with a mean age of approximately 66.0 years (± 7.5 years) in AAA patients [11]. Previous studies have shown a steady increase in prevalence of AAA among elderly patients from the age of 65 – 79 years [102, 118]. One group screened 10,328 men over the age of 50 and found a linear correlation between prevalence and age of the individual [119]. AAA rises to the 12th leading cause of death in individuals aged 65 – 74 years as compared to 17th leading cause in all age groups [120]. Additionally, the mortality rate of AAA increases with age, with one study reporting 84% of AAA deaths to occur in persons over the age of 65 [121].

3.1.4. Caucasian ethnicity

Most cardiovascular diseases, such as atherosclerosis, are more prevalent in the African American than Caucasian population. In contrast, the prevalence of AAA is higher in Caucasian than African American men [36, 121, 122]. A large 5-year retrospective case-control study on femoral bypass and abdominal aortic aneurysmectomy was performed using hospital discharge information from 1984 to 1988 in Massachusetts [122]. During this time, 4,682 abdominal aortic aneurysmectomies were performed. The number of procedures was low in both African American and Caucasian women, but slightly higher in Caucasian women. Caucasian men accounted for 80% of the aneurysmectomies and the African American/Caucasian odds ratio for an AAA was 0.29. Additionally, in the large cohort study by Lederle and colleagues [36] African American race was negatively associated with AAA, with an OR = 0.72 (95% CI: 0.59 – 0.87) for small aneurysms (3.0 – 3.9 cm) and OR = 0.49 (95% CI: 0.35 – 0.69) for larger aneurysms (>4.0 cm) (Figure 3).

3.1.5. Family history

The genetic nature of a disease is, in part, supported by familial aggregation. The first evidence of the genetic involvement in AAA was reported in 1977 by Clifton when he operated on three brothers with AAAs. His insightful comment was: "The chance occurrence of this condition in three brothers is remote and constitutional and hereditary factors must be looked to for an explanation" [14]. Since then several reports interviewing first-degree relatives of patients with AAA have been published, showing a strong indication of AAA clustering in families (Table 1). One such study by Powell and colleagues [123] observed 60 AAA patients, 25 with a positive family history, and concluded that the genetic component of AAA contributed to approximately 70% of the disease. Combined analysis of studies based on patient interviews showed that approximately 13% of AAA patients acknowledge a positive family history of the disease (Table 1).

To date, one of the largest ultrasonography screening studies was conducted in 1997 when over 70,000 veterans between the ages of 50 – 79 years were examined for AAA and detailed information on risk factor profile was collected. Approximately 3,300 individuals had an infrarenal aortic diameter of at least 3.0 cm, which is characteristically defined as an AAA. Analysis of the results using multiple logistic regression concluded that family history was a risk factor for AAA with OR = 1.96 (95% CI: 1.68 – 2.28) (Figure 3) [36]. Many other studies have reported screening of family members of AAA patients by abdominal ultrasonography, revealing a high prevalence of AAA in brothers (19.5%) and in sisters (5.7%) (Table 2). When comparing the prevalence of AAA among siblings of patients with AAA to the prevalence of AAA among spouses' siblings based on an ultrasonography screening an eight-fold higher prevalence in siblings of AAA patients was found [124].

Table 1. Familial prevalence of AAA based on interviews

	Patients (N)		
Study	Surveyed	Positive History	Familial Prevalence (%)
Norrgård et al. 1984 [234]	87	16	18.4
Johansen and Koepsell 1986 [235]	250	48	19.2
Powell and Greenhalgh 1987 [123]	56	20	35.7
Johnston and Scobie 1988 [108]	666	41	6.1
Cole et al. 1989 [236]	305	34	11.1
Darling et al. 1989 [128]	542	82	15.1
Majumder et al. 1991 [15]	91	13	14.3
Verloes et al. 1995 [17]	313	39	12.5
Lederle et al. 1997 [36]	985	91	9.2
Lawrence et al. 1998 [237]	86	19	22.1
Salkowski et al. 1999 [238]	72	19	26.4
Rossaak et al. 2001 [239]	248	48	19.4
Total	3701	470	
Combined Prevalence			12.7

Modified with permission from Kuivaniemi & Tromp, 2000 [233].

3.2. Segregation Analysis: A Formal Test for Genetic Inheritance

Complex segregation analysis using statistical methods can answer two important questions about a disease: 1) is the disease genetic; and 2) what is the most likely mode of inheritance [125]. In order to carry out a proper segregation analysis, the patients must be sampled in an unbiased manner, e.g. collecting information from every AAA patient during a specific time period. Using an existing collection of AAA families is therefore, not an appropriate starting point for segregation analysis. The first step in segregation analysis involves testing whether a genetic model can explain the aggregation of the disease in families. Segregation analysis can also be used to examine which mode of inheritance best fits with the data by determining the proportion of affected to unaffected individuals, also known as the segregation ratio. In diseases with an autosomal recessive pattern, the segregation ratio should be 1 in 4. However, the analysis becomes more complicated for non-Mendelian complex traits. Here, different genetic models for disease are fit to the data under a maximum likelihood framework to determine which model fits best [126].

Early reports on collections of families discussed the possibility of both a single gene effect and a multifactorial mode of inheritance for AAA [16, 123]. In 1991, Majumder and colleagues [15] were the first group to perform a formal segregation analysis for AAA, where data on first-degree relatives was collected for 91 AAA patients. The possibility of a non-genetic model was rejected in this study with the data demonstrating statistically significant evidence for a genetic model, in which the multifactorial model had minimal effect. They found that an autosomal recessive model for a major gene fit best with their data [15].

Verloes and colleagues [17] also performed a segregation analysis on 313 pedigrees and concluded that an autosomal dominant model for a major gene was the best fit for the familial aggregation of AAA in their sample. They suggested that the morbid allele frequency was 1:250, with an age-related penetrance of 0.4 [17]. It is worth noting that both studies agreed on a major gene effect, and that the evidence for autosomal dominant and autosomal recessive models was almost equal. This can occur when there is genetic heterogeneity, so that the model that fits best differs between samples. The AAA segregation results [15, 17] may therefore be interpreted as AAA is a disease with a major gene effect and heterogeneity.

Table 2. Prevalence of AAA among first-degree family members based on ultrasonography screening

Study	Country	Brothers[1] (%)	Sisters[1] (%)	Other[1] (%)
Bengtsson et al. 1989 [240]	Sweden	10/35 (28.6)	3/52 (5.8)	
Collin & Walton 1989 [241]	UK	4/16 (25.0)	0/15 (0)	
Webster et al. 1991 [242]	USA	5/24 (20.8)	2/30 (6.7)	7/103 (6.8)
Adamson et al. 1992 [129]	UK	5/25 (20.0)	3/28 (10.7)	
Bengtsson et al. 1992 [243]	Sweden			9/62 (14.5)
van der Lugt et al. 1992 [244]	Netherlands	16/56 (28.6)	3/52 (5.8)	
Adams et al. 1993 [245]	UK	4/23 (17.4)	1/28 (3.6)	6/23 (26.1)
Moher et al. 1994 [246]	Canada	9/48 (18.8)		
Fitzgerald et al. 1995 [247]	Ireland	13/60 (21.7)	2/65 (3.1)	
Larcos et al. 1995 [248]	Australia			0/52 (0)
Baird et al. 1995 [130]	Canada	7/26 (26.9)	3/28 10.7)	
Jaakkola et al. 1996 [249]	Finland	4/45 (8.9)	1/78 (1.3)	
van der Graaf et al. 1998 [250]	Netherlands	26/210 (12.4)		
Salo et al. 1999 [251]	Finland			11/238 (4.6)
Rossaak et al. 2001 [239]	New Zealand			4/49 (8.2)
Frydman et al. 2003 [252]	Australia	64/150 (42.7)	20/126 (15.9)	
Ogata et al. 2005 [124]	Canada	11/98 (11.2)	4/147 (2.7)	0/31 (0)
Badger et al. 2007 [253]	Northern Ireland	8/136 (5.8)	2/122 (1.6)	0/42 (0)
Total		186/952 (19.5)	44/771 (5.7)	37/638 (5.7)

[1]Number of individuals identified with AAA/number of individuals examined by ultrasonography. Other refers to relatives other than sisters and brothers of the AAA-patient, or the categories of relatives were not specified. Modified with permission from Kuivaniemi & Tromp, 2000 [233].

When investigating collections of AAA families, many studies have produced evidence of multifactorial inheritance for AAA. Multifactorial inheritance hypothesis assumes that multiple genetic loci and environmental factors contribute to disease pathogenesis, and the genetic risk factors are usually not inherited in either a dominant or recessive pattern. A key characteristic of a multifactorial disease is that if the two sexes have different probabilities of getting the disease and the less likely sex is affected, then they are more likely to produce affected offspring and the disease can occur at an earlier age and be more severe [126]. Considering that familial cases of AAAs are often younger and have more affected women, the multifactorial model is plausible [123]. A large collection of AAA families with 233 multiplex families (Figure 7) found that 72% of the AAA families were consistent with an autosomal recessive pattern, while 25% showed an autosomal dominant pattern of inheritance [13]. Since no single mode of inheritance is consistently identified, it suggests that AAA is a multifactorial disease with multiple genetic and environmental factors playing a role in the disease pathogenesis (Figure 5).

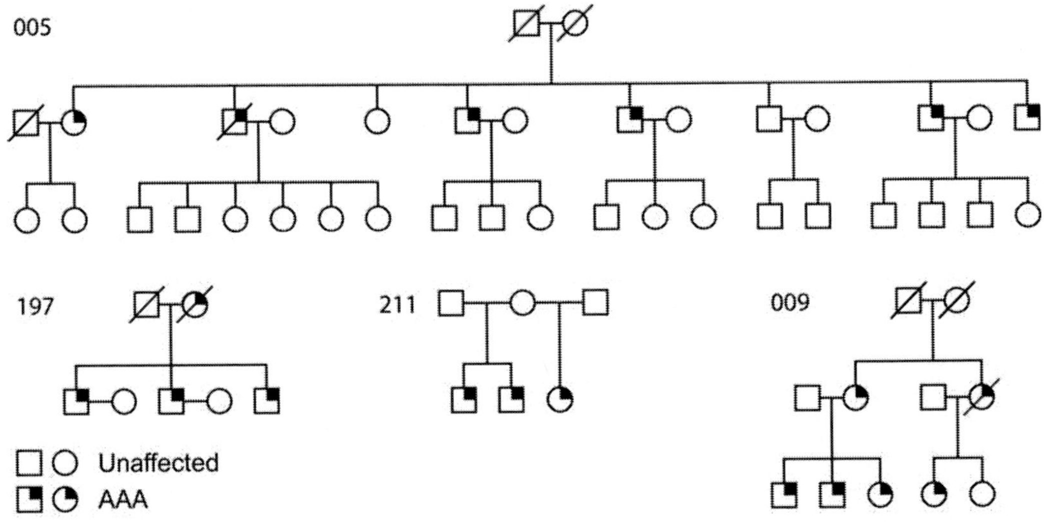

Figure 7. Four multiplex AAA families. Representative AAA families from our collection of 233 families [13]. Slash across symbol means death. Squares and circles with the upper right quadrant darkened indicate male and female members, respectively, diagnosed with AAA. Reproduced with permission from Lillvis et al. 2009 [231].

3.3. Clinical Differences between Familial AAA (FAAA) and Sporadic AAA (SAAA)

The genetic nature of AAA is further supported by differences between the disease in familial and sporadic cases. More severe disease in familial cases or an earlier age at onset (age at diagnosis) is considered additional evidence for the genetic nature of disease since either or both suggest an increased risk attributed to the genetic component. Similarly, the genetic nature of disease is supported when younger patients have more affected relatives than older patients. These conditions follow from the Falconer threshold model for disease [127].

In 1989, Darling and colleagues [128] conducted a 9-year study with over 500 patients to observe differences in familial AAA (FAAA) patients who had at least one first-degree relative with an AAA, compared to sporadic AAA (SAAA), with no family history of AAA. Their results demonstrated that the FAAA group was more likely to have affected women (35% compared to 14%) than the SAAA group. Also, men with FAAA were generally 5 years younger than SAAA cases. However, there were no differences in the anatomical features of AAA between the two groups [128]. Adamson and colleagues [129] also reported that the younger the patient was, the greater the familial component. Furthermore, other studies confirmed that age at onset, as well as age at rupture, was younger in FAAA [17, 130], and that the prevalence of rupture was significantly higher in the FAAA group compared to the SAAA group, with rates of 99% and 32% ($p < 0.001$), respectively [17].

Additional evidence for the genetic nature of disease may be supplied by anticipation: the phenomenon of decreasing age at onset, or increased severity, in successive generations. One of the most well known examples of anticipation is Huntington disease, where the disease can sometimes occur 24 years earlier in offspring than parent [131, 132]. Origuchi and colleagues [133] studied seven AAA families, with 15 affected individuals and found that the age at onset was much younger in the 2nd generation as compared to the 1st (mean age of 55 ± 10.5 vs. 69.6 ± 7.4 years, respectively). No further studies have, however, reported anticipation in AAA; in part because formal proof of anticipation requires taking into consideration a substantial sampling bias in parent-child samples (the child cannot be older than the parent). Additionally, because of the improved diagnostics, any proposed anticipation must be interpreted with caution. It could simply be the result of increased clinical scrutiny among family members of AAA patients to identify the AAAs before they rupture.

3.4. Genome-Wide Linkage Analysis to Identify Susceptibility Loci for AAA

DNA linkage analysis is an unbiased genome-wide method used to identify susceptibility loci by following inheritance patterns of the disease of interest in a family through the use of genetic markers. Typically, linkage between a specific marker, or several markers, and the disease of interest can be determined [134]. Such studies require large collections of multigenerational families. AAA is a difficult disease to study using the traditional family-based DNA linkage approach due to the fact that it is a disease of the aging and information on parents or children is limited. The parents of most AAA patients have already died by the time the patient is diagnosed with an AAA, and their children are not yet old enough to show the disease. An alternative approach is affected-relative-pairs (ARP) linkage analysis, which is a robust method used to determine shared chromosomal segments in families. In this analysis, an assumption is made that related individuals share alleles identity-by-descent (IBD) from a common ancestor, e.g., sibling pairs are expected to share 0, 1, or 2 parental haplotypes with the probabilities of ¼, ½, ¼, respectively. If both sibs are affected, it is more likely that they will share at least one parental risk allele or haplotype at the disease risk locus [126, 135]. This analysis makes the null hypothesis assumption that the recombination events are independent on the same chromosome and that the marker and disease allele are in linkage equilibrium. If a marker and disease risk allele are linked, ARPs are expected to share more alleles IBD than by chance [135].

Shibamura and colleagues [136] studied 119 AAA families using an ARP approach with sex and number of affected relatives, and their interactions as covariates, allowing for genetic heterogeneity. As outlined in Figure 8, clinical data and blood samples were collected from AAA patients as well as their relatives. Using a 2-phase, 2-stage study design, a whole genome scan was completed using approximately 400 microsatellite markers. The first phase analyzed 36 multiplex families with 78 ARPs using sex and the number of first-degree relatives as covariates. Twelve regions on eight chromosomes (3, 4, 5, 6, 9, 14, 19, 21) were identified as being worthy of follow-up with $p < 0.05$. The second stage of phase 1 was to genotype additional markers in regions giving positive results. Phase 2 included testing of positive markers in 83 new multiplex families, which included 157 ARPs. After detailed follow up analysis with a combined set of 235 ARPs, significant linkage was found on chromosomes 4q31 (LOD score = 3.73, p = 0.0012) and 19q13 (LOD score = 4.75, p = 0.00014) (Figure 9). These genomic regions have been designated as AAA2 and AAA1 susceptibility loci, respectively, in the Online Mendelian Inheritance in Man (OMIM) [137]. In addition, a second locus on chromosome 4, at 4q12, had a LOD of 3.13 (p = 0.0042; [136]; Figure 8). Although the LOD score and the parameter estimates provide less support for this locus than for the other two loci, it would be worth performing follow-up studies, provided that the results are replicated in another population [136].

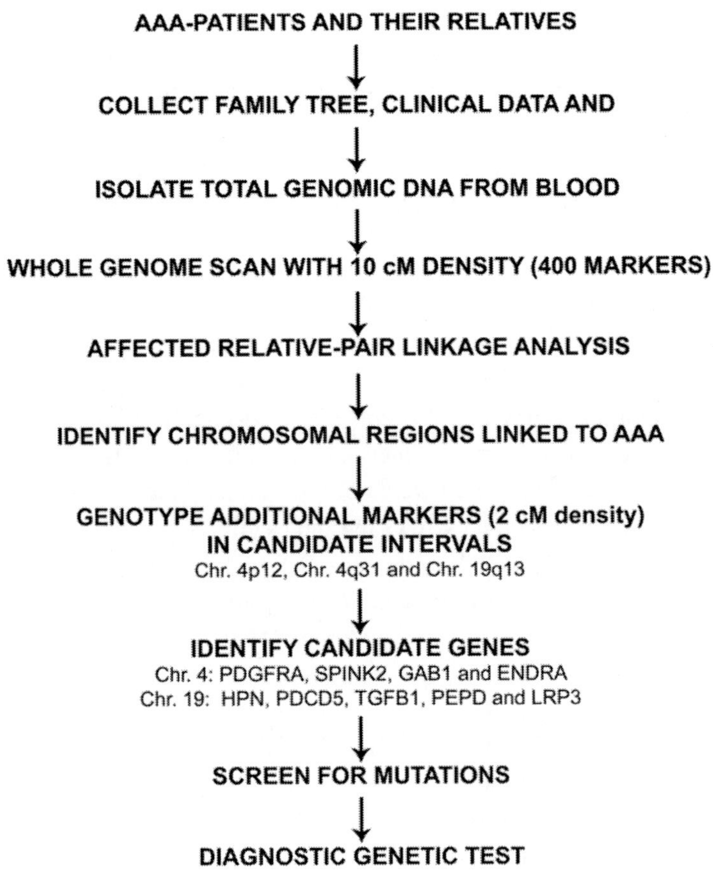

Figure 8. Outline of steps needed to identify susceptibility gene(s) for AAA using affected relative pair – DNA linkage analysis. As discussed in the text, including only the relatives who have been diagnosed with AAA will improve the accuracy of the analysis, since AAA is a late-age-at-onset disease. For details, see Shibamura et al. 2004 [136]. Reproduced with permission from Kuivaniemi et al. 2006 [232].

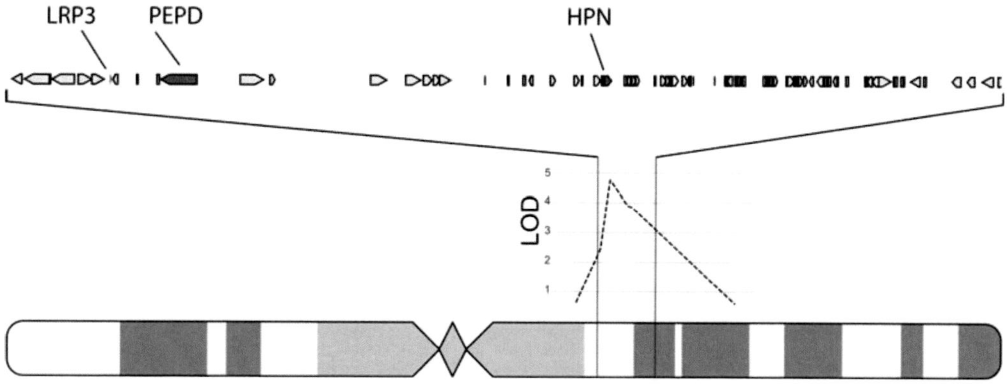

Figure 9. Genetic susceptibility locus on chromosome 19 for AAA. This genetic region was identified in a genome-wide DNA linkage study using affected relative pair approach [136]. The bottom of the figure shows chromosome 19 with the linked region bracketed. The middle plot shows the logarithm of odds (LOD) score within the region. At the top of the figure, the locations of genes in the region are indicated by arrows. The locations of three candidate genes, low density lipoprotein receptor-related protein 3 (*LRP3*), peptidase D (*PEPD*), and hepsin (*HPN*), are indicated. Reproduced with permission from Lillvis et al. 2009 [231].

The candidate intervals contain a large number of plausible candidate genes related to cardiovascular pathology and physiology. Examples include low density lipoprotein receptor-related protein 3 (*LRP3)*, peptidase D (*PEPD)*, and hepsin (*HPN)* located on the chromosome 19q13 AAA1 locus [136]. The 4q31 candidate interval (AAA2 locus) contains such plausible candidate genes as interleukin 15 (*IL15)*, GRB2-associated binding protein 1 (*GAB1)* and endothelin receptor type A (*EDNRA)*. Further analysis of these candidate genes is needed to determine their potential role in AAA pathogenesis.

Interestingly, another group studying three Dutch families with at least four affected siblings was able to replicate linkage to 19q13 [138]. Their analysis used different statistical methods, without covariates, and the 19q13 linkage was slightly more telomeric compared to the Shibamura report [138]. Nevertheless, there is strong evidence of linkage to the region of 19q13 and further studies are needed to narrow the candidate interval.

3.5. DNA linkage studies on other forms of aneurysms: IA and TAAD

DNA linkage analyses have also been carried out in other types of aneurysms (Figure 10). Genome-wide studies on IA have identified nine susceptibility loci, 1p34.4-p36.16 [139], 5p15.2-p14.3 [140], 5q22-q31 [141], 7q11 [141], 11q24-q25 [142], 14q22,q23-31 [141, 142], 17 cen [143], 19q13 [143-145], and Xp22 [135, 143]. Notably, the 19q13 region shares a linkage signal for IA and AAA, suggesting that there may be a common vascular risk factor important in aneurysm formation on this locus. Interestingly, another cardiovascular disease, Kawasaki disease has also been linked to 19q13 [146], as well as to other susceptibility loci. To follow up the linkage results, an association study with over 1,200 SNPs in the 19q13 region was performed in Kawasaki patients and controls. The gene, inositol 1,4,5-trisphosphate 3-kinase C (*ITPKC)* was studied further, based on its biological role in T-cell signaling and is the most likely positional candidate gene for Kawasaki disease [146].

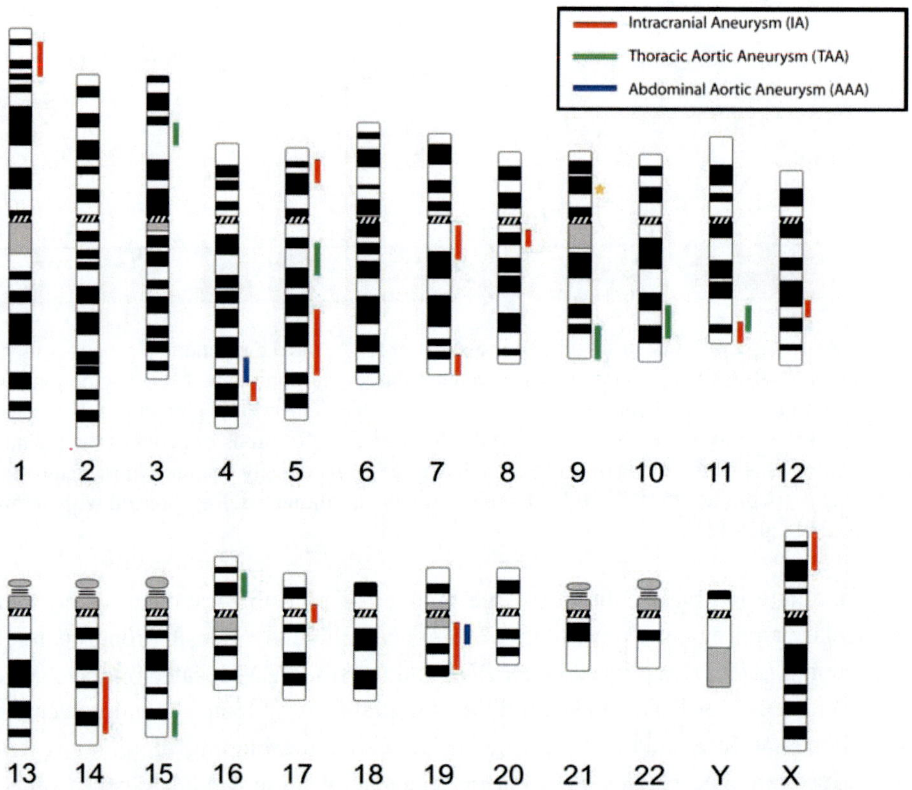

Figure 10. Chromosomal locations of the genetic susceptibility loci for AAA, IA and TAAD. Altogether two, thirteen and seven loci for AAA (blue), IA (red) and TAAD (green), have been reported in the literature. The chromosome 9p21 region which contains the genetic variant rs10757278 associated with CAD, AAA and IA [194] is indicated with a yellow star. For details see text. The ideograms can be obtained from "Idiogram Album: Human" (copyright © 1994 David Adler, University of Washington, Department of Pathology) at http://www.pathology.washington.edu/research/cytopages/idiograms/human/.

Seven loci have been identified for TAAD (Figure 10): 3p22 [147], 5q13-q14 [148], 9q33-q34 [149], 10q23-24 [150], 11q23.3-q24 [151], 15q24-26 [40], and 16p13.13-p13.12 [152]. Interestingly, there is an overlap region on chromosome 11q24 that is linked to both IA and TAAD. In four of the TAAD loci, the candidate gene has been identified and mutations in TAAD patients have been found in the genes *TGFBR1* and *TGFBR2* [149], *MYH11* [150], and *ACTA2* [153], which together account for an estimated 20% of TAAD.

Detailed analysis of the shared genetic regions could prove beneficial if there is an underlying common vascular component involved in multiple types of aneurysms, as has been discussed in a meta-analysis of whole-genome linkage studies on AAA, IA and TAAD [154]. AAA and TAAD sometimes coexist in patients or families [155, 156] and there have also been reports of AAA and IA coexisting in the same patients or in the same families [17, 157, 158].

3.6. Candidate Gene Analysis

Two of the most commonly used approaches to study candidate genes are DNA sequencing and genetic association. Typically, DNA sequencing is performed for a limited number of individuals, whereas association requires large samples of individuals. DNA sequencing is useful when there are many different risk alleles in a locus (allelic heterogeneity), whereas genetic association relies on a common risk allele inherited IBD by a substantial fraction of the cases. The common allele is usually detected by a polymorphic marker allele which is tightly correlated with the risk allele (the correlation is called linkage disequilibrium). While a limited number of genes have been sequenced in AAA patients, a large number of genes have been tested in genetic association studies using known polymorphisms. Table 3 lists all the candidate gene studies for AAA.

Table 3. Candidate genes studied in AAA

Gene Symbol	Full Gene Name	Chromosomal Location	Number of Studies [References]
Group 1: Structural and Remodeling			
ABCC6	ATP-binding cassette, sub-family C (CFTR/MRP), member 6	16p13.1	1 [254]
COL3A1	Collagen, type III, alpha 1	2q31	10 [129, 159-162, 168, 255-258]
ELN	Elastin	7q11.23	2 [168, 259]
FBLN2	Fibulin 2	3p25.1	1 [163]
FBN1	Fibrillin 1	15q21.1	2 [257, 260]
MMP1	Matrix metallopeptidase 1 (interstitial collagenase)	11q22.3	1 [168]
MMP10	Matrix metallopeptidase 10 (stromelysin 2)	11q22.3	1 [168]
MMP12	Matrix metallopeptidase 12 (macrophage elastase)	11q22.3	3 [168, 169, 261]
MMP13	Matrix metallopeptidase 13 (collagenase 3)	11q22.3	1 [168]
MMP2	Matrix metallopeptidase 2 (gelatinase A)	16q13-q21	4 [168, 169, 261, 262]
MMP3	Matrix metallopeptidase 3 (stromelysin 1)	11q22.3	5 [168, 169, 261, 263, 264]
MMP9	Matrix metallopeptidase 9 (gelatinase B)	20q11.2-q13.1	6 [167-169, 261, 263, 265]
SERPINA1	Serpin peptidase inhibitor, clade A, member 1	14q32.1	3 [266-268]
SERPINE1	Serpin peptidase inhibitor, clade E, member 1	7q21.3-q22	5 [169, 261, 263, 269, 270]
SPP1	Secreted phosphoprotein 1 (osteopontin)	4q21-q25	1 [271]
TIMP1	TIMP metallopeptidase inhibitor 1	Xp11.3-p11.23	4 [164, 168, 261, 272]
TIMP2	TIMP metallopeptidase inhibitor 2	17q25	2 [164, 168]
TIMP3	TIMP metallopeptidase inhibitor 3	22q12.3	1 [168]

Table 3. (Continued)

Gene Symbol	Full Gene Name	Chromosomal Location	Number of Studies [References]
XYLT1	Xylosyltransferase1	16p12.3	1 [273]
Group 2: Cardiovascular Genes			
ACE	Angiotensin I converting enzyme (peptidyl-dipeptidase A) 1	17q23.3	5 [172-175, 274]
AGT	Angiotensinogen	1q42-q43	1 [175]
AGTR1	Angiotensin II receptor, type 1	3q21-q25	2 [174, 175]
APOB	Apolipoprotein B (including Ag(x) antigen)	2p24-p23	1 [257]
APOE	Apolipoprotein E	19q13.2	1 [275]
BDKRB2	Bradykinin receptor	14q32.1-q32.2	1 [175]
CETP	Cholesteryl ester transfer protein, plasma	16q21	3 [276-278]
F2	Coagulation factor II (thrombin)	11p11	1 [181]
F5	Coagulation factor V (proaccelerin, labile factor)	1q23	1 [181]
MTHFR	5,10-methylenetetrahydrofolate reductase	1p36.3	7 [178-181, 279-281]
NOS3	Nitric oxide synthase 3 (endothelial cell)	7q36	1 [282]
Group 3: Immunity			
CCR5	Chemokine (C-C motif) receptor 5	3p21.31	1 [283]
HLA@	Human leukocyte antigen locus	6p21.3	10 [185, 187-190, 284-288]
IL10	Interleukin 10	1q31-q32	1 [289]
IL1A	Interleukin 1, alpha	2q14	1 [290]
IL1B	Interleukin 1, beta	2q14	2 [289, 290]
IL1RN	Interleukin 1 receptor antagonist	2q14.2	1 [290]
IL6	Interleukin 6 (interferon, beta 2)	7p21	2 [289, 291]
PLA2G7	Phospholipase A2, group VII	6p21.2-p12	1 [292]
TNF	Tumor necrosis factor (TNF superfamily, member 2)	6p21.3	1 [289]
Group 4: Signaling			
ESR1	Estrogen receptor 1	6q25.1	1 [259]
ESR2	Estrogen receptor 2 (ER beta)	14q23.2	1 [259]
PGR	Progesterone receptor	11q22-q23	1 [259]
TGFB1	Transforming growth factor, beta 1	19q13.1	2 [168, 259]
Group 5: Other			
CST3	Cystatin C (amyloid angiopathy and cerebral hemorrhage)	20p11.21	1 [293]
HMOX1	Heme oxygenase (decycling) 1	22q13.1	1 [294]
HP	Haptoglobin	16q22.1	2 [129, 276]

Gene symbols are those approved by the HGNC and were obtained from http://www.genenames.org/ [41]. Genes were studied either by sequencing for mutations or by association (linkage disequilibrium mapping).

3.6.1. Sequencing of candidate genes

DNA sequencing is a common approach to identify candidate genes in AAA. Typically a gene with biologically plausible function to vascular biology is chosen and its sequence is analyzed in AAA patients to determine if the gene harbors mutations. One of the first genes studied was *COL3A1* which encodes a structural protein, located mainly in the wall of arteries. Mutations in *COL3A1* cause the type IV variant of EDS, the vascular form of EDS, making *COL3A1* a biologically relevant candidate gene to study for AAA. One such study found a glycine to arginine substitution at amino acid 619 (G619R) when investigating the coding sequence of *COL3A1*. The mutation segregated with arterial rupture in the family and was found to alter the protein structure by making it more susceptible to proteinase digestion, strongly implying its significance [159]. The G619R mutation was tested in different families by two additional groups and no association was found, suggesting that this is a rare mutation [129, 160, 161]. When the coding region of *COL3A1* was sequenced in a large number of AAA patients, only two sequence variations, P501T and G136R, were found [162]. Based on these findings mutations in the *COL3A1* gene only occur in a minor subset of AAA families (~2%) [162].

Fibulin-2 (*FBLN2*), an ECM protein gene, was sequenced in eleven AAA patients and two controls and fourteen single nucleotide variations in the sequence were detected. Only two of these variants (1203G>A and 1295C>T) were undetected in 102 additional controls, however the 1203G>A mutation was neutral. The 1295C>T mutation was screened in the AAA patient's two sisters who also had AAAs, but found not to segregate with the disease [163].

Other biologically plausible candidate genes which have been analyzed by DNA sequencing in AAA patients include the genes for TIMP1 and TIMP2 [164]. There is a decreased level of TIMPs in AAA patients and a higher ratio of MMPs to TIMPs in AAA tissue compared to a control aorta [49, 165]. Two variations in both *TIMP1* and *TIMP2* were discovered; however, these were all neutral changes that did not affect amino acids, and therefore are unlikely to contribute to AAA [164].

3.6.2. Genetic association studies

Genetic association studies are used to determine if a particular allele or variant is associated with the disease of interest by occurring significantly more often in individuals with the disease than in the general population [126]. Typically the candidate gene is chosen based on biological function. Numerous studies have been published testing over 40 candidate genes thought to be involved in AAA pathogenesis (Figure 5). These genes can be grouped into five categories: structural and remodeling, cardiovascular, immunity, signaling and other (Table 3).

Several genes for structural components of the aorta, such as COL3A1, ELN and FBN1, were studied assuming that variants in these genes would be involved in AAA pathogenesis (Table 3). Genes for matrix remodeling proteases, particularly MMPs, and their inhibitors (TIMPs) were similarly regarded as plausible targets (Table 3). The T allele of a C/T SNP (rs3918242) in the promoter sequence of *MMP9* was reported to increase activity of the protein by 1.5-fold compared to the C allele [166], and it was tested for association in 414 AAA patients and 375 controls. The frequency distribution of the genotypes in AAA cases was significantly different ($p = 0.0026$) from controls, however the allelic frequencies of the SNP (C vs. T) did not differ [167]. In an attempt to replicate these findings, Ogata and colleagues [168] studied the same SNP in a set of 397 cases and 425 controls, and found no significant differences between cases and controls, indicating that this SNP in the *MMP9* gene was not associated with AAA. An additional study investigated the role of this SNP in the growth of small AAAs. A group of 455 patients with small AAAs were followed for approximately 2.6 years to monitor AAA growth. There were no differences in the growth rates of the patients with different genotypes [169].

Genes involved in the cardiovascular system constitute another group of genes investigated for their role in AAA. One gene that has been investigated closely is angiotensin I converting enzyme 1 (*ACE*). *ACE*, located on chromosome 17q23.3, has an insertion(I)/deletion(D) (indel) polymorphism in an Alu repeat in intron 16. This indel correlates with plasma levels of *ACE*, and homozygotes with the deletion have an approximate two-fold increase in *ACE* levels [170, 171]. One case-control study found no association between *ACE* and AAA in either genotypic or allelic frequencies between cases and controls [172]. Another group compared genotypes of *ACE* with the growth rate of small AAAs. The study used a small case-control group and found no significant association with the *ACE* genotype and the expansion rate of AAA [173]. A larger case-control study (n=250/250) on *ACE*, found an association with the deletion (D) allele, where 63% of AAA patients compared to 49% of the controls had this allele, and the DD genotype was significantly enriched in AAA patients ($p = 0.002$). In a multivariable analysis with the known risk factors for AAA, the DD genotype was independently associated with AAA risk [174]. This study also investigated the role of an A to C polymorphism in the 3' untranslated region of angiotensin II receptor, type 1 (*AGTR1*), but found no association between *AGTR1* and AAA in either the allelic or genotypic frequencies [174].

Recently, Jones and colleagues [175] conducted a genetic association study on *ACE*, angiotensinogen (*AGT*), *AGTR1*, and bradykinin receptor (*BDKRB2*), using a total of 1,226 AAA patients and 1,723 controls from three geographical regions in New Zealand, the United Kingdom and Australia. The T allele of the *AGT* 268C>T SNP in exon 2 was associated with AAA in the New Zealand group; however, the association could not be replicated in the other two populations. The *ACE* indel did not associate with AAA in any of the individual cohorts, but did when the three geographical regions were combined with an OR = 1.31 (95% CI: 1.04 – 1.65). The most significant association was found with the 1166A>C SNP in *AGTR1* with AAA in all three geographical regions, both independently and combined with an OR = 1.60 (95% CI: 1.32 – 1.93; $p = 1.1 \times 10^{-6}$) [175]. Although this study suggested that polymorphisms in the genes *AGTR1* and *ACE* are associated with AAA pathogenesis, further analyses are needed due to other contradictory reports.

Another cardiovascular candidate gene investigated for an association with AAA is 5,10-methylenetetrahydrofolate reductase (*MTHFR*), which is located on chromosome 1p36.3 and involved in homocysteine metabolism [176]. In particular, analyses have focused on the SNP rs1801133 (677C>T). This alanine to valine substitution results in a 70% reduction in enzymatic activity *in vitro* [177]. Early studies using small sample sizes of cases and controls found that the alleles, but not the genotypes, had an association with AAA [178, 179]. In another study the CT individuals instead of TT individuals had an increased risk (OR = 4.43, 95% CI: 2.11 – 9.34) [178]. Two larger case-control studies examining the role of rs1801133 in AAA patients, concluded that there was no association between this variant and AAA [180, 181].

Meta-analysis is an excellent method by which data from numerous candidate gene association studies can be combined with the aim of generating a more robust and reliable estimate of the OR, and of providing stronger evidence to accept or reject the hypothesis of association. There are limitations in meta-analysis and of particular concern is the inability to account for heterogeneity between and within the original studies [182, 183]. Recently, Thompson and colleagues [183], published a meta-analysis of 26 case-control and 5 aneurysm expansion studies investigating 78 different SNPs in 34 AAA candidate genes. Only six SNPs were studied in more than one case-control study: *ACE* I/D, *MTHFR* 677C>T, *IL1B* 3953C>T, *TIMP1* 434C>T, *NOS3* 4a/4b and *MMP9* 1562C>T, and could, therefore, be included in the meta-analysis. In the combined analysis, no significant associations were found with the SNPs studied in *TIMP1*, *IL1B*, or *NOS3*. Associations, however, were found between the variants *ACE* I/D, (RR = 1.37; 95% CI: 1.23 – 1.52), *MTHFR* 677C>T (RR = 1.14; 95% CI: 1.08 – 1.21), and *MMP9* 1562C>T (RR = 1.09; 95% CI: 1.01 – 1.18) in AAA [183]. Even when combining studies, the sample sizes were still small for genetic studies on complex diseases such as AAAs.

Evidence of the immune system's role in AAA has led to the investigation of human leukocyte antigen (HLA) class II genes for their involvement in AAA. HLAs are known for their involvement in many autoimmune diseases, such as rheumatoid arthritis [184]. One of the first studies found that HLA-DR B1*15 and HLA-DR B1*0404 were associated with AAA [185]. Since then, additional studies have found associations with HLA-DQ3, HLA-DR B1*02, and HLA-DR B1*04 [186-188]. These studies, however, used fewer than 150 cases and 150 controls and genetic association studies with such small sample sizes are prone to type I error. More recent publications regarding HLA variants had significantly larger numbers of cases and controls. One group studied HLA variants in two different geographical groups, Belgian and Canadian, and found association with only one variant, HLA DQA*0102, in the Belgian population only [189]. Another group, using a population from Northern Ireland, studied variants HLA-A, HLA-B and HLA-DR and found no association with AAA [190]. Since the HLA locus has a large number of different alleles, none of the studies were appropriately powered to give reliable answers.

A more recent approach to studying complex diseases is a genome-wide association study (GWAS). To date, no GWAS has been completed on AAA, however a large consortium has tested a variant, rs10757278, discovered from another GWAS involving CAD [191-193], in five different vascular phenotypes: CAD, peripheral arterial disease (PAD), atherosclerotic stroke, IA and AAA. This study analyzed AAA and control samples from seven different geographical regions: Belgium, Finland, Italy, the Netherlands, New Zealand, the United Kingdom and the United States [194]. The SNP rs10757278 was associated with AAA ($p = 1.2 \times 10^{-12}$, OR = 1.31, 95% CI: 1.22 – 1.42) and IA ($p = 2.5 \times 10^{-6}$, OR = 1.29, 95% CI: 1.16 – 1.43) (Table 4; Figure 10). This is the first genetic variant associated with both AAA and IA and it suggests a common pathway involved in vascular disease etiology

[194]. The SNP rs10757278 is located on chromosome 9p21 in a gene called *ANRIL*. The function of *ANRIL*, a non-coding RNA, is not known, however it is expressed in vascular endothelial cells, monocyte-derived macrophages, and coronary SMCs [195]. It is of interest that another SNP, rs10811661, known to be associated with type 2 diabetes and located only 10 kbp way from rs10757278, was not associated with AAA or IA [194]. This finding is in agreement with epidemiological data demonstrating that diabetes is not a risk factor for AAA (Figure 3).

Table 4. Common genetic variant (rs10757278-G) on chromosome 9p21 is associated with AAA

Study Population	Controls	Cases	OR (95% CI)	P-value
Iceland	14,259	398	1.37 (1.18–1.58)	2.6×10^{-5}
Belgium	267	176	1.21 (0.92–1.58)	0.18
Canada	150	206	1.29 (0.96–1.74)	0.097
PA, USA	447	101	1.39 (1.02–1.89)	0.037
The Netherlands	915	476	1.31 (1.12–1.53)	0.00078
UK	252	478	1.35 (1.09–1.68)	0.0064
New Zealand	442	588	1.25 (1.05–1.50)	0.012
Total	16,732	2,836	1.31 (1.22–1.42)	1.2×10^{-12}

The original study was reported by Helgadottir et al. 2008 [194].

4. Animal Models for AAA

Animal models have greatly advanced the study of human diseases with AAA being no exception [2]. The use of a living animal allows the complexities of an entire organism to be involved in the disease process, granting otherwise unattainable insights into the disease. It is important to keep in mind, however, the differences between a particular animal model and human disease when interpreting the results. Although currently there are no animal models for AAA, which replicate the pathology in all aspects seen in human AAA, studies including mouse [196], rat [38], and pig models [197] have been used in surgical research. The most widely used in the research on the pathogenesis of AAAs are the three mouse models described below (Figure 11).

A distinct advantage of using an animal model to study AAA is the ability to control the genetic background of the animal. As mentioned previously, Caucasians are more prone to have AAAs than African Americans most likely due to variations in their genetic risk factors [36] (Figure 3). Furthermore, in the industrialized world, relocation and intermarriage are common making genetically homogenous populations more difficult to find. Additionally, collecting an adequate number of samples from such a restricted group can be burdensome. Therefore, studying genetic effects in animals, particularly in well established mouse lines, is an effective way to control for population stratification [198, 199].

Another advantage of using an animal model is the availability of tissue samples. Due to the progressive nature of the degeneration involved in an AAA, as well as the risks associated with the open repair of an aneurysm, human tissue samples from early stages of AAA development are not available for study. Additionally, the number of open repair operations compared to endovascular repairs is limited, making harvesting tissue difficult.

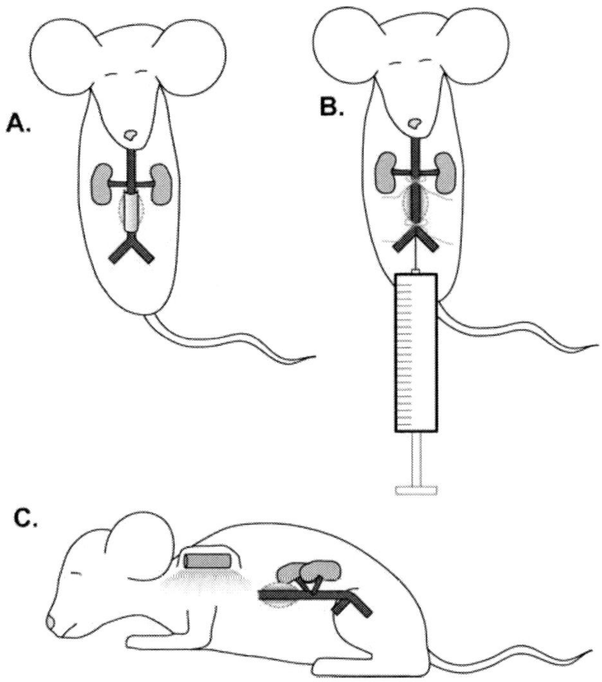

Figure 11. Mouse models of AAA. Schematic representation of A) the periarterial application of calcium chloride to the abdominal aorta, which will then give rise to a dilatation at the site of application; B) the elastase perfusion model of AAA, where the abdominal aorta is isolated and then perfused transiently under pressure with elastase to induce the aneurysm; and C) the angiotensin II infusion model of AAA, where a mini-osmotic pump is placed under the skin of mice deficient in apolipoprotein E (*Apoe*$^{-/-}$) to release angiotensin II continuously. A dilatation eventually forms in the supra-renal location of the aorta of the animal.

4.1. Three Different Methods to Induce AAA in Mouse Models

There are some naturally occurring mouse mutants that have aortic dissection or general vascular instability as a phenotype, but they do not accurately resemble the human AAA. Similarly, several knockout mice deficient in genes that code for the structural components, such as collagen, in the vasculature [200-202] or lysyl oxidase [203], an enzyme important in the crosslinking of collagen and elastin, have shown a vascular phenotype, but not AAA. The exceptions are mice with mutations in a heat-shock protein that is involved in the proper deposition of some of the structural components of the vasculature [204], and a mouse strain with altered copper metabolism which affects the ability of lysyl oxidase to crosslink collagen [205].

There are three experimental techniques commonly used to induce aortic aneurysms in mice: elastase perfusion, $CaCl_2$ application, and AngII infusion (Figure 11) [196]. The last method only produces aneurysms consistently if applied to mice that are knockouts for the apolipoprotein E gene (*Apoe*$^{-/-}$). As seen in Table 5, these three techniques have been used to discern many of the genes now thought to be involved in AAA.

Table 5. Use of gene knock-outs in AAA mouse models

	Gene Knocked Out		
AAA Model	Symbol(s)	Gene ID(s)	AAA Susceptibility [Reference]
AngII infusion	*Apoe*	11816	Increased [209, 210]
	Apoe / Alox5	11816 / 11689	No Change [295]
	Apoe / Ccr2	11816 / 12772	Decreased [296]
	Apoe / Ltb4r1	11816 / 16995	Decreased [297]
	Apoe / Ncf1	11816 / 17969	Decreased [298]
	Apoe / Plau	11816 / 11792	Decreased [210]
	Apoe / Spp1	11816 / 20750	Decreased [299]
	Ldlr / Agtr1a	16835 / 11607	Decreased [300]
	Ldlr / Ptgs2	16835 / 9225	Decreased [301]
	Nox1	237038	Decreased [302]
	Plau	11792	Decreased [210]
	Ptgs2	19225	Decreased [303]
CaCl perfusion	*Ccr2*	12772	Decreased [304]
	Ccr5	12774	No Change [304]
	Cd4	12504	Decreased [221]
	Cxcr3	12766	No Change [304]
	Ifng	15978	Decreased [221]
	Mmp12	17381	Decreased [216]
	Mmp2	17390	Decreased [215]
	Mmp9	17395	Decreased [215]
	Timp2	21858	Decreased [218]
Elastase perfusion	*Ctsc*	13032	Decreased [305]
	Mmp12	17381	No Change [207]
	Mmp8	17394	No Change [220]
	Mmp9	17395	Decreased [207]
	Nos2	18126	Increased [306]
	Sell	20343	Decreased [219]
	Selp	20344	Decreased [307]
	Timp1	21857	Increased [217]

See Figure 11 and text for detailed description of the models. The column "AAA Susceptibility" indicates the result in the knockout mouse compared to the wild type mouse (same strain background).

In the elastase perfusion model, which is probably the most widely used method, the abdominal aorta is isolated and the lumen of the vessel is perfused for a short period with crude elastase, usually derived from porcine pancreatic tissue, leading to a local dilatation of the aorta after about 14 days. This model was first developed in rats [206], and later adapted for use in the mouse [207] to take advantage of mouse genetics. The elastase model resembles the human AAA histology in that chronic inflammatory response is seen in the aortic wall [38]. Initial dilatation is also seen with heat-inactivated elastase controls, presumably due to the prolonged elevated and static pressure that the aorta is subjected to during the initial perfusion. Histological analysis of tissue taken immediately after the perfusion indicates that the internal elastic lamellae are intact and it is later, typically after 14 days, that the exposed sections of the aortas from the experimental group undergo SMC depletion, elastin degradation, and develop a full grown aneurysm.

Another model of AAA in which the aneurysm is induced by exposure of the aorta to an exogenous chemical is the $CaCl_2$ model [208]. Here, the $CaCl_2$ is applied periarterially, making it less invasive and technically demanding than the elastase model. Like the elastase model, the mice used in these experiments develop aneurysms gradually, with an increase of 100% in the diameter, seen at the end of the third week [208]. Again the dilatation seems to result from a chronic inflammatory response initiated by the application of the calcium salt solution, with no such response being elicited in controls treated with sodium chloride [208].

In the Ang II infusion model biologically active Ang II is infused into hyperlipidemic mice deficient in the gene for apolipoprotein E (*Apoe*$^{-/-}$) or the low density lipoprotein receptor (*Ldlr*$^{-/-}$) using a subcutaneous, osmotic mini-pump for approximately four weeks. This model mimics the actions of the renin/angiotensin system, in which renin cleaves angiotensin I to form Ang II. In these mice the aneurysms develop in the suprarenal region of the aorta, often preceded by a dissection [209]. One study showed that although the Apoe deficiency enhances the rate of AAA formation it is not necessary for the formation of aneurysms [210]. The histology of these aneurysms is somewhat different from that seen in human AAA with more intact elastin. Despite these limitations, the Ang II model is the least invasive and simplest of the three models to employ from a technical standpoint. Even with the differences between classical human AAA and the AngII model, this method has quickly gained acceptance and is becoming the predominant model of AAA research.

4.2. Findings from AAA Models

One striking feature of human AAA is that males are much more prone to AAA than females (Figure 3). Interestingly, this disparity is seen also in animal models for AAA, with the propensity for aneurysms to form much more often in male than female animals (82% vs. 29%) [115]. This difference in prevalence has been investigated further in mouse and rat models using a number of approaches involving hormone treatment, orchiectomy and ovariectomy [115, 211-213]. Current thinking about the sex bias in AAA is that sex hormones influence immune infiltration [212], or the production and activation of MMPs [213]. However, results from a study using orchiectomy and ovariectomy in the AngII model indicated that it is the presence of the androgens which contribute to AAA formation rather than the estrogens having a protective effect against it [211].

Animal models, particularly mouse models, are useful in determining the contributions of the genetic background and, by proxy, genetic heterogeneity to the risk of developing AAA. Examination of the effect of genetic background on the formation of aneurysms using eight different mouse strains and the elastase perfusion method produced intriguing results [214]. Although there was no difference in the initial aortic diameter between the different mice strains, the aortic diameters immediately post-perfusion and at the end of the experiment differed greatly, most notably between the 129/SvEv (0.98 ± 0.02 mm; n=41) and the C57BL/6J (1.38 ± 0.03 mm; n=66). These mice are now being used in an outcross experiment to determine the genetic contributions to the susceptibility to elastase-induced aneurysm [214].

As in other areas of AAA research, the MMPs and the TIMPs are among the most studied in animal models (Table 5). *Mmp9* has been shown to be important for the formation of AAA in both the elastase and the $CaCl_2$ model, and in both models the resistance to the formation of the aneurysm could be eliminated by bone marrow transplantation of *Mmp9* wild-type cells [207, 215]. *Mmp12* also was tested in both the elastase [207] and the $CaCl_2$ [216] models, but with mixed results. In the elastase study there was no change in susceptibility to AAA in the *Mmp12* knockout mice while the $CaCl_2$ model demonstrated that *Mmp12* was important for AAA formation. Although both studies used 129/SvJ mice, such discrepancy between the different AAA models is not unexpected due to the different methods used to initiate AAA. The role of TIMPs in the susceptibility to AAA has also been investigated using the various mouse models. The deletion of TIMP1 showed the expected phenotype of an increase in the size of the aneurysms generated in the elastase model for the knockout mice [217]. Surprisingly, *Timp2* deletion resulted in a decreased susceptibility to $CaCl_2$ induced aneurysms [218]. This is yet another example of the complex interplay between MMPs and TIMPs.

A wide variety of knockout mice have been generated and tested using the AAA models to elucidate the role of immune-related genes in AAA pathology (Table 5). The overwhelming trend in these studies is that a fully functioning immune system is necessary for the formation of an experimental aneurysm. For example, it was shown that the L-selectin protein and gene were involved in experimental aneurysm formation in rats. Subsequently knockout mice were shown to be resistant to dilatation in the elastase model [219]. Several studies have also investigated the effects of knock-down or knockout animals deficient in particular types of immune cells on AAA development. Some of the cells studied include neutrophils [220], mast-cells [91], and $CD4^+$ T-cells [221]. All of these studies point to the critical roles of these cell types in the formation of experimental AAA.

In humans smoking is the most important environmental risk factor for AAA (Figure 3). To elucidate the mechanism on how smoking contributes to the disease, Bergoeing and colleagues [222] exposed mice to tobacco smoke in the context of the elastase perfusion model. Animals were exposed to tobacco smoke for two weeks prior to elastase perfusion and two weeks after perfusion (a total of four weeks). There was no difference in the initial enlargement of the aorta between the animals exposed to tobacco smoke and those not exposed. Two weeks later, however, the animals exposed to smoke had approximately 60%

larger aortas and more elastin degradation compared to animals not exposed to smoke, but Mmp9 and Mmp12 levels were not different. The enlargement in aortic diameter was seen only in animals perfused with smaller amounts of elastase, whereas when larger amounts of elastase were used, there was no difference between the two groups. These results suggest that smoking worsened the disease outcome in a synergistic manner, but that when the elastase-induced damage was already extensive, smoking had no effect [222].

AAA models have also been used for the analysis of gene expression in the aorta [223, 224]. While these studies generally support much of what is known about gene expression in human AAA disease [71], there are distinct differences inherent in working with animal models which make direct comparisons difficult at best. One example is the study of simvastatin in the inhibition of AAA in an elastase induced rat model [223]. The expression of genes known to be related to inflammation, ECM remodeling and oxidative stress (i.e. *Mmp9*, *Nfkb*) was decreased in the simvastatin group. Further comparisons, however, are limited as the annotation for rat genes is much more limited than for human and mouse. Additional limitations include the abrupt nature of the elastase model for AAA compared to the decades-long degeneration which occurs in humans, and the inability to compare treated human tissue with those from treated models to verify similarity. Despite these limitations, the remarkable similarities seen between human gene expression studies [71] and those done on various animal models lend great support to the claim that these animal models are indeed good surrogates for the human disease.

A considerable advantage to having animal models of a disease is the ability to test treatment options for the disease. In the case of AAA, since the etiology of the initiation of the disease might be quite different between experimental aneurysms and what is seen in humans, treating the initial trigger for AAA is not yet feasible. However, since the expansion, including histological features, of the aneurysm in both the animal model and the human disease are so similar, research to prevent the expansion and rupture of AAA in animals could prove useful in humans. With varying degrees of success, statins, ACE inhibitors, and anti-inflammatory drugs have been used to prevent or slow down the growth of experimental aneurysms; therefore, these are potential pharmacological treatments in humans as well [225-228]. Since these drugs have been approved for use in humans for other diseases it will not be necessary to prove safety and tolerance; it will only be necessary to determine efficacy and dosage. In addition to existing drugs, novel compounds more specific to AAA are being investigated. An example is the chemical compound pentagalloyl glucose (PGG) used to protect elastin from degradation. PGG was applied periadventitially prior to $CaCl_2$ application in the rat model in the treatment group. A single treatment was enough to inhibit elastin degeneration and limit the development of the AAA [229]. PGG had no effect on the levels of MMP and inflammatory infiltration; an interesting twist to preventing the progression of an aneurysm in an environment that would otherwise lead to degeneration.

5. Conclusion

We have summarized above the current knowledge on AAA pathobiology with a special emphasis on what is known about the genetic predisposition to AAAs. Common complex diseases, such as AAAs, are likely to have many genetic risk factors each with a small effect size. The challenge lies, therefore, in the identification of these genetic risk factors. Thus far, the most significant findings in AAA genetics have been accomplished using DNA linkage studies in which two susceptibility loci, named AAA1 and AAA2, have been found. Additionally, a SNP on chromosome 9p21, which is associated with up to 70% increase in risk for AAA and IA has been discovered using a case-control study approach. This variant, which is common at a 40% frequency in the population and also confers risk for CAD, was the first described variant that predisposes a person to AAA or IA, or both, and applies to several Caucasian populations.

Unraveling the pathophysiology of AAA and identifying the specific risk factors for AAA will require interdisciplinary approaches. Identification of susceptibility genes, in which sequence variants confer risk to the AAA phenotype, can be accomplished through the integration of expression, linkage and genetic association analyses (Figure 12). Furthermore, genome-wide studies with large sample sizes are needed to identify additional genetic factors which contribute to the development, growth and rupture of AAA. The identified risk factors could provide the basis for genetic testing to identify individuals harboring AAA before the rupture occurs and leads to sudden death. Identification of the AAA susceptibility gene(s) will also allow us to develop animal models for testing new therapies.

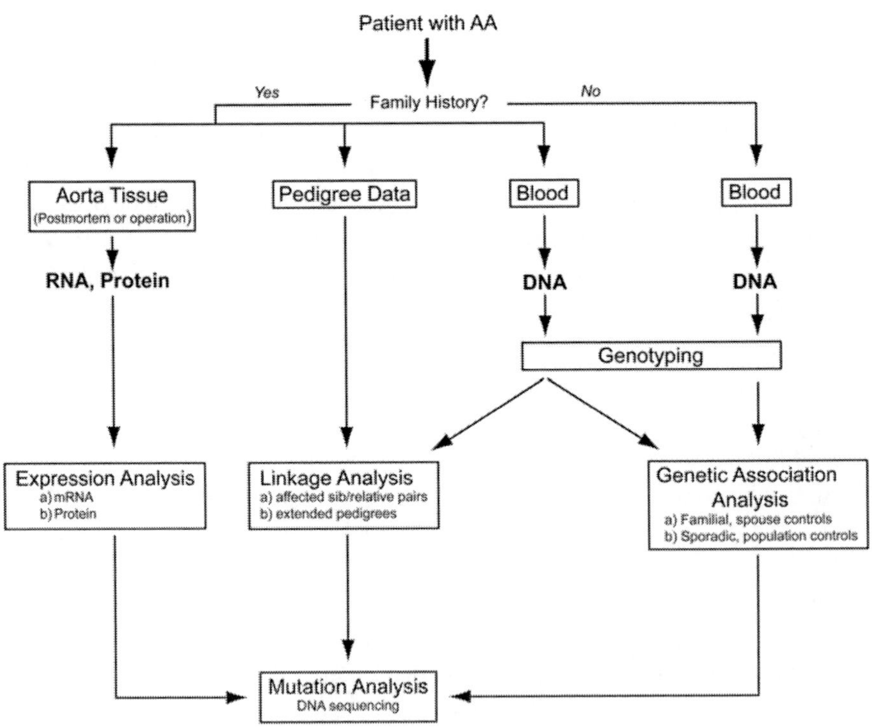

Figure 12. How to study the pathogenesis and risk factors of AAA in humans? Schematic drawing of the approaches used to identify genetic risk factors of aortic aneurysms (AA) and biological processes involved in AA are shown demonstrating how information from one approach can facilitate another approach. Multidisciplinary approaches are needed to elucidate which genes are involved in aneurysm formation, growth and rupture. Modified with permission from Kuivaniemi and Tromp, 2000 [233].

6. Acknowledgements

The original work carried out in the Kuivaniemi laboratory was funded in part by the National Heart, Lung, and Blood Institute of the NIH (grants HL045996 and HL064310 to H.K.), as well as by the Office of the Vice President for Research and by Department of Surgery of Wayne State University. The study was also supported in part by a grant from the NCHGR (HG001577), and a grant from the NCRR (RR003655). Some of the results were obtained using S.A.G.E., which is also supported by RR003655. J.H.L. is a recipient of a Predoctoral Fellowship from the National Institute on Aging, NIH (AG030900), and in 2005-2007 G.M.L. was a recipient of a Predoctoral Fellowship from the American Heart Association (0510063Z and 0710099Z). We gratefully acknowledge the dedicated collaboration of many vascular surgeons, molecular biologists and geneticists who are shown as coauthors in the original publications listed in the reference section. The authors thank Marc Nischan for Figure 1 and Yoshiki Kyo for Figure 2.

References

[1] Fleming, C; Whitlock, EP; Beil, TL; Lederle, FA: Screening for abdominal aortic aneurysm: a best-evidence systematic review for the U.S. Preventive Services Task Force. *Ann Intern Med*, 2005, 142, 203-11.

[2] Golledge, J; Muller, J; Daugherty, A; Norman, P: Abdominal aortic aneurysm: pathogenesis and implications for management. *Arterioscler Thromb Vasc Biol*, 2006, 26, 2605-13.

[3] Vande, Geest, JP; Di Martino, ES; Bohra, A; Makaroun, MS; Vorp, DA: A biomechanics-based rupture potential index for abdominal aortic aneurysm risk assessment: demonstrative application. *Ann N Y Acad Sci.*, 2006, 1085, 11-21.

[4] Suy, RME: Arterial Aneurysms: a historical review. Sint-Genesius-Rode, Belgium: *DEMOL Printing*, 2004.

[5] Livesay, JJ; Messner, GN; Vaughn, WK: Milestones in the treatment of aortic aneurysm: Denton A. Cooley, MD, and the Texas Heart Institute. *Tex Heart Inst J.*, 2005, 32, 130-4.

[6] Chandler, JJ: The Einstein sign: the clinical picture of acute cholecystitis caused by ruptured abdominal aortic aneurysm. *N Engl J Med.*, 1984, 310, 1538.

[7] Cohen, JR; Graver, LM. The ruptured abdominal aortic aneurysm of Albert Einstein. *Surg Gynecol Obstet*, 1990, 170, 455-8.

[8] Centers for Disease Control. [cited March 14, 2008]. Available from: http://www.cdc.gov/.

[9] Ernst, CB. Abdominal aortic aneurysm. *N Engl J Med.*, 1993, 328, 1167-72.

[10] Alcorn, HG; Wolfson, SK; Jr., Sutton-Tyrrell, K; Kuller, LH; O'Leary D. Risk factors for abdominal aortic aneurysms in older adults enrolled in The Cardiovascular Health Study. *Arterioscler Thromb Vasc Biol.*, 1996, 16, 963-70.

[11] Lederle, FA; Johnson, GR; Wilson, SE; Chute, EP; Hye, RJ; Makaroun, MS; Barone, GW; Bandyk, D; Moneta, GL; Makhoul, RG: The aneurysm detection and management

study screening program: validation cohort and final results. Aneurysm Detection and Management Veterans Affairs Cooperative Study Investigators. *Arch Intern Med.*, 2000, 160, 1425-30.

[12] Lederle, FA; Johnson, GR; Wilson, SE: Abdominal aortic aneurysm in women. *J Vasc Surg.*, 2001, 34, 122-6.

[13] Kuivaniemi, H; Shibamura, H; Arthur, C; Berguer, R; Cole, CW; Juvonen, T; Kline, RA; Limet, R; Mackean, G; Norrgård, Ö; Pals, G; Powell, JT; Rainio, P; Sakalihasan, N; Van Vlijmen-van Keulen, C; Verloes, A; Tromp, G. Familial abdominal aortic aneurysms: collection of 233 multiplex families. *J Vasc Surg.*, 2003, 37, 340-5.

[14] Clifton, MA. Familial abdominal aortic aneurysms. *Br J Surg.*, 1977, 64, 765-6.

[15] Majumder, PP; St Jean, PL; Ferrell, RE; Webster, MW; Steed, DL. On the inheritance of abdominal aortic aneurysm. *Am J Hum Genet*, 1991, 48, 164-70.

[16] Tilson, MD; Seashore, MR. Fifty families with abdominal aortic aneurysms in two or more first-order relatives. *Am J Surg.*, 1984, 147, 551-3.

[17] Verloes, A; Sakalihasan, N; Koulischer, L; Limet, R: Aneurysms of the abdominal aorta: familial and genetic aspects in three hundred thirteen pedigrees. *J Vasc Surg.*, 1995, 21, 646-55.

[18] Brady, AR; Thompson, SG; Fowkes, FG; Greenhalgh, RM; Powell, JT. Abdominal aortic aneurysm expansion: risk factors and time intervals for surveillance. *Circulation*, 2004, 110, 16-21.

[19] Lederle, FA; Simel, DL. The rational clinical examination. Does this patient have abdominal aortic aneurysm? *JAMA*, 1999, 281, 77-82.

[20] Wilmink, ABM; Forshaw, M; Quick, CRG; Hubbard, CS; Day, NE. Accuracy of serial screening for abdominal aortic aneurysms by ultrasound. *J Med Screen*, 2002, 9, 125-7.

[21] Isselbacher EM: Thoracic and abdominal aortic aneurysms. Circulation, 2005, 111, 816-28.

[22] Lederle, FA; Wilson, SE; Johnson, GR; Reinke, DB; Littooy, FN; Acher, CW; Messina, LM; Ballard, DJ; Ansel, HJ. Variability in measurement of abdominal aortic aneurysms. Abdominal Aortic Aneurysm Detection and Management Veterans Administration Cooperative Study Group. *J Vasc Surg.*, 1995, 21, 945-52.

[23] Freiberg, MS; Arnold, AM; Newman, AB; Edwards, MS; Kraemer, KL; Kuller, LH. Abdominal aortic aneurysms, increasing infrarenal aortic diameter, and risk of total mortality and incident cardiovascular disease events: 10-year follow-up data from the Cardiovascular Health Study. *Circulation*, 2008, 117, 1010-7.

[24] Hirsch, AT; Haskal, ZJ; Hertzer, NR; Bakal, CW; Creager, MA; Halperin, JL; Hiratzka, LF; Murphy, WR; Olin, JW; Puschett, JB; Rosenfield, KA; Sacks, D; Stanley, JC; Taylor, LM; Jr.; White, CJ; White, J; White, RA; Antman, EM; Smith, SC; Jr.; Adams, CD; Anderson, JL; Faxon, DP; Fuster, V; Gibbons, RJ; Hunt, SA; Jacobs, AK; Nishimura R; Ornato, JP; Page, RL; Riegel, B. ACC/AHA 2005 Practice Guidelines for the management of patients with peripheral arterial disease (lower extremity, renal, mesenteric, and abdominal aortic): a collaborative report from the American Association for Vascular Surgery/Society for Vascular Surgery, Society for Cardiovascular Angiography and Interventions, Society for Vascular Medicine and

Biology, Society of Interventional Radiology, and the ACC/AHA Task Force on Practice Guidelines (Writing Committee to Develop Guidelines for the Management of Patients With Peripheral Arterial Disease): endorsed by the American Association of Cardiovascular and Pulmonary Rehabilitation; National Heart, Lung, and Blood Institute; Society for Vascular Nursing; TransAtlantic Inter-Society Consensus; and Vascular Disease Foundation. *Circulation*, 2006, 113, 463-654.

[25] The United Kingdom Small Aneurysm Trial Participants: Long-term outcomes of immediate repair compared with surveillance of small abdominal aortic aneurysms. *N Engl J Med.*, 2002, 346, 1445-52.

[26] Lederle, FA; Wilson, SE; Johnson, GR; Reinke, DB; Littooy, FN; Acher, CW; Ballard, DJ; Messina, LM; Gordon, IL; Chute, EP; Krupski, WC; Busuttil, SJ; Barone, GW; Sparks, S; Graham, LM; Rapp, JH; Makaroun, MS; Moneta, GL; Cambria, RA; Makhoul, RG; Eton, D; Ansel, HJ; Freischlag, JA; Bandyk, D. Immediate repair compared with surveillance of small abdominal aortic aneurysms. *N Engl J Med.*, 2002, 346, 1437-44.

[27] Powell, JT; Brown, LC; Forbes, JF; Fowkes, FG; Greenhalgh, RM; Ruckley, CV; Thompson, SG. Final 12-year follow-up of surgery versus surveillance in the UK Small Aneurysm Trial. *Br J Surg.*, 2007, 94, 702-8.

[28] The UK Small Aneurysm Trial Participants: Mortality results for randomised controlled trial of early elective surgery or ultrasonographic surveillance for small abdominal aortic aneurysms. *The Lancet*, 1998, 352, 1649-1655.

[29] Greenhalgh, RM; Powell, JT. Endovascular repair of abdominal aortic aneurysm. *N Engl J Med.*, 2008, 358, 494-501.

[30] Schermerhorn, ML; O'Malley, AJ; Jhaveri, A; Cotterill, P; Pomposelli, F; Landon, BE. Endovascular vs. open repair of abdominal aortic aneurysms in the Medicare population. *N Engl J Med.*, 2008, 358, 464-74.

[31] EVAR trial participants: Endovascular aneurysm repair versus open repair in patients with abdominal aortic aneurysm (EVAR trial 1): randomised controlled trial. *The Lancet*, 2005, 365, 2179-2186.

[32] Visser, JJ; Van Sambeek, MR; Hamza, TH; Hunink, MG; Bosch, JL. Ruptured, abdominal aortic aneurysms: endovascular repair versus open surgery--systematic review. *Radiology*, 2007, 245, 122-9.

[33] Blankensteijn, JD; De Jong, SE; Prinssen, M; Van Der Ham, AC; Buth, J; Van Sterkenburg, SM; Verhagen, HJ; Buskens, E; Grobbee, DE. Two-year outcomes after conventional or endovascular repair of abdominal aortic aneurysms. *N Engl J Med.*, 2005, 352, 2398-405.

[34] EVAR trial participants: Endovascular aneurysm repair and outcome in patients unfit for open repair of abdominal aortic aneurysm (EVAR trial 2): randomised controlled trial. *The Lancet*, 2005, 365, 2187-2192.

[35] Schoen, FJ: Blood vessels. In: Kumar, V; Abbas, AK; Fausto, N; eds. Robbins and Cotran Pathologic Basis of Disease. *Philadelphia: Elsevier/Saunders*; 2005, 511-54.

[36] Lederle, FA; Johnson, GR; Wilson, SE; Chute, EP; Littooy, FN; Bandyk, D; Krupski, WC; Barone, GW; Acher, CW; Ballard, DJ: Prevalence and associations of abdominal aortic aneurysm detected through screening. Aneurysm Detection and Management

(ADAM) Veterans Affairs Cooperative Study Group. *Ann Intern Med.*, 1997, 126, 441-9.

[37] Beckman, L. Aortic Aneurysms: pathophysiology, epidemiology, and prognosis. In: Creager MA; Dzau VJ; Loscalzo J; eds. Vascular Medicine: a companion to Braunwald's heart disease. Philadelpia: *Saunders Elsevier*, 2006.

[38] Thompson, RW; Geraghty, PJ; Lee, JK. Abdominal aortic aneurysms: basic mechanisms and clinical implications. *Curr Probl Surg.*, 2002, 39, 110-230.

[39] Topouzis, S; Majesky, MW. Smooth muscle lineage diversity in the chick embryo. Two types of aortic smooth muscle cell differ in growth and receptor-mediated transcriptional responses to transforming growth factor-β. *Dev Biol.*, 1996, 178, 430-45.

[40] Pannu, H; Avidan, N; Tran-Fadulu, V; Milewicz, DM. Genetic basis of thoracic aortic aneurysms and dissections: potential relevance to abdominal aortic aneurysms. *Ann N Y Acad Sci.*, 2006, 1085, 242-55.

[41] Bruford, EA; Lush, MJ; Wright, MW; Sneddon, TP; Povey, S; Birney, E. The HGNC Database in 2008: a resource for the human genome. *Nucleic Acids Res.*, 2007, 36, D445-8.

[42] Dobrin, PB; Baker, WH; Gley, WC. Elastolytic and collagenolytic studies of arteries. Implications for the mechanical properties of aneurysms. *Arch Surg.*, 1984, 119, 405-9.

[43] Kuivaniemi, H; Tromp, G; Prockop, DJ: Mutations in collagen genes: causes of rare and some common diseases in humans. *FASEB J*, 1991, 5, 2052-60.

[44] Bou-Gharios, G; Ponticos, M; Rajkumar, V; Abraham, D. Extra-cellular matrix in vascular networks. *Cell Prolif.*, 2004, 37, 207-20.

[45] Keeling, WB; Armstrong, PA; Stone, PA; Bandyk, DF; Shames, ML. An overview of matrix metalloproteinases in the pathogenesis and treatment of abdominal aortic aneurysms. *Vasc Endovascular Surg.*, 2005, 39, 457-64.

[46] Raffetto, JD; Khalil, RA. Matrix metalloproteinases and their inhibitors in vascular remodeling and vascular disease. *Biochem Pharmacol*, 2008, 75, 346-59.

[47] Knox, JB; Sukhova, GK; Whittemore, AD; Libby, P. Evidence for altered balance between matrix metalloproteinases and their inhibitors in human aortic diseases. Circulation, 1997, 95, 205-12.

[48] Nishimura, K; Ikebuchi, M; Kanaoka, Y; Ohgi, S; Ueta, E; Nanba, E; Ito H. Relationships between matrix metalloproteinases and tissue inhibitor of metalloproteinases in the wall of abdominal aortic aneurysms. Int Angiol, 2003, 22, 229-38.

[49] Elmore, JR; Keister, BF; Franklin, DP; Youkey, JR; Carey, DJ. Expression of matrix metalloproteinases and TIMPs in human abdominal aortic aneurysms. *Ann Vasc Surg.*, 1998, 12, 221-8.

[50] Yamashita, A; Noma, T; Nakazawa, A; Saito, S; Fujioka, K; Zempo, N; Esato, K. Enhanced expression of matrix metalloproteinase-9 in abdominal aortic aneurysms. *World J Surg*, 2001, 25, 259-65.

[51] Sakalihasan, N; Delvenne, P; Nusgens, BV; Limet, R; Lapière, CM. Activated forms of MMP2 and MMP9 in abdominal aortic aneurysms. *Journal of Vascular Surgery*, 1996, 24, 127-133.
[52] Davis, V; Persidskaia, R; Baca-Regen, L; Itoh, Y; Nagase, H; Persidsky, Y; Ghorpade, A; Baxter, BT. Matrix metalloproteinase-2 production and its binding to the matrix are increased in abdominal aortic aneurysms. *Arterioscler Thromb Vasc Biol.*, 1998, 18, 1625-33.
[53] Crowther, M; Goodall, S; Jones, JL; Bell, PR; Thompson, MM. Localization of matrix metalloproteinase 2 within the aneurysmal and normal aortic wall. *Br J Surg.*, 2000, 87, 1391-400.
[54] Newman, KM; Jean-Claude, J; Li, H; Scholes, JV; Ogata, Y; Nagase, H; Tilson, MD. Cellular localization of matrix metalloproteinases in the abdominal aortic aneurysm wall. *J Vasc Surg.*, 1994, 20, 814-20.
[55] Patel, MI; Melrose, J; Ghosh, P; Appleberg, M. Increased synthesis of matrix metalloproteinases by aortic smooth muscle cells is implicated in the etiopathogenesis of abdominal aortic aneurysms. *J Vasc Surg.*, 1996, 24, 82-92.
[56] Wilson, WR; Anderton, M; Schwalbe, EC; Jones, JL; Furness, PN; Bell, PR; Thompson MM. Matrix metalloproteinase-8 and -9 are increased at the site of abdominal aortic aneurysm rupture. *Circulation*, 2006, 113, 438-45.
[57] Watanabe, T; Sato, A; Sawai, T; Uzuki, M; Goto, H; Yamashita, H; Akamatsu, D; Sato, H; Shimizu, T; Miyama, N; Nakano, Y; Satomi, S. The elevated level of circulating matrix metalloproteinase-9 in patients with abdominal aortic aneurysms decreased to levels equal to those of healthy controls after an aortic repair. *Ann Vasc Surg.*, 2006, 20, 317-21.
[58] Eugster, T; Huber, A; Obeid, T; Schwegler, I; Gürke, L; Stierli, P. Aminoterminal propeptide of type III procollagen and matrix metalloproteinases-2 and -9 failed to serve as serum markers for abdominal aortic aneurysm. *Eur J Vasc Endovasc Surg.*, 2005, 29, 378-82.
[59] Goodall, S; Crowther, M; Hemingway, DM; Bell, PR; Thompson, MM. Ubiquitous elevation of matrix metalloproteinase-2 expression in the vasculature of patients with abdominal aneurysms. *Circulation*, 2001, 104, 304-9.
[60] Johnson, C; Galis, ZS. Matrix metalloproteinase-2 and -9 differentially regulate smooth muscle cell migration and cell-mediated collagen organization. *Arterioscler Thromb Vasc Biol.*, 2004, 24, 54-60.
[61] Goodall, S; Porter, KE; Bell, PR; Thompson, MM. Enhanced invasive properties exhibited by smooth muscle cells are associated with elevated production of MMP-2 in patients with aortic aneurysms. *Eur J Vasc Endovasc Surg.*, 2002, 24, 72-80.
[62] Curci, JA; Liao, S; Huffman, MD; Shapiro, SD; Thompson, RW. Expression and localization of macrophage elastase (matrix metalloproteinase-12) in abdominal aortic aneurysms. *J Clin Invest*, 1998, 102, 1900-10.
[63] Annabi, B; Shédid, D; Ghosn, P; Kenigsberg, RL; Desrosiers, RR; Bojanowski, MW; Beaulieu, E; Nassif, E; Moumdjian, R, Béliveau, R. Differential regulation of matrix metalloproteinase activities in abdominal aortic aneurysms. *J Vasc Surg.*, 2002, 35, 539-46.

[64] Ramos-DeSimone, N; Hahn-Dantona, E; Sipley, J; Nagase, H; French, DL; Quigley, JP. Activation of matrix metalloproteinase-9 (MMP-9) via a converging plasmin/stromelysin-1 cascade enhances tumor cell invasion. *J Biol Chem.*, 1999, 274, 13066-76.
[65] Carrell, TW; Burnand, KG; Wells, GM; Clements, JM; Smith, A. Stromelysin-1 (matrix metalloproteinase-3) and tissue inhibitor of metalloproteinase-3 are overexpressed in the wall of abdominal aortic aneurysms. *Circulation*, 2002, 105, 477-82.
[66] Nollendorfs, A; Greiner, TC; Nagase, H; Baxter, BT. The expression and localization of membrane type-1 matrix metalloproteinase in human abdominal aortic aneurysms. J *Vasc Surg*, 2001, 34, 316-22.
[67] Sukhova, GK; Shi, GP; Simon, DI; Chapman, HA; Libby, P. Expression of the elastolytic cathepsins S and K in human atheroma and regulation of their production in smooth muscle cells. *J Clin Invest*, 1998, 102, 576-83.
[68] Liu, J; Sukhova, GK; Yang, JT; Sun, J; Ma, L; Ren, A; Xu, WH, Fu, H, Dolganov, GM, Hu C, Libby, P, Shi, GP. Cathepsin L expression and regulation in human abdominal aortic aneurysm, atherosclerosis, and vascular cells. *Atherosclerosis*, 2006, 184, 302-11.
[69] Kuivaniemi, H; Platsoucas, CD; Tilson MD; 3rd: Aortic aneurysms: an immune disease with a strong genetic component. *Circulation*, 2008, 117, 242-52.
[70] Koch, AE; Haines, GK; Rizzo, RJ; Radosevich, JA; Pope, RM; Robinson, PG; Pearce WH. Human abdominal aortic aneurysms. Immunophenotypic analysis suggesting an immune-mediated response. *Am J Pathol*, 1990, 137, 1199-213.
[71] Lenk, GM; Tromp, G; Weinsheimer, S; Gatalica, Z; Berguer, R; Kuivaniemi, H. Whole genome expression profiling reveals a significant role for immune function in human abdominal aortic aneurysms. *BMC Genomics*, 2007, 8, 237.
[72] Maiellaro, K; Taylor, WR. The role of the adventitia in vascular inflammation. *Cardiovasc Res*. 2007, 75, 640-8.
[73] Hynecek, RL; DeRubertis, BG; Trocciola, SM; Zhang, H; Prince, MR; Ennis, TL; Kent, KC; Faries, PL. The creation of an infrarenal aneurysm within the native abdominal aorta of swine. *Surgery*, 2007, 142, 143-9.
[74] Ocana, E; Bohórquez, JC; Pérez-Requena, J; Brieva, JA; Rodríguez, C. Characterisation of T and B lymphocytes infiltrating abdominal aortic aneurysms. *Atherosclerosis*, 2003, 170, 39-48.
[75] Forester, ND; Cruickshank, SM; Scott, DJ; Carding, SR. Functional characterization of T cells in abdominal aortic aneurysms. *Immunology*, 2005, 115, 262-70.
[76] Wen, J; Wang, P; Smith, SV; Haller, CA; Chaikof, EL. Syndecans are differentially expressed during the course of aortic aneurysm formation. *J Vasc Surg*. 2007, 46, 1014-25.
[77] Cheuk, BL; Cheng, SW. Differential secretion of prostaglandin E(2), thromboxane A(2) and interleukin-6 in intact and ruptured abdominal aortic aneurysms. *Int J Mol Med*. 2007, 20, 391-5.
[78] Bobryshev, YV; Lord, RS. Vascular-associated lymphoid tissue (VALT) involvement in aortic aneurysm. *Atherosclerosis*, 2001, 154, 15-21.

[79] Galle, C; Schandené, L; Stordeur, P; Peignois, Y; Ferreira, J; Wautrecht, JC; Dereume, JP; Goldman, M. Predominance of type 1 $CD4^+$ T cells in human abdominal aortic aneurysm. *Clin Exp Immunol*, 2005, 142, 519-27.

[80] Schönbeck, U; Sukhova, GK; Gerdes, N; Libby, P. T_H2 predominant immune responses prevail in human abdominal aortic aneurysm. *Am J Pathol*, 2002, 161, 499-506.

[81] Shimizu, K; Mitchell, RN; Libby, P. Inflammation and cellular immune responses in abdominal aortic aneurysms. *Arterioscler Thromb Vasc Biol.*, 2006, 26, 987-94.

[82] Lindeman, JH; Abdul-Hussien, H; Schaapherder, AF; Van Bockel, JH; Von Der Thüsen JH; Roelen, DL; Kleemann, R. Enhanced expression and activation of pro-inflammatory transcription factors distinguish aneurismal from atherosclerotic aorta: IL-6 and IL-8 dominated inflammatory responses prevail in the human aneurysm. *Clin Sci., (Lond)*, 2008, 114, 687-97.

[83] Middleton, RK; Lloyd, GM; Bown, MJ; Cooper NJ; London NJ; Sayers RD. The pro-inflammatory and chemotactic cytokine microenvironment of the abdominal aortic aneurysm wall: a protein array study. *J Vasc Surg.*, 2007, 45, 574-80.

[84] Bobryshev, YV; Lord, RS; Parsson, H. Immunophenotypic analysis of the aortic aneurysm wall suggests that vascular dendritic cells are involved in immune responses. *Cardiovasc Surg.*, 1998, 6, 240-9.

[85] Rasmussen, TE; Hallett, JW; Jr.: Inflammatory aortic aneurysms. A clinical review with new perspectives in pathogenesis. *Ann Surg.*, 1997, 225, 155-64.

[86] Gregory, AK; Yin, NX; Capella, J; Xia, S; Newman, KM; Tilson, MD. Features of autoimmunity in the abdominal aortic aneurysm. *Arch Surg.*, 1996, 131, 85-8.

[87] Platsoucas, CD; Lu, S; Nwaneshiudu, I; Solomides, C; Agelan, A; Ntaoula, N; Purev, E; Li, LP; Kratsios, P; Mylonas, E; Jung, W-J; Evans, K; Roberts, S; Lu, Y; Layvi, R; Lin, WL; Zhang, X; Gaughan, J; Monos, DS; Oleszak, EL; White, JV. Abdominal aortic aneurysm is a specific antigen-driven T cell disease. *Ann N Y Acad Sci.*, 2006, 1085, 224-35.

[88] Yen, HC; Lee, FY; Chau, LY. Analysis of the T cell receptor Vβ repertoire in human aortic aneurysms. *Atherosclerosis*, 1997, 135, 29-36.

[89] Porqueddu, M; Spirito, R; Parolari, A; Zanobini, M; Pompilio, G; Polvani, G; Alamanni, F; Stangalini, D; Tremoli, E; Biglioli, P. Lack of association between serum immunoreactivity and Chlamydia pneumoniae detection in the human aortic wall. Circulation, 2002, 106, 2647-8.

[90] Chew, DK; Knoetgen, J; Xia, S; Tilson, MD. The role of a putative microfibrillar protein (80 kDa) in abdominal aortic aneurysm disease. *J Surg Res.*, 2003, 114, 25-9.

[91] Sun, J; Sukhova, GK; Yang, M; Wolters, PJ; MacFarlane, LA; Libby, P; Sun, C; Zhang, Y; Liu, J; Ennis, TL; Knispel, R; Xiong, W; Thompson, RW; Baxter, BT; Shi GP. Mast cells modulate the pathogenesis of elastase-induced abdominal aortic aneurysms in mice. *J Clin Invest*, 2007, 117, 3359-68.

[92] Tsuruda, T; Kato, J; Hatakeyama, K; Yamashita, A; Nakamura, K; Imamura, T; Kitamura, K; Onitsuka, T; Asada, Y; Eto, T. Adrenomedullin in mast cells of abdominal aortic aneurysm. *Cardiovasc*, Res., 2006, 70, 158-64.

[93] Holmes, DR; Lõpez-Candales, A; Liao, S; Thompson, RW. Smooth muscle cell apoptosis and p53 expression in human abdominal aortic aneurysms. *Ann N Y Acad, Sci.*, 1996, 800, 286-7.

[94] Chan, WL; Pejnovic, N; Liew, TV; Hamilton, H. Predominance of Th2 response in human abdominal aortic aneurysm: mistaken identity for IL-4-producing NK and NKT cells? *Cell Immunol*, 2005, 233, 109-14.

[95] Henderson, EL; Geng, YJ; Sukhova, GK; Whittemore, AD; Knox, J; Libby, P. Death of smooth muscle cells and expression of mediators of apoptosis by T lymphocytes in human abdominal aortic aneurysms. *Circulation*, 1999, 99, 96-104.

[96] Chan, WL; Pejnovic, N; Hamilton, H; Liew, TV; Popadic, D; Poggi, A; Khan, SM. Atherosclerotic abdominal aortic aneurysm and the interaction between autologous human plaque-derived vascular smooth muscle cells, type 1 NKT, and helper T cells. *Circ Res.*, 2005, 96, 675-83.

[97] Moran, CS; McCann, M; Karan, M; Norman, P; Ketheesan, N; Golledge, J. Association of osteoprotegerin with human abdominal aortic aneurysm progression. *Circulation*, 2005, 111, 3119-25.

[98] Leuner, K; Pantel, J; Frey, C; Schindowski, K; Schulz, K; Wegat, T; Maurer, K; Eckert, A; Müller, WE. Enhanced apoptosis, oxidative stress and mitochondrial dysfunction in lymphocytes as potential biomarkers for Alzheimer's disease. *J Neural Transm Suppl*,, 2007, 207-15.

[99] Sun, Y. Oxidative stress and cardiac repair/remodeling following infarction. *Am J Med Sci.*, 2007, 334, 197-205.

[100] McCormick, ML; Gavrila, D; Weintraub, NL. Role of oxidative stress in the pathogenesis of abdominal aortic aneurysms. *Arterioscler Thromb Vasc Biol.*, 2007, 27, 461-9.

[101] Manea, A; Manea, SA; Gafencu, AV; Raicu, M; Simionescu, M. AP-1-dependent transcriptional regulation of NADPH oxidase in human aortic smooth muscle cells. Role of p22phox subunit. *Arterioscler Thromb Vasc Biol.*, 2008, 28, 878-85.

[102] Auerbach, O; Garfinkel, L. Atherosclerosis and aneurysm of aorta in relation to smoking habits and age. *Chest.*, 1980, 78, 805-9.

[103] Wilmink, TBM; Quick CRG; Day NE. The association between cigarette smoking and abdominal aortic aneurysms. *J Vasc Surg.*, 1999, 30, 1099-105.

[104] Lindholt, JS; Heegaard, NHH; Vammen, S; Fasting, H; Henneberg, EW; Heickendorff, L: Smoking, but not lipids, lipoprotein(a) and antibodies against oxidised LDL, is correlated to the expansion of abdominal aortic aneurysms. *European Journal of Vascular and Endovascular Surgery*, 2001, 21, 51-56.

[105] Pleumeekers, HJ; Hoes, AW; Van Der Does, E; Van Urk, H; Hofman, A; De Jong, PT; Grobbee, DE. Aneurysms of the abdominal aorta in older adults. The Rotterdam Study. *Am J Epidemiol*, 1995, 142, 1291-9.

[106] Scott, RA; Bridgewater, SG; Ashton, HA. Randomized clinical trial of screening for abdominal aortic aneurysm in women. *Br J Surg.*, 2002, 89, 283-5.

[107] Semmens, JB; Norman, PE; Lawrence-Brown, MM; Holman, CD. Influence of gender on outcome from ruptured abdominal aortic aneurysm. *Br J Surg.*, 2000, 87, 191-4.

[108] Johnston, KW; Scobie, TK. Multicenter prospective study of nonruptured abdominal aortic aneurysms. I. Population and operative management. *J Vasc Surg.*, 1988, 7, 69-81.

[109] Norman, PE; Jamrozik, K; Lawrence-Brown, MM; Le, MTQ; Spencer CA; Tuohy RJ; Parsons RW; Dickinson JA. Population based randomised controlled trial on impact of screening on mortality from abdominal aortic aneurysm. *BMJ*, 2004, 329, 1259.

[110] Lindholt, JS; Juul, S; Fasting, H; Henneberg, EW. Screening for abdominal aortic aneurysms. single centre randomised controlled trial. *BMJ*, 2005, 330, 750.

[111] Wanhainen, A; Lundkvist, J; Bergqvist, D; Björck, M. Cost-effectiveness of screening women for abdominal aortic aneurysm. *J Vasc Surg.*, 2006, 43, 908-14.

[112] Stenbaek, J; Granath, F; Swedenborg, J. Outcome after abdominal aortic aneurysm repair. Difference between men and women. *Eur J Vasc Endovasc Surg.*, 2004, 28, 47-51.

[113] Forbes, TL; Lawlor, DK; DeRose, G; Harris, KA. Gender differences in relative dilatation of abdominal aortic aneurysms. *Ann Vasc Surg.*, 2006, 20, 564-8.

[114] Sonesson, B; Hansen, F; Stale, H; Lanne, T. Compliance and diameter in the human abdominal aorta--the influence of age and sex. *Eur J Vasc Surg.*, 1993, 7, 690-7.

[115] Ailawadi, G; Eliason, JL; Roelofs, KJ; Sinha, I; Hannawa, KK; Kaldjian, EP; Lu, G; Henke, PK; Stanley, JC; Weiss, SJ; Thompson, RW; Upchurch, GR. Jr.: Gender differences in experimental aortic aneurysm formation. *Arterioscler Thromb Vasc Biol.*, 2004, 24, 2116-22.

[116] Kent, S. Hormones and heart disease. *Geriatrics*, 1979, 34, 97-102.

[117] La Vecchia, C; Decarli, A; Franceschi, S; Gentile, A; Negri, E; Parazzini, F. Menstrual and reproductive factors and the risk of myocardial infarction in women under fifty-five years of age. *Am J Obstet Gynecol*, 1987, 157, 1108-12.

[118] Vardulaki, KA; Walker, NM; Day, NE; Duffy, SW; Ashton, HA; Scott, RA. Quantifying the risks of hypertension, age, sex and smoking in patients with abdominal aortic aneurysm. *Br J Surg.*, 2000, 87, 195-200.

[119] Wilmink, ABM; Quick, CRG. Epidemiology and potential for prevention of abdominal aortic aneurysm. *Br J Surg.*, 1998, 85, 155-62.

[120] Centers for Disease Control and Prevention, National Center for Injury Prevention and Control: Web-based Injury Statistics Query and Reporting System (WISQARS) [online]. 2004. [cited March 14, 2008]. Available from: http://www.cdc.gov/ncipc/wisqars.

[121] Gillum, RF. Epidemiology of aortic aneurysm in the United States. *J Clin Epidemiol*, 1995, 48, 1289-98.

[122] LaMorte, WW; Scott, TE; Menzoian, JO. Racial differences in the incidence of femoral bypass and abdominal aortic aneurysmectomy in Massachusetts: relationship to cardiovascular risk factors. *J Vasc Surg.*, 1995, 21, 422-31.

[123] Powell, JT; Greenhalgh, RM. Multifactorial inheritance of abdominal aortic aneurysm. *Eur J Vasc Surg.*, 1987, 1, 29-31.

[124] Ogata, T; MacKean, GL; Cole, CW; Arthur, C; Andreou, P; Tromp, G; Kuivaniemi, H. The lifetime prevalence of abdominal aortic aneurysms among siblings of aneurysm

patients is eightfold higher than among siblings of spouses: an analysis of 187 aneurysm families in Nova Scotia; Canada. *J Vasc Surg.*, 2005, 42, 891-7.

[125] Majumder, P. Segregation Analysis, Classical. In: Elston R, Olson J, Palmer L, eds. Biostatistical Genetics and Genetic Epidemiology. West Sussex, England: *John Wiley & Sons Ltd.*, 2002.

[126] Strachan, T; Read, AP. Human Molecular Genetics 3. Independence, KY: Garland Science/Taylor & Francis Group, 2004.

[127] Falconer, DS. Introduction to Quantitative Genetics. Essex, England: *Longman Scientific & Technical*, 1981.

[128] Darling, RC; 3rd, Brewster, DC; Darling, RC; LaMuraglia, GM; Moncure, AC; Cambria, RP; Abbott, WM. Are familial abdominal aortic aneurysms different? *J Vasc Surg.*, 1989, 10, 39-43.

[129] Adamson, J; Powell, JT; Greenhalgh, RM. Selection for screening for familial aortic aneurysms. *Br J Surg.*, 1992, 79, 897-8.

[130] Baird, PA; Sadovnick, AD; Yee, IM; Cole, CW; Cole, L. Sibling risks of abdominal aortic aneurysm. *Lancet*, 1995, 346, 601-4.

[131] Myers, RH; Madden, JJ; Teague, JL; Falek, A. Factors related to onset age of Huntington disease. *Am J Hum Genet*, 1982, 34, 481-8.

[132] Ridley, RM; Frith, CD; Crow, TJ; Conneally, PM. Anticipation in Huntington's disease is inherited through the male line but may originate in the female. *J Med Genet*, 1988, 25, 589-95.

[133] Origuchi, N; Shigematsu, H; Hatakeyama, T; Nunokawa, M; Yasuhara, H; Muto, T. A clinicopathological study of familial abdominal aortic aneurysms. *Int Angiol*, 1996, 15, 26-32.

[134] Olson, JM; Witte, JS; Elston, RC. Genetic mapping of complex traits. *Stat Med.*, 1999, 18, 2961-81.

[135] Olson, JM; Vongpunsawad, S; Kuivaniemi, H; Ronkainen, A; Hernesniemi, J; Ryynänen, M; Kim, LL; Tromp, G. Search for intracranial aneurysm susceptibility gene(s) using Finnish families. *BMC Med Genet.*, 2002, 3, 7.

[136] Shibamura, H; Olson, JM; Van Vlijmen-Van Keulen, C; Buxbaum, SG; Dudek, DM; Tromp, G; Ogata, T; Skunca, M; Sakalihasan, N; Pals, G; Limet, R; MacKean, GL; Defawe, O; Verloes, A; Arthur, C; Lossing, AG; Burnett, M; Sueda, T; Kuivaniemi, H. Genome scan for familial abdominal aortic aneurysm using sex and family history as covariates suggests genetic heterogeneity and identifies linkage to chromosome 19q13. *Circulation*, 2004, 109, 2103-8.

[137] McKusick, VA. Online Mendelian Inheritance in Man, OMIM™. 2006. [cited March 14, 2008]. Available from: http://www.ncbi.nlm.nih.gov/omim/.

[138] Van Vlijmen-Van Keulen, CJ; Rauwerda, JA; Pals, G. Genome-wide linkage in three Dutch families maps a locus for abdominal aortic aneurysms to chromosome 19q13.3. *Eur J Vasc Endovasc Surg.*, 2005, 30, 29-35.

[139] Nahed, BV; Seker, A; Guclu, B; Ozturk, AK; Finberg, K; Hawkins, AA; DiLuna, ML; State, M; Lifton, RP; Gunel, M. Mapping a Mendelian form of intracranial aneurysm to 1p34.3-p36.13. *Am J Hum Genet*, 2005, 76, 172-9.

[140] Verlaan, DJ; Dubé, MP; St-Onge, J; Noreau, A; Roussel, J; Satgé, N; Wallace, MC; Rouleau, GA. A new locus for autosomal dominant intracranial aneurysm, ANIB4, maps to chromosome 5p15.2-14.3. *J Med Genet*, 2006, 43, 31.
[141] Onda, H; Kasuya, H; Yoneyama, T; Takakura, K; Hori, T; Takeda, J; Nakajima, T; Inoue, I. Genomewide-linkage and haplotype-association studies map intracranial aneurysm to chromosome 7q11. *Am J Hum Genet*, 2001, 69, 804-19.
[142] Ozturk, AK, Nahed, BV; Bydon, M; Bilguvar, K; Goksu, E; Bademci, G; Guclu, B; Johnson, MH; Amar, A; Lifton, RP; Gunel, M. Molecular genetic analysis of two large kindreds with intracranial aneurysms demonstrates linkage to 11q24-25 and 14q23-31. *Stroke*, 2006, 37, 1021-7.
[143] Yamada, S; Utsunomiya, M; Inoue, K; Nozaki, K; Inoue, S; Takenaka, K; Hashimoto, N; Koizumi, A. Genome-wide scan for Japanese familial intracranial aneurysms: linkage to several chromosomal regions. *Circulation*, 2004, 110, 3727-33.
[144] Van Der Voet, M; Olson, JM; Kuivaniemi, H; Dudek, DM; Skunca, M; Ronkainen A; Niemelä, M; Jääskeläinen, J; Hernesniemi, J; Helin, K; Leinonen, E; Biswas, M; Tromp, G. Intracranial aneurysms in Finnish families: confirmation of linkage and refinement of the interval to chromosome 19q13.3. *Am J Hum Genet*, 2004, 74, 564-71.
[145] Mineharu, Y; Inoue, K; Inoue, S; Yamada, S; Nozaki, K; Hashimoto, N; Koizumi, A. Model-based linkage analyses confirm chromosome 19q13.3 as a susceptibility locus for intracranial aneurysm. *Stroke*, 2007, 38, 1174-8.
[146] Onouchi, Y; Gunji, T; Burns, JC; Shimizu, C; Newburger, JW; Yashiro, M; Nakamura, Y; Yanagawa, H; Wakui, K; Fukushima, Y; Kishi, F; Hamamoto, K; Terai, M; Sato, Y; Ouchi, K; Saji, T; Nariai, A; Kaburagi, Y; Yoshikawa, T; Suzuki, K; Tanaka, T; Nagai, T; Cho, H; Fujino, A; Sekine, A; Nakamichi, R; Tsunoda, T; Kawasaki, T; Nakamura, Y; Hata, A. ITPKC functional polymorphism associated with Kawasaki disease susceptibility and formation of coronary artery aneurysms. *Nat Genet,* 2008, 40, 35-42.
[147] Hasham, SN; Willing, MC; Guo, DC; Muilenburg, A; He, R; Tran VT; Scherer SE; Shete SS; Milewicz DM. Mapping a locus for familial thoracic aortic aneurysms and dissections (TAAD2) to 3p24-25. *Circulation*, 2003, 107, 3184-90.
[148] Guo, D; Hasham, S; Kuang, SQ; Vaughan, CJ; Boerwinkle, E; Chen, H; Abuelo, D; Dietz, HC; Basson, CT; Shete, SS; Milewicz, DM. Familial thoracic aortic aneurysms and dissections: genetic heterogeneity with a major locus mapping to 5q13-14. *Circulation*, 2001, 103, 2461-8.
[149] Mátyás, G; Arnold, E; Carrel, T; Baumgartner, D; Boileau, C; Berger, W; Steinmann, B. Identification and in silico analyses of novel TGFBR1 and TGFBR2 mutations in Marfan syndrome-related disorders. *Hum Mutat*, 2006, 27, 760-9.
[150] Guo, DC; Pannu, H; Tran-Fadulu, V; Papke, CL; Yu, RK; Avidan, N; Bourgeois, S; Estrera, AL; Safi, HJ; Sparks, E; Amor, D; Ades, L; McConnell, V; Willoughby, CE; Abuelo, D; Willing, M; Lewis, RA; Kim, DH; Scherer, S; Tung, PP; Ahn, C; Buja, LM; Raman, CS; Shete, SS; Milewicz, DM. Mutations in smooth muscle α-actin (ACTA2) lead to thoracic aortic aneurysms and dissections. *Nat Genet*, 2007, 39, 1488-93.
[151] Vaughan, CJ; Casey, M; He, J; Veugelers, M; Henderson, K; Guo, D; Campagna, R; Roman, MJ; Milewicz, DM; Devereux, RB; Basson, CT. Identification of a

chromosome 11q23.2-q24 locus for familial aortic aneurysm disease, a genetically heterogeneous disorder. *Circulation*, 2001, 103, 2469-75.

[152] Khau Van Kien, P; Mathieu, F; Zhu, L; Lalande, A; Betard, C; Lathrop, M; Brunotte, F; Wolf, JE; Jeunemaitre, X. Mapping of familial thoracic aortic aneurysm/dissection with patent ductus arteriosus to 16p12.2-p13.13. *Circulation*, 2005, 112, 200-6.

[153] Zhu, L; Vranckx, R; Khau Van Kien, P; Lalande, A; Boisset, N; Mathieu, F; Wegman, M; Glancy, L; Gasc, JM; Brunotte, F; Bruneval, P; Wolf, JE; Michel, JB; Jeunemaitre, X, Mutations in myosin heavy chain 11 cause a syndrome associating thoracic aortic aneurysm/aortic dissection and patent ductus arteriosus. *Nat Genet*, 2006, 38, 343-9.

[154] Ruigrok, YM; Elias, R; Wijmenga, C; Rinkel, GJ. A comparison of genetic chromosomal loci for intracranial, thoracic aortic, and abdominal aortic aneurysms in search of common genetic risk factors. *Cardiovasc Pathol*, 2008, 17, 40-7.

[155] Crawford, ES; Cohen, ES. Aortic aneurysm: a multifocal disease. Presidential address. *Arch Surg*, 1982, 117, 1393-400.

[156] Pressler, V; McNamara, JJ. Aneurysm of the thoracic aorta. Review of 260 cases. *J Thorac Cardiovasc Surg.*, 1985, 89, 50-4.

[157] Norrgård, Ö; Angqvist, KA; Fodstad, H; Forssell, A; Lindberg, M. Co-existence of abdominal aortic aneurysms and intracranial aneurysms. *Acta Neurochir (Wien)*, 1987, 87, 34-9.

[158] Kim, DH; Van Ginhoven, G; Milewicz, DM. Familial aggregation of both aortic and cerebral aneurysms: evidence for a common genetic basis in a subset of families. *Neurosurgery*, 2005, 56, 655-61, discussion 655-61.

[159] Kontusaari, S; Tromp, G; Kuivaniemi, H; Romanic, AM; Prockop, DJ. A mutation in the gene for type III procollagen (COL3A1) in a family with aortic aneurysms. *J Clin Invest*, 1990, 86, 1465-73.

[160] Powell, JT; Adamson, J; MacSweeney, ST; Greenhalgh, RM; Humphries, SE; Henney, A. Genetic variants of collagen III and abdominal aortic aneurysm. *Eur J Vasc Surg*, 1991, 5, 145-8.

[161] Powell, JT; Adamson, J; MacSweeney, ST; Greenhalgh, RM; Humphries, SE; Henney, AM. Influence of type III collagen genotype on aortic diameter and disease. *Br J Surg*, 1993, 80, 1246-8.

[162] Tromp, G; Wu, Y; Prockop, DJ; Madhatheri, SL; Kleinert, C; Earley, JJ; Zhuang, J, Norrgård, Ö; Darling, RC; Abbott, WM; Cole, CW; Jaakkola, P; Ryynänen, M; Pearce, WH; Yao, JST; Majamaa, K; Smullens, SN; Gatalica, Z; Ferrell, RE; Jiminez, SA; Jackson, CE; Michels, VV; Kaye, M; Kuivaniemi, H. Sequencing of cDNA from 50 unrelated patients reveals that mutations in the triple-helical domain of type III procollagen are an infrequent cause of aortic aneurysms. *J Clin Invest*, 1993, 91, 2539-45.

[163] Kuivaniemi, H; Marshall, A; Ganguly, A; Chu, ML; Abbott, WM, Tromp, G. Fibulin-2 exhibits high degree of variability, but no structural changes concordant with abdominal aortic aneurysms. *Eur J Hum Genet*, 1998, 6, 642-6.

[164] Wang, X; Tromp, G; Cole, CW; Verloes, A; Sakalihasan, N; Yoon, S; Kuivaniemi, H, Analysis of coding sequences for tissue inhibitor of metalloproteinases 1 (TIMP1) and 2 (TIMP2) in patients with aneurysms. *Matrix Biol.*, 1999, 18, 121-4.

[165] Tamarina, NA; McMillan, WD; Shively, VP; Pearce, WH. Expression of matrix metalloproteinases and their inhibitors in aneurysms and normal aorta. Surgery, 1997, 122, 264-71; discussion 271-2.

[166] Zhang, B; Ye, S; Herrmann, SM; Eriksson, P; De Maat, M; Evans, A; Arveiler, D; Luc, G; Cambien, F; Hamsten, A; Watkins, H; Henney, AM. Functional polymorphism in the regulatory region of gelatinase B gene in relation to severity of coronary atherosclerosis. *Circulation*, 1999, 99, 1788-94.

[167] Jones, GT; Phillips, VL; Harris, EL; Rossaak, JI; Van Rij, AM. Functional matrix metalloproteinase-9 polymorphism (C-1562T) associated with abdominal aortic aneurysm. *J Vasc Surg*., 2003, 38, 1363-7.

[168] Ogata, T; Shibamura, H; Tromp, G; Sinha, M; Goddard, KA; Sakalihasan, N; Limet, R; MacKean, GL; Arthur, C; Sueda, T; Land, S; Kuivaniemi, H. Genetic analysis of polymorphisms in biologically relevant candidate genes in patients with abdominal aortic aneurysms. *J Vasc Surg*., 2005, 41, 1036-42.

[169] Eriksson, P; Jormsjö-Pettersson, S; Brady, AR; Deguchi, H; Hamsten, A; Powell, JT. Genotype-phenotype relationships in an investigation of the role of proteases in abdominal aortic aneurysm expansion. *Br J Surg*., 2005, 92, 1372-6.

[170] Rigat, B; Hubert, C; Alhenc-Gelas, F; Cambien, F; Corvol, P; Soubrier, F. An insertion/deletion polymorphism in the angiotensin I-converting enzyme gene accounting for half the variance of serum enzyme levels. *J Clin Invest*, 1990, 86, 1343-6.

[171] Rigat, B; Hubert, C; Corvol, P; Soubrier, F. PCR detection of the insertion/deletion polymorphism of the human angiotensin converting enzyme gene (DCP1) (dipeptidyl carboxypeptidase 1). *Nucleic Acids Res*., 1992, 20, 1433.

[172] Hamano, K; Ohishi, M; Ueda, M; Fujioka, K; Katoh, T; Zempo, N; Fujimura, Y; Okamura, A; Rakugi, H; Higaki, J; Ogihara, T; Esato, K. Deletion polymorphism in the gene for angiotensin-converting enzyme is not a risk factor predisposing to abdominal aortic aneurysm. *Eur J Vasc Endovasc Surg*., 1999, 18, 158-61.

[173] Yeung, JM, Heeley, M; Gray, S; Lingam, MK; Manning, G; Nash, JR; Donnelly, R. Does the angiotensin-converting enzyme (ACE) gene polymorphism affect rate of abdominal aortic aneurysm expansion? *Eur J Vasc Endovasc Surg*., 2002, 24, 69-71.

[174] Fatini, C; Pratesi, G; Sofi, F; Gensini, F; Sticchi, E; Lari, B; Pulli, R; Dorigo, W; Azas, L, Pratesi, C; Gensini, GF; Abbate, R. ACE DD genotype: a predisposing factor for abdominal aortic aneurysm. *Eur J Vasc Endovasc Surg*., 2005, 29, 227-32.

[175] Jones, GT; Thompson, AR; Van Bockxmeer, FM; Hafez, H; Cooper, JA; Golledge, J, Humphries, SE; Norman, PE; Van Rij AM. Angiotensin II type 1 receptor 1166C polymorphism is associated with abdominal aortic aneurysm in three independent cohorts. *Arterioscler Thromb Vasc Biol*., 2008, 28, 764-70.

[176] Goyette, P; Sumner, JS; Milos, R; Duncan, AM; Rosenblatt, DS; Matthews, RG; Rozen, R. Human methylenetetrahydrofolate reductase: isolation of cDNA, mapping and mutation identification. *Nat Genet*, 1994, 7, 195-200.

[177] Sharp, L; Little, J. Polymorphisms in genes involved in folate metabolism and colorectal neoplasia: a HuGE review. *Am J Epidemiol*, 2004, 159, 423-43.

[178] Strauss, E; Waliszewski, K; Gabriel, M; Zapalski, S; Pawlak, AL. Increased risk of the abdominal aortic aneurysm in carriers of the MTHFR 677T allele. *J Appl Genet*, 2003, 44, 85-93.

[179] Brunelli, T; Prisco, D; Fedi, S; Rogolino, A; Farsi, A; Marcucci, R; Giusti, B; Pratesi, C; Pulli, R; Gensini, GF; Abbate, R; Pepe, G. High prevalence of mild hyperhomocysteinemia in patients with abdominal aortic aneurysm. *J Vasc Surg.*, 2000, 32, 531-6.

[180] Jones, GT; Harris, EL; Phillips, LV; Van Rij, AM. The methylenetetrahydrofolate reductase C677T polymorphism does not associate with susceptibility to abdominal aortic aneurysm. *Eur J Vasc Endovasc Surg.*, 2005, 30, 137-42.

[181] Sofi, F; Marcucci, R; Giusti, B; Pratesi, G; Lari, B; Sestini, I; Lo Sapio, P; Pulli, R; Pratesi, C; Abbate, R; Gensini, GF. High levels of homocysteine, lipoprotein (a) and plasminogen activator inhibitor-1 are present in patients with abdominal aortic aneurysm. *Thromb Haemost*, 2005, 94, 1094-8.

[182] Noble, JH; Jr.: Meta-analysis: Methods, strengths, weaknesses, and political uses. *J Lab Clin Med.*, 2006, 147, 7-20.

[183] Thompson, AR; Drenos, F; Hafez, H; Humphries, SE. Candidate gene association studies in abdominal aortic aneurysm disease: a review and meta-analysis. *Eur J Vasc Endovasc Surg.*, 2008, 35, 19-30.

[184] Gregersen, PK; Silver, J; Winchester, RJ. The shared epitope hypothesis. An approach to understanding the molecular genetics of susceptibility to rheumatoid arthritis. *Arthritis Rheum*, 1987, 30, 1205-13.

[185] Rasmussen, TE; Hallett, JW; Jr.; Metzger, RL; Richardson, DM; Harmsen, WS; Goronzy, JJ; Weyand, CM. Genetic risk factors in inflammatory abdominal aortic aneurysms: polymorphic residue 70 in the HLA-DR B1 gene as a key genetic element. *J Vasc Surg*, 1997, 25, 356-64.

[186] Hirose, H; Tilson, MD. Abdominal aortic aneurysm as an autoimmune disease. *Ann N Y Acad Sci.*, 2001, 947, 416-8.

[187] Rasmussen, TE; Hallett, JW; Jr.; Schulte, S; Harmsen, WS; O'Fallon, WM; Weyand, CM. Genetic similarity in inflammatory and degenerative abdominal aortic aneurysms: a study of human leukocyte antigen class II disease risk genes. *J Vasc Surg.*, 2001, 34, 84-9.

[188] Rasmussen, TE; Hallett, JW; Jr., Tazelaar, HD; Miller, VM; Schulte, S; O'Fallon, WM; Weyand, CM. Human leukocyte antigen class II immune response genes, female gender, and cigarette smoking as risk and modulating factors in abdominal aortic aneurysms. *J Vasc Surg.*, 2002, 35, 988-93.

[189] Ogata, T; Gregoire, L; Goddard, KA; Skunca, M; Tromp, G; Lancaster, WD; Parrado, AR; Lu, Q; Shibamura, H; Sakalihasan, N; Limet, R; MacKean, GL; Arthur, C; Sueda, T; Kuivaniemi, H. Evidence for association between the HLA-DQA locus and abdominal aortic aneurysms in the Belgian population: a case control study. *BMC Med Genet*, 2006, 7, 67.

[190] Badger, SA; Soong, CV; O'Donnell, ME; Middleton, D. The role of human leukocyte antigen genes in the formation of abdominal aortic aneurysms. *J Vasc Surg.*, 2007, 45, 475-80.

[191] Saxena, R; Voight, BF; Lyssenko, V; Burtt, NP; De Bakker, PIW; Chen, H; Roix, JJ; Kathiresan, S; Hirschhorn, JN; Daly, MJ; Hughes, TE; Groop, L; Altshuler, D; Almgren, P; Florez, JC; Meyer, J; Ardlie, K; Bengtsson Boström, K; Isomaa, B; Lettre, G; Lindblad, U; Lyon, HN; Melander, O; Newton-Cheh, C; Nilsson, P; Orho-Melander, M; Råstam, L, Speliotes, EK; Taskinen, MR; Tuomi, T; Guiducci, C; Berglund, A; Carlson J; Gianniny, L; Hackett, R; Hall, L; Holmkvist, J; Laurila, E; Sjögren, M; Sterner, M; Surti, A; Svensson, M; Svensson, M; Tewhey, R; Blumenstiel, B; Parkin, M; Defelice, M; Barry, R; Brodeur, W; Camarata, J; Chia, N; Fava, M; Gibbons, J; Handsaker, B; Healy, C; Nguyen, K; Gates, C; Sougnez, C; Gage, D; Nizzari, M; Gabriel, SB; Chirn, GW; Ma, Q; Parikh, H; Richardson, D; Ricke, D; Purcell, S. Genome-wide association analysis identifies loci for type 2 diabetes and triglyceride levels. *Science*, 2007, 316, 1331-6.

[192] Scott, LJ; Mohlke, KL; Bonnycastle, LL; Willer, CJ; Li, Y; Duren, WL; Erdos, MR; Stringham, HM; Chines, PS; Jackson, AU; Prokunina-Olsson, L; Ding, C-J; Swift, AJ; Narisu, N; Hu, T; Pruim, R; Xiao, R; Li, XY; Conneely, KN; Riebow, NL; Sprau, AG; Tong, M; White, PP; Hetrick, KN; Barnhart, MW; Bark, CW; Goldstein, JL; Watkins, L; Xiang, F; Saramies, J; Buchanan, TA; Watanabe, RM; Valle, TT; Kinnunen, L; Abecasis, GR; Pugh, EW; Doheny, KF; Bergman, RN; Tuomilehto, J; Collins, FS; Boehnke, M. A genome-wide association study of type 2 diabetes in Finns detects multiple susceptibility variants. *Science*, 2007, 316, 1341-5.

[193] Zeggini, E; Weedon, MN; Lindgren, CM; Frayling, TM; Elliott, KS; Lango, H; Timpson, NJ; Perry, JR; Rayner, NW; Freathy, RM; Barrett, JC; Shields, B; Morris, AP; Ellard, S; Groves, CJ; Harries, LW; Marchini, JL; Owen, KR; Knight, B; Cardon, LR; Walker, M; Hitman, GA; Morris, AD; Doney, AS; McCarthy, MI; Hattersley, AT. Replication of genome-wide association signals in UK samples reveals risk loci for type 2 diabetes. *Science*, 2007, 316, 1336-41.

[194] Helgadottir, A; Thorleifsson, G; Magnusson, KP; Grétarsdottir, S; Steinthorsdottir, V; Manolescu, A; Jones, GT; Rinkel, GJ; Blankensteijn, JD; Ronkainen, A; Jääskeläinen, JE; Kyo, Y; Lenk, GM; Sakalihasan, N; Kostulas, K; Gottsäter, A; Flex, A; Stefansson, H; Hansen, T; Andersen, G; Weinsheimer, S; Borch-Johnsen, K; Jorgensen, T; Shah, SH; Quyyumi, AA; Granger, CB; Reilly, MP; Austin, H; Levey, AI; Vaccarino, V; Palsdottir, E; Walters, GB; Jonsdottir, T; Snorradottir, S; Magnusdottir, D; Gudmundsson, G; Ferrell, RE; Sveinbjornsdottir, S; Hernesniemi, J; Niemelä, M; Limet, R; Andersen, K; Sigurdsson, G; Benediktsson, R; Verhoeven, EL; Teijink, JA; Grobbee, DE; Rader, DJ; Collier, DA; Pedersen, O; Pola, R; Hillert, J; Lindblad, B; Valdimarsson, EM; Magnadottir, HB; Wijmenga, C; Tromp, G; Baas, AF; Ruigrok, YM; Van Rij, AM; Kuivaniemi, H; Powell, JT; Matthiasson, SE; Gulcher, JR; Thorgeirsson, G; Kong, A; Thorsteinsdottir, U; Stefansson, K. The same sequence variant on 9p21 associates with myocardial infarction, abdominal aortic aneurysm and intracranial aneurysm. *Nat Genet*, 2008, 40, 217-24.

[195] Broadbent, HM; Peden, JF; Lorkowski, S; Goel, A; Ongen, H; Green, F; Clarke, R; Collins, R; Franzosi, MG; Tognoni, G; Seedorf, U; Rust, S; Eriksson, P; Hamsten, A; Farrall, M; Watkins, H. Susceptibility to coronary artery disease and diabetes is

encoded by distinct; tightly linked SNPs in the ANRIL locus on chromosome 9p. *Hum Mol Genet*, 2008, 17, 806-14.

[196] Daugherty, A; Cassis, LA. Mouse models of abdominal aortic aneurysms. *Arterioscler Thromb Vasc Biol.*, 2004, 24, 429-34.

[197] Maynar, M; Qian, Z; Hernandez, J; Sun, F; DeMiguel, C; Crisostomo, V; Uson, J; Pineda, LF; Espinoza, CG; Castañeda, WR. An animal model of abdominal aortic aneurysm created with peritoneal patch: technique and initial results. *Cardiovasc Intervent Radiol*, 2003, 26, 168-76.

[198] Taft, RA; Davisson, M; Wiles, MV. Know thy mouse. Trends Genet; 2006, 22, 649-53.

[199] Wade CM, Daly MJ. Genetic variation in laboratory mice. *Nat Genet*, 2005, 37, 1175-80.

[200] Li, DY; Faury, G; Taylor, DG; Davis, EC; Boyle, WA; Mecham, RP; Stenzel, P; Boak, B; Keating, MT. Novel arterial pathology in mice and humans hemizygous for elastin. *J Clin Invest*, 1998, 102, 1783-7.

[201] Liu, X; Wu, H; Byrne, M; Krane, S; Jaenisch, R. Type III collagen is crucial for collagen I fibrillogenesis and for normal cardiovascular development. *Proc Natl Acad Sci.,* USA, 1997, 94, 1852-6.

[202] Pereira, L; Lee, SY; Gayraud, B; Andrikopoulos, K; Shapiro, SD; Bunton, T; Biery, NJ; Dietz, HC; Sakai, LY; Ramirez, F. Pathogenetic sequence for aneurysm revealed in mice underexpressing fibrillin-1. *Proc Natl Acad Sci.*, USA, 1999, 96, 3819-23.

[203] Mäki, JM; Räsänen, J; Tikkanen, H; Sormunen, R; Mäkikallio, K; Kivirikko, KI; Soininen, R. Inactivation of the lysyl oxidase gene Lox leads to aortic aneurysms, cardiovascular dysfunction, and perinatal death in mice. *Circulation*, 2002, 106, 2503-9.

[204] Nagai, N; Hosokawa, M; Itohara, S; Adachi, E; Matsushita, T; Hosokawa, N; Nagata, K. Embryonic lethality of molecular chaperone hsp47 knockout mice is associated with defects in collagen biosynthesis. *J Cell Biol.*, 2000, 150, 1499-506.

[205] Brophy, CM; Tilson, JE; Braverman, IM; Tilson, MD. Age of onset, pattern of distribution, and histology of aneurysm development in a genetically predisposed mouse model. *J Vasc Surg.*, 1988, 8, 45-8.

[206] Anidjar, S; Salzmann, JL; Gentric, D; Lagneau, P; Camilleri, JP; Michel, JB. Elastase-induced experimental aneurysms in rats. *Circulation*, 1990, 82, 973-81.

[207] Pyo, R; Lee, JK; Shipley, JM; Curci, JA; Mao, D; Ziporin, SJ; Ennis, TL; Shapiro, SD, Senior, RM; Thompson, RW. Targeted gene disruption of matrix metalloproteinase-9 (gelatinase B) suppresses development of experimental abdominal aortic aneurysms. *J Clin Invest*, 2000, 105, 1641-9.

[208] Chiou, AC; Chiu, B; Pearce, WH. Murine aortic aneurysm produced by periarterial application of calcium chloride. *J Surg Res.*, 2001, 99, 371-6.

[209] Daugherty, A; Manning, MW; Cassis, LA. Angiotensin II promotes atherosclerotic lesions and aneurysms in apolipoprotein E-deficient mice. *J Clin Invest,* 2000, 105, 1605-12.

[210] Deng, GG; Martin-McNulty, B; Sukovich, DA; Freay, A; Halks-Miller, M; Thinnes T; Loskutoff, DJ; Carmeliet, P; Dole, WP; Wang, YX. Urokinase-type plasminogen

activator plays a critical role in angiotensin II-induced abdominal aortic aneurysm. *Circ Res.*, 2003, 92, 510-7.

[211] Henriques, TA; Huang, J; D'Souza, SS; Daugherty, A; Cassis, LA. Orchidectomy, but not ovariectomy, regulates angiotensin II-induced vascular diseases in apolipoprotein E-deficient mice. *Endocrinology*, 2004, 145, 3866-72.

[212] Sinha, I; Cho, BS; Roelofs, KJ; Stanley, JC; Henke, PK; Upchurch, GR. Jr.: Female gender attenuates cytokine and chemokine expression and leukocyte recruitment in experimental rodent abdominal aortic aneurysms. *Ann N Y Acad Sci.*, 2006, 1085, 367-79.

[213] Woodrum, DT; Ford, JW; Ailawadi, G; Pearce, CG; Sinha, I; Eagleton, MJ; Henke, PK; Stanley, JC; Upchurch, GR. Jr.: Gender differences in rat aortic smooth muscle cell matrix metalloproteinase-9. *J Am Coll Surg.*, 2005, 201, 398-404.

[214] Thompson, RW; Curci, JA; Ennis, TL; Mao, D; Pagano, MB; Pham, CT. Pathophysiology of abdominal aortic aneurysms: insights from the elastase-induced model in mice with different genetic backgrounds. *Ann N Y Acad Sci.*, 2006, 1085, 59-73.

[215] Longo, GM; Xiong, W; Greiner, TC; Zhao, Y; Fiotti, N; Baxter, BT. Matrix, metalloproteinases 2 and 9 work in concert to produce aortic aneurysms. *J Clin Invest*, 2002, 110, 625-32.

[216] Longo, GM; Buda, SJ; Fiotta, N; Xiong, W; Griener, T; Shapiro, S; Baxter, BT. MMP-12 has a role in abdominal aortic aneurysms in mice. *Surgery*, 2005, 137, 457-62.

[217] Eskandari, MK; Vijungco, JD; Flores, A; Borensztajn, J; Shively, V; Pearce, WH. Enhanced abdominal aortic aneurysm in TIMP-1-deficient mice. *J Surg Res.*, 2005, 123, 289-93.

[218] Xiong, W; Knispel, R; Mactaggart, J; Baxter, BT. Effects of tissue inhibitor of metalloproteinase 2 deficiency on aneurysm formation. *J Vasc Surg.*, 2006, 44, 1061-6.

[219] Hannawa, KK; Eliason, JL; Woodrum, DT; Pearce, CG; Roelofs, KJ; Grigoryants, V; Eagleton, MJ; Henke, PK; Wakefield, TW; Myers, DD; Stanley, JC; Upchurch, GR. Jr.: L-selectin-mediated neutrophil recruitment in experimental rodent aneurysm formation. *Circulation*, 2005, 112, 241-7.

[220] Eliason, JL; Hannawa, KK; Ailawadi, G; Sinha, I; Ford, JW; Deogracias, MP; Roelofs, KJ; Woodrum, DT; Ennis, TL; Henke, PK; Stanley, JC; Thompson, RW; Upchurch, GR. Jr.: Neutrophil depletion inhibits experimental abdominal aortic aneurysm formation. *Circulation*, 2005, 112, 232-40.

[221] Xiong, W, Zhao, Y; Prall, A; Greiner, TC; Baxter, BT. Key roles of $CD4^+$ T cells and IFN-γ in the development of abdominal aortic aneurysms in a murine model. *J Immunol*, 2004, 172, 2607-12.

[222] Bergoeing, MP; Arif, B; Hackmann, AE; Ennis, TL; Thompson, RW; Curci, JA. Cigarette smoking increases aortic dilatation without affecting matrix metalloproteinase-9 and -12 expression in a modified mouse model of aneurysm formation. *J Vasc Surg.*, 2007, 45, 1217-1227.

[223] Kalyanasundaram, A; Elmore, JR; Manazer, JR; Golden, A; Franklin, DP; Galt, SW. Zakhary, EM; Carey, DJ. Simvastatin suppresses experimental aortic aneurysm expansion. *J Vasc Surg.*, 2006, 43, 117-24.

[224] Van Vickle-Chavez, SJ; Tung, WS; Absi, TS; Ennis, TL; Mao, D; Cobb, JP; Thompson, RW. Temporal changes in mouse aortic wall gene expression during the development of elastase-induced abdominal aortic aneurysms. *J Vasc Surg.*, 2006, 43, 1010-20.
[225] Diehm, N; Dick, F; Schaffner, T; Schmidli, J; Kalka, C; Di Santo, S; Voelzmann, J; Baumgartner, I. Novel insight into the pathobiology of abdominal aortic aneurysm and potential future treatment concepts. *Prog Cardiovasc Dis.*, 2007, 50, 209-17.
[226] Aoki, H; Yoshimura, K; Matsuzaki, M. Turning back the clock: regression of abdominal aortic aneurysms via pharmacotherapy. *J Mol Med.*, 2007, 85, 1077-88.
[227] Golledge, J; Powell, JT. Medical management of abdominal aortic aneurysm. *Eur J Vasc Endovasc Surg.*, 2007, 34, 267-73.
[228] Thompson, RW; Baxter, BT. MMP inhibition in abdominal aortic aneurysms. Rationale for a prospective randomized clinical trial. *Ann N Y Acad Sci.*, 1999, 878, 159-78.
[229] Isenburg, JC; Simionescu, DT; Starcher, BC; Vyavahare, NR. Elastin stabilization for treatment of abdominal aortic aneurysms. *Circulation*, 2007, 115, 1729-37.
[230] Boddy, AM; Lenk, GM; Lillvis, JH; Nischan, J; Kyo, Y; Kuivaniemi, H. Basic research studies to understand aneurysm disease. *Drug News Perspect*, 2008, 21, 142-8.
[231] Lillvis, JH; Lenk, GM; Kuivaniemi, H. Genetics of Abdominal Aortic Aneurysms. In: Upchurch G; Criado E; eds. Aortic Aneurysms: pathogenesis and treatment. Totowa, NJ: *Humana Press Inc.*, 2009, 1-26.
[232] Kuivaniemi, H; Kyo, Y; Lenk, G; Tromp, G. Genome-wide approach to finding abdominal aortic aneurysm susceptibility genes in humans. *Ann N Y Acad Sci.*, 2006, 1085, 270-81.
[233] Kuivaniemi, H; Tromp, G. Search for the aneurysm susceptibility gene(s). In: Keen RR, Dobrin PB; eds. Development of Aneurysms. Georgetown: *Landes Bioscience*; 2000, 219-233.
[234] Norrgård, Ö; Rais, O; Ängquist, KA. Familial occurrence of abdominal aortic aneurysms. *Surgery*, 1984, 95, 650-6.
[235] Johansen, K; Koepsell, T. Familial tendency for abdominal aortic aneurysms. *Jama*, 1986, 256, 1934-6.
[236] Cole, CW; Barber, GG; Bouchard, AG; McPhail, NV; Roberge, C; Waddell, WG; Wellington, JL. Abdominal aortic aneurysm: consequences of a positive family history. *Can J Surg.*, 1989, 32, 117-20.
[237] Lawrence, PF; Wallis, C; Dobrin, PB; Bhirangi, K; Gugliuzza, N; Galt, S; Kraiss, L. Peripheral aneurysms and arteriomegaly: is there a familial pattern? *J Vasc Surg.*, 1998, 28, 599-605.
[238] Salkowski, A; Greb, A; Al-Aouar, R; Tromp, G; Berguer, R; Olson, JM; Kuivaniemi, H. Familial incidence of abdominal aortic aneurysms. *J Genet Couns*, 1999, 8, 407.
[239] Rossaak, JI; Hill, TM; Jones, GT; Phillips, LV; Harris, EL; Van Rij AM, Familial abdominal aortic aneurysms in the Otago region of New Zealand. *Cardiovasc Surg.*, 2001, 9, 241-8.
[240] Bengtsson, H; Norrgård, Ö; Ängquist, KA; Ekberg, O; Öberg, L; Bergqvist, D. Ultrasonographic screening of the abdominal aorta among siblings of patients with abdominal aortic aneurysms. *Br J Surg.*, 1989, 76, 589-91.

[241] Collin, J; Walton, J. Is abdominal aortic aneurysm familial? *BMJ*, 1989, 299, 493.
[242] Webster, MW; St Jean, PL; Steed, DL; Ferrell, RE; Majumder, PP. Abdominal aortic aneurysm: results of a family study. *J Vasc Surg*., 1991, 13, 366-72.
[243] Bengtsson, H; Sonesson, B; Lanne, T; Nilsson, P; Solvig, J; Loren, I; Bergqvist, D. Prevalence of abdominal aortic aneurysm in the offspring of patients dying from aneurysm rupture. *Br J Surg*., 1992, 79, 1142-3.
[244] Van Der Lugt, A; Kranendonk, SE; Baars, AM. [Screening for familial occurrence of abdominal aortic aneurysm]. *Ned Tijdschr Geneeskd,* 1992, 136, 1910-3.
[245] Adams, DC; Tulloh, BR; Galloway, SW; Shaw, E; Tulloh, AJ; Poskitt, KR. Familial abdominal aortic aneurysm: prevalence and implications for screening. *Eur J Vasc Surg*., 1993, 7, 709-12.
[246] Moher, D, Cole, CW; Hill, GB. Definition and management of abdominal aortic aneurysms: results from a Canadian survey. *Can J Surg*., 1994, 37, 29-32.
[247] Fitzgerald, P; Ramsbottom, D; Burke, P; Grace, P; McAnena, O; Croke, DT; Collins, P; Johnson, A; Bouchier-Hayes, D. Abdominal aortic aneurysm in the Irish population: a familial screening study. *Br J Surg*., 1995, 82, 483-6.
[248] Larcos, G; Gruenewald, SM; Fletcher, JP. Ultrasound screening of families with abdominal aortic aneurysm. *Australas Radiol*, 1995, 39, 254-6.
[249] Jaakkola, P; Kuivaniemi, H; Partanen, K; Tromp, G; Liljeström, B; Ryynänen, M. Familial abdominal aortic aneurysms: screening of 71 families. *Eur J Surg*., 1996, 162, 611-7.
[250] Van Der Graaf, Y; Akkersdijk, GJ; Hak, E; Godaert, GL; Eikelboom, BC. Results of aortic screening in the brothers of patients who had elective aortic aneurysm repair. *Br J Surg*., 1998, 85, 778-80.
[251] Salo, JA; Soisalon-Soininen, S; Bondestam, S; Mattila, PS. Familial occurrence of abdominal aortic aneurysm. *Ann Intern Med*., 1999, 130, 637-42.
[252] Frydman, G; Walker, PJ; Summers, K; West, M; Xu, D; Lightfoot, T; Codd, C; Dique, T; Nataatmadja, M. The value of screening in siblings of patients with abdominal aortic aneurysm. *Eur J Vasc Endovasc Surg*., 2003, 26, 396-400.
[253] Badger, SA; O'Donnell, ME; Boyd, CS; Hannon, RJ; Lau, LL; Lee, B; Soong, CV. The low prevalence of abdominal aortic aneurysm in relatives in Northern Ireland. *Eur J Vasc Endovasc Surg*, 2007, 34, 163-8.
[254] Schulz, V; Hendig, D; Schillinger, M; Exner, M; Domanovits, H; Raith, M; Szliska, C; Kleesiek, K; Götting, C. Analysis of sequence variations in the ABCC6 gene among patients with abdominal aortic aneurysm and pseudoxanthoma elasticum. *J Vasc Res*., 2005, 42, 424-32.
[255] Anderson, DW; Edwards, TK; Ricketts, MH; Kuivaniemi, H; Tromp, G; Stolle, CA; Deak, SB; Boyd, CD. Multiple defects in type III collagen synthesis are associated with the pathogenesis of abdominal aortic aneurysms. *Ann N Y Acad Sci*., 1996, 800, 216-28.
[256] Kontusaari, S; Tromp, G; Kuivaniemi, H; Ladda, RL; Prockop, DJ. Inheritance of an RNA splicing mutation ($G^{+1\ IVS20}$) in the type III procollagen gene (COL3A1) in a family having aortic aneurysms and easy bruisability: phenotypic overlap between familial arterial aneurysms and Ehlers-Danlos syndrome type IV. *Am J Hum Genet*, 1990, 47, 112-20.

[257] MacSweeney, ST; Skidmore, C; Turner, RJ; Sian, M; Brown, L; Henney, AM. Greenhalgh, RM; Powell, JT. Unravelling the familial tendency to aneurysmal disease: popliteal aneurysm, hypertension and fibrillin genotype. *Eur J Vasc Endovasc Surg.*, 1996, 12, 162-6.

[258] Powell, J. Greenhalgh, RM. Cellular, enzymatic, and genetic factors in the pathogenesis of abdominal aortic aneurysms. *J Vasc Surg.*, 1989, 9, 297-304.

[259] Massart, F; Marini, F; Menegato, A; Del Monte, F; Nuti, M; Butitta, F; Ferrari, M; Balbarini, A; Brandi, ML. Allelic genes involved in artery compliance and susceptibility to sporadic abdominal aortic aneurysm. *J Steroid Biochem Mol Biol.*, 2004, 92, 413-8.

[260] Powell, JT; MacSweeney, ST; Greenhalgh, RM; Turner, RJ; Henney, AM. Interaction between fibrillin genotype and blood pressure and the development of aneurysmal disease. *Ann N Y Acad Sci.*, 1996, 800, 198-207.

[261] Powell, JT. Genes predisposing to rapid aneurysm growth. *Ann N Y Acad Sci.*, 2006, 1085, 236-41.

[262] Hinterseher, I; Bergert, H; Kuhlisch, E; Bloomenthal, A; Pilarsky, C; Ockert, D; Schellong, S; Saeger, HD; Krex, D. Matrix metalloproteinase 2 polymorphisms in a caucasian population with abdominal aortic aneurysm. *J Surg Res.*, 2006, 133, 121-8.

[263] Yoon, S; Tromp, G; Vongpunsawad, S; Ronkainen, A; Juvonen, T; Kuivaniemi, H. Genetic analysis of MMP3, MMP9, and PAI-1 in Finnish patients with abdominal aortic or intracranial aneurysms. *Biochem Biophys Res Commun*, 1999, 265, 563-8.

[264] Deguara, J; Burnand, KG; Berg, J; Green, P; Lewis, CM; Chinien, G; Waltham, M; Taylor, P; Stern, RF; Solomon, E; Smith, A. An increased frequency of the 5A allele in the promoter region of the MMP3 gene is associated with abdominal aortic aneurysms. *Hum Mol Genet*, 2007, 16, 3002-7.

[265] Armani, C; Curcio, M; Barsotti, MC; Santoni, T; Di Stefano, R; Dell'omodarme, M; Brandi, ML; Ferrari, M; Scatena, F; Carpi, A; Balbarini, A. Polymorphic analysis of the matrix metalloproteinase-9 gene and susceptibility to sporadic abdominal aortic aneurysm. *Biomed Pharmacother*, 2007, 61, 268-71.

[266] Schardey, HM; Hernandez-Richter, T; Klueppelberg, U; Tutsch-Bauer, E; Lauterjung, L. Alleles of the alpha-1-antitrypsin phenotype in patients with aortic aneurysms. *J Cardiovasc Surg (Torino)*, 1998, 39, 535-9.

[267] St Jean, P; Hart, B; Webster, M; Steed, D; Adamson, J; Powell, J; Ferrell, R. α_1-antitrypsin deficiency in aneurysmal disease. *Hum Hered*, 1996, 46, 92-7.

[268] Tilson, MD; Roberts, MP. Molecular diversity in the abdominal aortic aneurysm phenotype. *Arch Surg.*, 1988, 123, 1202-6.

[269] Jones, K; Powell, J; Brown, L; Greenhalgh, R; Jormsjö, S; Eriksson, P. The influence of 4G/5G polymorphism in the plasminogen activator inhibitor-1 gene promoter on the incidence, growth and operative risk of abdominal aortic aneurysm. *Eur J Vasc Endovasc Surg.*, 2002, 23, 421-5.

[270] Rossaak, JI; Van, Rij, AM; Jones, GT; Harris, EL. Association of the 4G/5G polymorphism in the promoter region of plasminogen activator inhibitor-1 with abdominal aortic aneurysms. *J Vasc Surg*, 2000, 31, 1026-32.

[271] Golledge, J; Muller, J; Shephard, N; Clancy, P; Smallwood, L; Moran, C; Dear, AE; Palmer, LJ; Norman, PE. Association between osteopontin and human abdominal aortic aneurysm. *Arterioscler Thromb Vasc Biol.*, 2007, 27, 655-60.
[272] Tilson, MD; Reilly, JM; Brophy, CM; Webster, EL; Barnett, TR. Expression and sequence of the gene for tissue inhibitor of metalloproteinases in patients with abdominal aortic aneurysms. *J Vasc Surg.*, 1993, 18, 266-70.
[273] Götting, C; Prante, C; Schillinger, M; Exner, M; Domanovits, H; Raith, M; Kuhn, J; Kleesiek, K. Xylosyltransferase I variants and their impact on abdominal aortic aneurysms. *Clin Chim Acta*, 2008, 391, 41-5.
[274] Pola, R; Gaetani, E; Santoliquido, A; Gerardino, L; Cattani, P; Serricchio, M; Tondi, P; Flore, R; Grande, M; Carbonin, P; Fadda, G; Pola, P. Abdominal aortic aneurysm in normotensive patients: association with angiotensin-converting enzyme gene polymorphism. *Eur J Vasc Endovasc Surg.*, 2001, 21, 445-9.
[275] Gerdes, LU, Lindholt, JS; Vammen, S; Henneberg, EW; Fasting, H. Apolipoprotein E genotype is associated with differential expansion rates of small abdominal aortic aneurysms. *Br J Surg.*, 2000, 87, 760-5.
[276] Powell, JT; Bashir, A; Dawson, S; Vine, N; Henney, AM; Humphries, SE; Greenhalgh, RM. Genetic variation on chromosome 16 is associated with abdominal aortic aneurysm. Clin Sci (Lond), 1990, 78, 13-6.
[277] Ramsbottom, D; Fitzgerald, P; Grace, PA; McAnena, O; Burke, P; Collins, P; Johnson, A; Croke, DT; Bouchier-Hayes, D. Biochemical and molecular genetic studies of abdominal aortic aneurysm in an Irish population. *Eur J Vasc Surg.*, 1994, 8, 716-22.
[278] Ramsbottom, D; O'Neill, A; Sexton, DM; Gafoor, RA; Bouchier-Hayes, D; Croke, DT. The cholesteryl ester transfer protein (CETP) locus as a candidate gene in abdominal aortic aneurysm. *Clin Genet*, 1997, 51, 241-5.
[279] Ferrara, F; Novo, S; Grimaudo, S; Raimondi, F; Meli, F; Amato, C; Amodeo, G; Lo Presti, R; Caimi, G. Methylenetetrahydrofolate reductase mutation in subjects with abdominal aortic aneurysm subdivided for age. *Clin Hemorheol Microcirc*, 2006, 34, 421-6.
[280] Peeters, AC; Van Landeghem, BA; Graafsma, SJ; Kranendonk, SE; Hermus, AR; Blom, HJ; Den Heijer, M. Low vitamin B6; and not plasma homocysteine concentration, as risk factor for abdominal aortic aneurysm: a retrospective case-control study. *J Vasc Surg.*, 2007, 45, 701-5.
[281] Strauss, E; Waliszewski, K; Pawlak, AL. [The normotensive carriers of the MTHFR 677T allele, displaying the increased risk of development of the abdominal aortic aneurysm (AAA), occur at the highest frequency among the smoking patients]. *Przegl Lek*, 2004, 61, 1086-9.
[282] Kotani, K; Shimomura, T; Murakami, F; Ikawa, S; Kanaoka, Y; Ohgi, S; Adachi, K; Nanba, E. Allele frequency of human endothelial nitric oxide synthase gene polymorphism in abdominal aortic aneurysm. *Intern Med.*, 2000, 39, 537-9.
[283] Ghilardi, G; Biondi, ML; Battaglioli, L; Zambon, A; Guagnellini, E; Scorza, R. Genetic risk factor characterizes abdominal aortic aneurysm from arterial occlusive disease in human beings: CCR5 Δ32 deletion. *J Vasc Surg.*, 2004, 40, 995-1000.

[284] Hirose, H; Takagi, M; Miyagawa, N; Hashiyada, H; Noguchi, M; Tada, S; Kugimiya, T; Tilson, MD. Genetic risk factor for abdominal aortic aneurysm: HLA-DR2(15), a Japanese study. *J Vasc Surg.*, 1998, 27, 500-3.
[285] Hirose, H; Tilson, MD. Negative genetic risk factor for abdominal aortic aneurysm: HLA-DQ3, a Japanese study. *J Vasc Surg.*, 1999, 30, 959-60.
[286] Moñux, G; Serrano, FJ; Vigil, P; De La Concha, EG. Role of HLA-DR in the pathogenesis of abdominal aortic aneurysm. *Eur J Vasc Endovasc Surg.*, 2003, 26, 211-4.
[287] Sugimoto, T; Sada, M; Miyamoto, T; Yao, H. Genetic analysis on HLA loci in Japanese patients with abdominal aortic aneurysm. *Eur J Vasc Endovasc Surg.*, 2003, 26, 215-8.
[288] Tromp, G; Ogata, T; Gregoire, L; Goddard, KA; Skunca, M; Lancaster, WD; Parrado, AR; Lu, Q; Shibamura, H; Sakalihasan, N; Limet, R; Mackean, GL; Arthur, C; Sueda, T; Kuivaniemi, H. HLA-DQA is associated with abdominal aortic aneurysms in the Belgian population. *Ann N Y Acad Sci.*, 2006, 1085, 392-5.
[289] Bown, MJ; Burton, PR; Horsburgh, T; Nicholson, ML; Bell, PR; Sayers, RD. The role of cytokine gene polymorphisms in the pathogenesis of abdominal aortic aneurysms: a case-control study. *J Vasc Surg.*, 2003, 37, 999-1005.
[290] Marculescu, R; Sodeck, G; Domanovits, H; Hobusch, G; Exner, M; Heinzl, H; Huber, K; Mannhalter, C; Minar, E; Wagner, O; Schillinger, M. Interleukin-1 gene cluster variants and abdominal aortic aneurysms. *Thromb Haemost*, 2005, 94, 646-50.
[291] Jones, KG; Brull, DJ; Brown, LC; Sian, M; Greenhalgh, RM; Humphries, SE; Powell, JT. Interleukin-6 (IL-6) and the prognosis of abdominal aortic aneurysms. *Circulation*, 2001, 103, 2260-5.
[292] Unno, N, Nakamura, T; Mitsuoka, H; Uchiyama, T; Yamamoto, N; Saito, T; Sugatani, J; Miwa, M; Nakamura, S. Association of a G994 -->T missense mutation in the plasma platelet-activating factor acetylhydrolase gene with risk of abdominal aortic aneurysm in Japanese. *Ann Surg.*, 2002, 235, 297-302.
[293] Eriksson, P; Jones, KG; Brown, LC; Greenhalgh, RM; Hamsten, A; Powell, JT. Genetic approach to the role of cysteine proteases in the expansion of abdominal aortic aneurysms. *Br J Surg.*, 2004, 91, 86-9.
[294] Schillinger, M; Exner, M; Mlekusch, W; Domanovits, H; Huber, K; Mannhalter, C; Wagner, O; Minar, E. Heme oxygenase-1 gene promoter polymorphism is associated with abdominal aortic aneurysm. *Thromb Res.*, 2002, 106, 131-6.
[295] Cao, RY; Adams, MA; Habenicht, AJ; Funk, CD. Angiotensin II-induced abdominal aortic aneurysm occurs independently of the 5-lipoxygenase pathway in apolipoprotein E-deficient mice. *Prostaglandins Other Lipid Mediat*, 2007, 84, 34-42.
[296] Ishibashi, M; Egashira, K; Zhao, Q; Hiasa, K; Ohtani, K; Ihara, Y; Charo, IF; Kura, S; Tsuzuki, T; Takeshita, A; Sunagawa, K. Bone marrow-derived monocyte chemoattractant protein-1 receptor CCR2 is critical in angiotensin II-induced acceleration of atherosclerosis and aneurysm formation in hypercholesterolemic mice. *Arterioscler Thromb Vasc Biol.*, 2004, 24, 174-8.

[297] Ahluwalia, N; Lin, AY; Tager, AM; Pruitt, IE; Anderson, TJ; Kristo, F; Shen, D; Cruz, AR; Aikawa, M; Luster, AD; Gerszten, RE. Inhibited aortic aneurysm formation in BLT1-deficient mice. *J Immunol*, 2007, 179, 691-7.

[298] Thomas, M; Gavrila, D; McCormick, ML; Miller, FJ; Jr.; Daugherty, A; Cassis, LA; Dellsperger, KC; Weintraub, NL. Deletion of p47phox attenuates angiotensin II-induced abdominal aortic aneurysm formation in apolipoprotein E-deficient mice. *Circulation*, 2006, 114, 404-13.

[299] Bruemmer, D; Collins, AR; Noh, G; Wang, W; Territo, M; Arias-Magallona, S; Fishbein, MC; Blaschke, F; Kintscher, U; Graf, K; Law, RE; Hsueh, WA. Angiotensin II-accelerated atherosclerosis and aneurysm formation is attenuated in osteopontin-deficient mice. *J Clin Invest.*, 2003, 112, 1318-31.

[300] Cassis, LA; Rateri, DL; Lu, H; Daugherty, A. Bone marrow transplantation reveals that recipient AT1a receptors are required to initiate angiotensin II-induced atherosclerosis and aneurysms. *Arterioscler Thromb Vasc Biol.*, 2007, 27, 380-6.

[301] Wang, M; Lee, E; Song, W; Ricciotti, E; Rader, DJ; Lawson, JA; Puré, E; Fitzgerald, GA. Microsomal prostaglandin E synthase-1 deletion suppresses oxidative stress and angiotensin II-induced abdominal aortic aneurysm formation. *Circulation*, 2008, 117, 1302-9.

[302] Gavazzi, G; Deffert, C; Trocme, C; Schappi, M; Herrmann, FR; Krause, KH. NOX1 deficiency protects from aortic dissection in response to angiotensin II. *Hypertension*, 2007, 50, 189-96.

[303] Gitlin, JM; Trivedi, DB; Langenbach, R; Loftin, CD. Genetic deficiency of cyclooxygenase-2 attenuates abdominal aortic aneurysm formation in mice. *Cardiovasc Res.*, 2007, 73, 227-36.

[304] MacTaggart, JN; Xiong, W; Knispel, R; Baxter, BT. Deletion of CCR2 but not CCR5 or CXCR3 inhibits aortic aneurysm formation. *Surgery.*, 2007, 142, 284-8.

[305] Pagano, MB; Bartoli, MA; Ennis, TL; Mao, D; Simmons, PM; Thompson, RW; Pham, CT. Critical role of dipeptidyl peptidase I in neutrophil recruitment during the development of experimental abdominal aortic aneurysms. *Proc Natl Acad Sci.*, USA, 2007, 104, 2855-60.

[306] Lee, JK; Borhani, M; Ennis, TL; Upchurch, GR; Jr.; Thompson, RW. Experimental abdominal aortic aneurysms in mice lacking expression of inducible nitric oxide synthase. *Arterioscler Thromb Vasc Biol.*, 2001, 21, 1393-401.

[307] Hannawa, KK; Cho, BS; Sinha, I; Roelofs, KJ; Myers, DD; Wakefield, TJ; Stanley, JC; Henke, PK; Upchurch, GR. Jr.: Attenuation of experimental aortic aneurysm formation in P-selectin knockout mice. *Ann N Y Acad Sci.*, 2006, 1085, 353-9.

In: Aneurysms: Types, Risks, Formation and Treatment
Editors: Alain Laurent and Ethan Morel
ISBN: 978-1-60741-557-2
©2009 Nova Science Publishers, Inc.

Chapter 4

Aortic Aneurysms—Risk Factors, Pathogenesis, and Therapeutic Management: A Review

Ying Zhuge, Muddassir Aliniazee, and Omaida C. Velazquez*
Division of Vascular Surgery, DeWitt Daughtry Family Department of Surgery,
University of Miami Miller School of Medicine, Miami, FL, USA

Abstract

Abdominal aortic aneurysm (AAA) affects approximately 2—4% of the adult population and is the thirteenth leading cause of death in the United States. Patients are mostly asymptomatic but they can present with mild abdominal or back pain, distal embolization of thrombus, compression of ureters and hydronephrosis, pulsatile abdominal mass, as well as rupture, which is characterized by sudden-onset pain, hypotension, syncope, or sudden death. Risk factors for AAA formation and progression include cigarette smoking, hypertension, dyslipidemia, advancing age, male gender, and family history, while protective factors include African race, female gender, and diabetes mellitus. The pathophysiology of thoracic aortic aneurysms (TAA) is cystic medial degeneration, a non-inflammatory process. On the other hand, formation of AAA results from complex interactions between mural inflammation, proteolysis by matrix metalloproteinases, oxidative stress, apoptosis of smooth muscle cells, and neovascularization of the vasa vasorum. Ultrasonography is the method of choice for detection of AAA, while computerized tomography (CT) and magnetic resonance imaging (MRI) are the most frequently used methods for planning therapeutic strategies. Surgical treatment of AAA is generally reserved for larger (> 5 cm), rapidly expanding, or symptomatic aneurysms and consists of open versus endovascular aneurysm repair (EVAR). Although endovascular repair has lower short-term mortality, this does not translate into long-term survival difference. With increased understanding of the pathophysiology of AAA formation, new medications are being investigated for

* Corresponding Author: Omaida C. Velazquez, MD, Room 3016 Holtz Center - JMH East Tower, 1611 N.W. 12th Avenue, Miami, FL 33135, Tel: (305) 585-5284, Fax: (305) 585-8569, ovelazquez@med.miami.edu

prevention of AAA and their progression, including angiotensin II inhibitors and statins. This review summarizes current knowledge of the incidence, pathophysiology, risk factors, natural history, and treatment of this increasingly more common pathology.

Introduction

Abdominal aortic aneurysm (AAA) affects 5% of elderly men in the United States and causes death in 1—3% of men over the age of 65, mostly due to rupture, which is fatal in greater than 60% of cases (1-3). AAA is the thirteenth most common cause of mortality in the United States, accounting for 15,000 deaths per year (3-5). Approximately 40,000 repairs are performed each year and 150,000 hospital admissions are due to this problem (4). The typical patient to present with AAA is the elderly, cigarette smoking, hypertensive, non-diabetic man (1). The incidence of AAA has been increasing in the Western world, partly due to increasing age of the population, rising number of smokers, increased incidence of hypertension and heart disease, and improved diagnostic techniques (3, 5).

Infrarenal AAA accounts for 80% of all aortic aneurysms (3, 4). The diameter of the infrarenal aorta increases as one ages. The median diameter is 1.75 cm at 25 years of age and 2.25 cm at 55 years of age (6). AAA is defined as focal dilatation exceeding 150% of the normal aortic diameter (3, 7). Infrarenal AAAs reach a significant rupture risk and become clinically worthy of operative repair at diameters of 5 cm or larger or when the rate of growth is faster than 0.5 cm every 6 months (4). Risk of rupture increases as maximum diameter increases, and it is estimated that half of all patients with ruptured AAA die before reaching the hospital (8).

Due to the increasing incidence of AAA in recent years, especially of smaller aneurysms, intense research efforts have been undertaken to investigate the pathophysiology of AAA and trials have been performed to study medical treatment for small aneurysms to slow their progression and even bring about regression of disease. Prospective randomized trials have also been conducted to compare the traditional open surgical approach with the novel endovascular approach to repair AAA. This is a comprehensive review of current knowledge of the clinical presentation, epidemiology and risk factors, pathophysiology, diagnosis, and treatment of this disease process in adults. It also addresses new medical therapeutic strategies that are still under investigation for AAA.

Anatomy and Hemodynamics

Aortic aneurysms are described based on their location, i.e. thoracic versus abdominal, size, and morphologic appearance. Aortic aneurysms are usually either fusiform or saccular. Fusiform aneurysms are symmetrical, and involve dilation of the full circumference of the aortic wall. On the other, saccular aneurysms appear as outpouching of only a portion of the aorta. Due to the unequal pressure exerted on an aorta with a saccular aneurysm, it has increased likelihood of rupture. Therefore, most saccular aneurysms undergo surgical intervention when discovered. Fusiform aneurysms, which account for the majority of AAA, can be observed depending on its size, rate of expansion, or presence of symptoms.

The most important structural element of the aortic wall is the media, which is composed of elastin, collagen, and smooth muscle cells. Elastin and collagen determine the mechanical properties of the aorta: elastin is the principal load bearer at lower pressures and small distention; both elastin and collagen are load bearers at higher pressures and larger distension (9). Elastin is predominantly found in the ascending aorta where distension is necessary, and it is not synthesized in the abdominal aorta in adults (3). In the normal aorta, there is a gradual reduction in the number of medial elastin layers from the proximal thoracic aorta (60-80 layers) to the infrarenal aorta (28-32 layers) (1, 4). The infrarenal aorta is the only segment where the proportion of elastin decreases relative to collagen (1), which is the main component of abdominal aorta (9).

Hemodynamic forces on the infrarenal aorta results in increased stress, leading to potential weakening and dilatation. The localization of hemodynamic stress in the infrarenal aorta is due to three factors: distal tapering of the aorta, progressive stiffening of the aortic wall, and the additive effects of retrograde pressure waves reflecting from the iliac bifurcation combining with antegrade pressure wave (9). This, combined with the relative deficiency of elastic lamellae, predisposes this segment of aorta to aneurysm formation.

Clinical Presentation

Most small, unruptured AAAs remain asymptomatic, and are usually discovered incidentally in adult patients when the patient is being worked up for another reason, e.g. coronary artery disease, peripheral vascular disease, cerebrovascular disease, or intra-abdominal processes via computerized tomography. Aortic aneurysms in the neonatal and pediatric population are also recognized, though rare, clinical entities. The disease in adults is believed to be largely degenerative. Conversely, aortic aneurysms in children are a rare and puzzling heterogeneous group of disease, with a largely genetic component in their etiology. In this review, we focus on aneurysms in adults. When they are symptomatic, aneurysms present with pain as the most frequent complaint. It is usually described as "gnawing," lasts for many hours, and is located in the hypogastrium or lower back (3). The abdomen can be tender to palpation. Complications of unruptured AAA can lead to its diagnosis, such as distal embolization of thrombus leading to limb ischemia, hydronephrosis from compression of ureters, iliac vein compression leading to deep vein thrombosis, and intestinal obstruction (3, 5).

Ruptured AAAs, on the other hand, is always symptomatic, characterized by sudden-onset of abdominal or back pain, pulsatile abdominal mass, and hypotension or shock. Prognosis after a rupture depends on the location and the size of the rupture. Survival rates are higher for ruptures that occur into the retroperitoneum, where bleeding can be tamponaded, than for free intraperitoneal ruptures, where the mortality rate is 97% (3). Other more rare forms of rupture include a small tear that temporarily seals to be followed by a larger rupture, aorto-enteric fistulas, and aorto-caval fistulas (5).

Epidemiology and Risk Factors

The formation of AAA arises from complex interactions between structural properties of the infrarenal aortic wall and various risk factors such as atherosclerosis, cigarette smoking, arterial hypertension, aging, gender, and hemodynamic factors, as well as genetic component (1), leading to loss of tensile strength of the wall and resultant dilatation (10). Modifiable and non-modifiable risk factors for AAA formation are summarized in **Table 1**. Male gender, increasing age, and family history are non-modifiable risk factors of AAA. AAA affects men nine times more frequently than women, and it is diagnosed ten years earlier in men than women (2, 3). Also, men are three times more likely to die from aneurismal rupture than women (4). Clinically relevant AAAs are found in about 1% of men between 55 and 64 years of age, and the prevalence increases by 2—4% per decade to a peak of 5.9% at age 80 (3, 4, 6). Positive family history is present in 15-19% of patients diagnosed with AAA with an autosomal dominant pattern (4, 11). Aneurysms also affect white Europeans more often than they do Asians and Africans (12, 13). TAA also has some familial patterns, i.e. 21.5% of patients have a positive family history, and these patients present earlier with TAA that grow at faster rates than sporadic TAA. In addition, other aneurysms coexist in other portions of the aorta (14).

Table 1. Modifiable and Non-Modifiable Risk and Protective Factors for AAA Formation and Expansion

Modifiable
Cigarette smoking
Atherosclerosis
Hypertension
Genetic factors
Autoimmune disease
Chlamydial species
Non-modifiable
Male gender
Increasing age
Family history
Protective
Diabetes
Female gender
African race
Expansion
Aneurysm size
Rapid rate of growth

The strongest independent risk factor for the development and expansion of AAAs is cigarette smoking (1, 3, 5). 90% of patients with aneurysms have a history of smoking, either current or previous. The incidence of AAAs in smokers is six times higher than in non-smokers. Continued smoking is also a risk factor for AAA expansion and eventual rupture (5, 15). There is some evidence that cessation of smoking results in a slow decline of risk for developing AAAs (16). Therefore, smoking cessation is an important part of counseling for patients with AAAs.

A weaker risk factor for AAAs is atherosclerosis. While some studies show that a history of, or being treated for, high plasma cholesterol concentrations has been associated with increased risk of AAAs (12), other studies have not. The actual relationship is mostly likely one of co-existence, not causal. Risk factors that lead to the formation of AAA and development of atherosclerosis are likely the same, and the processes of inflammation are similar, potentially involving similar molecules and cytokines. However, the processes occur in different locations of the blood vessel. A main histologic difference between aneurismal and atherosclerotic lesions appears to be the localization of macrophages in the media of the AAA wall rather than the subintima in atherosclerosis (1). Another piece of evidence highlighting the difference between these two disease processes is the fact that diabetes is a risk factor for atherosclerosis, but not for AAAs (see below).

Hypertension is another risk factor for AAA formation, though the exact association is difficult to assess due to the use of antihypertensive medications. There are additional unknown genetic factors that predispose certain individuals to AAA formation. Studies have demonstrated loci mapped to 5q13-14, 19q13, and 4q31 to be involved in AAA formation, demonstrating some genetic heterogeneity (4). Candidate genes in these regions include interleukin (IL)-15, endothelin receptor A, programmed cell death 5, and LDL-receptor-related protein 3 (5, 17). Replication of these gene association studies, however, has been inconsistent. AAA have also been linked with various autoimmune diseases, including giant cell arteritis, systemic lupus erythematosus (SLE), Takayasu's arteritis, and antiphospholipid syndrome (4). The risk of AAA is increased by certain human leukocyte antigen (HLA) class II molecules, such as HLA DR B1 *0401 and HLA-DQA1 (18, 19). A final cause of AAA that has been extensively studied is infection, specifically *Chlamydia* species. Several studies hypothesized this organism as a possible source of vascular pathology and have detected *C. pneumonia* in aorta fragments that are aneurismal, especially ruptured aortic aneurysms (4).

The natural history of aneurysm formation is progressive degeneration and expansion of aneurysm until rupture (4). Conclusions regarding the natural history of AAA are mostly derived from population-based studies following patients with small aneurysms or patients unsuitable for surgery (20, 21). AAA undergoes periods of rapid expansion followed periods of quiescence (5). Various risk factors have been identified for the growth and eventual rupture of AAAs, and understanding these factors can identify secondary prevention strategies to slow progression of disease. Aneurysm size and maximal aortic diameter are the most important factors related to progression (20). Studies have shown that aneurysms smaller than 4 cm have a 0.3% annual risk of rupture, those 4 cm to 4.9 cm have 1.5% annual risk, those 5 to 5.9 cm have 6.5 to 8% risk of rupture per year, those 6 to 6.9 cm have 10% annual risk rupture, and aneurysms larger than 7 cm have 20% risk of rupture (20, 21). Other factors predisposing to rapid progression include a history of rapid rate of growth and continued cigarette smoking (3, 15). Cigarette smoking is associated with increased AAA expansion rate of 15 to 20% (1, 22).

There are also protective factors for the development of AAA, including African race, female gender, and diabetes mellitus. Diabetes shows an inverse association with development and expansion of AAAs. This could be explained by the fact that the high intravascular glucose levels associated with diabetes that causes modification and glycation of molecules in the body, including collagen, which makes them resistant to cleavage by metalloproteinases (see below) and other proteases.

Pathogenesis

The pathophysiology of thoracic aortic aneurysm (TAA) and AAA are considered to be different processes and should be evaluated separately. Histologically, AAA is characterized by elastin fragmentation and degeneration. Current evidence suggests that there are three major players in the formation and progression of AAA: aortic wall proteolysis and remodeling by matrix metalloproteinases (MMPs), transmural inflammation, and smooth muscle cell apoptosis (**Table 2**) (1, 3, 4, 9).

Table 2. Pathogenesis of AAAs

Aortic wall proteolysis		
	Elastase	
	Collagenase	
	Cysteine proteases (cathepsins)	
	Matrix metalloproteinases (from inflammatory cells)	
		MMP-2
		MMP-9 (gelatinase B)
		MMP-12
		Imbalance of TIMPs
		Neovascularization of arterial wall
Transmural inflammation		
	Cells	
		Monocytes/Macrophages
		Lymphocytes
		Plasma cells
	Mediators	
		Interleukins
		C-reactive proteins
		Tumor necrosis factor
		Interferon
		Angiotensin II
	Phases	
		Inflammatory
		Active
		Amorphous
Smooth muscle cell apoptosis		
	Causes decreased structural integrity	

The most important component of the aortic wall is the media, which depends on elastin and collagen for its structural integrity and hemodynamic function. Elastin provides arterial wall distensibility on pulse propagation and is the principal load-bearing element (1, 3). On the other hand, collagen contributes tensile strength and prevents over-distension (1). Proteolytic degradation of these compounds by collagenase and elastase is a key factor involved in AAA formation. Some studies show that elastin degradation causes aneurismal dilation, whereas collagen destruction is required for aneurysm rupture (23, 24). Both elastase and collagenase activity have been found in aortic aneurysms, and both positively correlated with aneurysm size (1, 25). One group of proteases known as cysteine proteases, particularly cathepsins S, K, and L, are important in AAA formation. Cathepsins are elastolytic and collagenolytic, and their natural inhibitor is cystatin C. Some studies show elevated levels of cathepsins combined with decreased levels of cystatin C in AAA, causing aortic wall degradation and degeneration (26). Another group of enzymes that have also been extensively studied have an even greater role in the destruction of aortic wall and subsequent development of aortic aneurysms is the matrix metalloproteinase (MMP) family.

MMPs are zinc-mediated enzymes produced by inflammatory cells such as neutrophils and macrophages, as well as mesenchymal cells such as fibroblasts (1, 10), and as a group they can degrade almost all structural proteins of the extracellular matrix (9). They are involved in a variety of normal and pathologic tissue remodeling processes, including embryonic development, wound healing, cancer, arthritis, and inflammation (10, 27). They are released in the inactive form as pro-MMPs and can be activated by proteinases, as well as other MMPs (10). MMP activity is regulated at multiple levels to prevent uncontrolled tissue destruction, such as transcription, activation, and by the presence of natural inhibitors (9). MMPs are normally expressed in extremely low levels in the normal endothelium, tightly policed by a family of tissue inhibitor of metalloproteinases (TIMPs).

Specific MMPs have been implicated in the pathogenesis of AAA. MMP-2 and MMP-9 are both prominent in AAAs, where they are primarily found in the aortic media, and degrade both elastin and collagen (28-30). Matrix metalloproteinase-2 is a type IV (basement membrane) collagenase, though it is capable of degrading elastin, and interstitial collagen. Studies have shown that large amounts of MMP-2 are bound to the extracellular matrix in aneurismal aortas, and that a large portion of this matrix-bound MMP-2 is in the activated form (31). It has been demonstrated that MMP-2 level correlates with AAA diameter (32, 33). Studies also show that MMP-2 levels are elevated in the circulation of patients with aneurismal disease (34). Some studies show that MMP-2 is particularly elevated in small AAAs (35), suggesting a potential role in the early stages of aneurysm formation.

MMP-9, also known as gelatinase B, is the most studied MMP in patients with AAA. It appears to be less prevalent in small aneurysms, and more responsible for the continued expansion and eventual rupture of aneurysms (28, 35, 36). The primary source of MMP-9 is inflammatory cells infiltrating the arterial adventitia, including macrophages, and the main substrates for MMP-9 include collagen type I, type IV, elastase, and fibrinogen (1, 9). The gene encoding MMP-9 demonstrates a 12-fold increase in expression within aortic aneurysm tissue when compared to normal tissue (10), which leads to increased production of MMP-9 by smooth muscle cells within aneurismal aortic media when compared to normal tissue (37). Elevated MMP-9 levels have been shown to occur in the circulation of patients with AAAs, and MMP-9 expression appears to be proportional to aneurysm size (28, 38, 39). In addition, mouse models with mice that are MMP-9-deficient exhibit statistically decreased tendency to form AAAs. Along the same lines, wild type mice that undergo bone marrow transplant from MMP-9-deficient mice show no evidence of development of AAAs, while MMP-9-deficiency mice that receive bone marrow transplant from wild type mice did develop AAAs (40). In 2002, Lorelli *et al.* found that serum levels of MMP-9 decreased significantly for the group of patients who received endovascular repair of AAAs, while MMP-9 levels remained elevated in patients who underwent open repair (41). This difference persisted out to 6 months follow-up (42). Of interest, it was demonstrated that the small number of patients who had endoleaks following EVAR had significantly higher levels of MMP-9 in their serum, and a correlation was found between increased serum MMP-9 levels and increase in sac size following endovascular repair (10).

Another MMP that has been implicated in AAA formation is MMP-12, which is prominently localized to elastin fiber fragments within aneurysm tissue (9). This unique localization suggests an important role for this enzyme in aneurismal progression.

As mentioned earlier, there are naturally occurring inhibitors of MMPs, known as tissue inhibitors of metalloproteinases (TIMPs). TIMP-1 is capable of inhibiting most MMPs; TIMP-2 is specific for MMP-2, and TIMP-3 exists primarily in association with the extracellular matrix (9). One of the proposed mechanisms of AAA formation is an imbalance of MMPs and TIMPs, i.e. an increased MMP to TIMP ratio (43). It has been shown that MMP-2/TIMP-1 and MMP-9/TIMP-1 ratios were increased in aneurismal aortic tissue, and TIMP-1-deficient mice developed significantly larger aneurysms than wild type mice (44, 45). It has also been demonstrated, however, that TIMPs are increased in aneurysm walls, reflecting endogenous regulation that slows progression of AAAs (9). Another process closely linked to MMPs is neovascularization of the arterial wall, which has been linked to formation and rupture of AAA (46-49). Healthy infrarenal aorta is devoid of significant vasa vasorum and neovascularization increases local inflammation by recruiting lymphocytes and monocytes to the aortic media (1). MMPs have been linked to this pathologic process, as well as thrombus formation in the aorta, which leads to hypoxic conditions, causing neovascularization (50).

Another major component of AAA formation and progression is chronic mural inflammation. Inflammatory cells are recruited from blood and from neovascularization processes in the media layer forming a lymphomonocytic infiltrate (47, 51). Inflammatory cells present in AAAs consist of monocytes, macrophages, T cells, B cells, and plasma cells (9). Monocytes are recruited to the outer aortic wall, where they differentiate into macrophages and secrete cytokines, which attract lymphocytes and additional monocytes. Curci *et al.* divide the changes in the media into three areas: inflammatory, active, and amorphous (52). Inflammatory media is characterized by high amounts of T and B cells with a few macrophages and neutrophils. Active media consists of fragmented elastic fibers with predominantly smooth muscle cells and macrophages. Amorphous media appears hypocellular and lack any organizational pattern (9). Although the specific stimulus for the initiation of inflammation in the aortic wall is largely unknown, once the process starts, inflammatory cytokines and chemokines sustain this process for many years. For example, maximal AAA diameter has been shown to positively correlate with inflammatory mediators such as interleukin (IL)-6 and C-reactive protein (53-56). IL-1β and tumor necrosis factor (TNF)-α have also been shown to be increased AAA (57). Interferon (INF)-γ is yet another mediator that has been shown to be elevated in human AAAs, and has been associated particularly with rapidly expanding AAAs (58). In addition to having a chemotactic effect on the influx of additional inflammatory cells, these cytokines also play important roles in modulating the transcription of MMPs, their inhibitors, and their activators (9). Conversely, MMPs also cleave these inflammatory mediators to more potent forms. For example, IL-8 can be enhanced by specific cleavage by MMP-9, making it ten times more potent as an inducer of inflammation and further MMP-9 release (59). This brings about a vicious cycle that results in the eventual formation of aneurismal aortas. Another inflammatory mediator is angiotensin II (AT-II), which exerts numerous effects on the cardiovascular system, including vascular hypertrophy, cell proliferation, induction of cytokines, production of extracellular matrix, and activation of macrophages (1). It has been shown that AT-II enhances inflammation and induces formation of AAA in mice (60). AT-II also promotes atherosclerotic lesions in these mice (61), thereby establishing an important link between intimal inflammation resulting in atherosclerotic lesions as well as medial inflammation leading to aneurismal degeneration.

While increased proteolytic breakdown is a major factor in the pathogenesis of AAA, impaired connective tissue repair is of equal importance. Since the stability of established AAAs depends on collagen production to withstand progression and rupture, the cells that produce collagen are pivotal in maintaining structural integrity of the infrarenal aorta. Adventitial fibroblasts and medial smooth muscle cells (SMCs) are the main cells that produce collagen and elastin and depletion of medial SMCs may also be important in aneurismal degeneration (9). Some studies have shown that up to 30% of SMCs in AAAs exhibit fragmented DNA, consistent with apoptosis (62, 63), while other studies report that remaining cells within the aneurysm wall do not replicate normally (64). Studies on human serum and tissue have assessed aortic histology, protein and gene expression and serum markers, and have shown that the above mechanisms, i.e. inflammatory cytokines, MMPs, and loss of extracellular matrix, are reproducible findings in human AAA biopsies (5). However, while these findings give clues to molecular biology behind end-stage AAA, the initiating pathways are still poorly understood.

Diagnosis

Since the physical examination has such a poor predictive value for the diagnosis of AAA, other modes of diagnosis are necessary. Ultrasonography is the method of choice for the detection of AAA with a sensitivity of 95% and specificity of 100% (65). Ultrasounds can be used for the initial diagnosis, as well as surveillance of the aneurysm to evaluate any changes in size or morphology. Part of the increased incidence of AAA in recent years has been due to improved ultrasonographic technology and increased usage for detection in asymptomatic patients. While studies have shown that ultrasound screening for AAAs decreases short-term mortality from this disease process, long-term mortality is not affected, and it is not cost effective for the general population (66). However, it is recommended for high-risk groups such as older men who have a smoke history (present or remote).

Other modes of imaging, such as computerized tomography and magnetic resonance imaging are used to plan therapeutic approaches in the treatment of AAAs. Angiography has traditionally also been used to visualize aneurysms that are difficult to characterize by other means, but now is mostly used in endovascular therapy of AAAs.

Studies are underway to determine the usefulness of certain biomarkers for AAA, which are protein, peptides, gene, or metabolic products that represent this particular biologic process and can be used as surrogate markers for aneurysm size and risk of rupture (67). An ideal circulating biomarker should be procured in a non-invasive manner, be reliable in their correlation with aneurysm size, and not be costly. For example, it was found that serum elastin peptide (SEP), degradation products of elastin, which also stimulate leukocyte recruitment and cytokine production, had a significant correlation with aneurysm growth and eventual rupture, though further studies are needed (67).

Therapeutic Management

Therapeutic management of AAAs depends on aneurysm size, rate of growth, and presence of clinical symptoms. For asymptomatic AAAs that are smaller than 4.5 cm, ultrasonographic surveillance every 6 months is necessary. For AAAs between 4.5 and 5 cm, surveillance every 3 to 6 months is recommended (3). Studies have shown that while screening decreases aneurysm-related deaths, it does not reduce overall mortality (68). In addition, randomized-controlled trials comparing surveillance with early elective surgery in asymptomatic aneurysms less than 5.5 cm demonstrate no difference in survival between the patient groups (69-71). The Aneurysm Detection and Management Veterans Affairs Cooperative (ADAM) study also showed no difference in survival in patients who received early surgery. However, certain patients groups should be contemplated for early surgery. Patients who are younger than 65 years of age should be contemplated for elective surgery due to their higher probability of needing surgery in the future. Other properties that may predispose a patient to earlier surgery include rapid growth of the aneurysm, saccular morphology, and low surgical risk (3). Asymptomatic AAA that is greater than 5.0 cm require surgical therapy. Also, symptomatic and/or ruptured AAAs require invasive therapy.

Until recently, open surgical therapy was the only method for repairing AAAs. Currently, endovascular repair by placement of a stent graft across the aneurysm and fixation of proximal and distal limbs to normal portions of the aorta and iliac arteries has revolutionized the treatment of this important disease process (72). Since their development, more than 25,000 patients worldwide have received aortic stent grafts (73). Open repair is associated with lower rate of graft failure, but endovascular therapy represents a less morbid approach and patients who would otherwise not tolerate open surgery can undergo repair.

Unfortunately, both approaches have their respective shortcomings. For example, open repair has a mortality rate of 2.7 to 5.5%, and while EVAR carries a lower peri-operative mortality rate, it has a 20% re-intervention rate at 5 years (5, 74, 75). The lower peri-operative mortality for endovascular therapies is likely due to decreased blood loss and transfusion requirements (76), reduce perioperative morbidity (77), and shorter initial hospital stay. Long-term complications of EVAR include aneurysm expansion, endoleaks, migration, graft limb thrombosis, and disruption of stent graft integrity (73). There is also a small risk of late rupture, ranging from 0.5% to 1% per year (73, 78, 79). Therefore, patients have to be radiologically monitored frequently and indefinitely after endovascular repair to monitor for these potential complications. The current recommendations for follow-up for patients without evidence of endoleaks suggest screening at 1, 6, and 12 months post-operative and then annual after that (80). The imaging modalities of choice for monitoring of AAAs after endovascular repair consist of computer tomography angiography (CTA). CTA has high accuracy for detecting endoleaks, determining aneurysm growth and stent migration, and it is also quick to perform (81).

The most well known complication of EVAR is an endoleak. The incidence of endoleak ranges from 15% to 25% within 30 days of surgery (73, 82). It is defined as persistent blood flow outside the lumen of the stent graft and within the aneurysm sac, and there are five categories of endoleaks based on the source of blood in-flow (83, 84). Type I endoleaks occurs when a persistent channel of blood flow develops due to inadequate seal at the graft ends, either proximal (1a), distal (1b), or non-occluded iliac artery in patients with aorto-uni-iliac (AUI) stent graft (1c) (73). Early intervention, usually at the time of surgery, is necessary to seal type I endoleaks due to high risk of rupture if it is not fixed. Treatment options include balloon remodeling of the stent and placement of extenders at the proximal or distal ends of the graft. Type II endoleaks are the most commonly encountered endoleaks after EVAR, with an overall incidence of 10.5% (73). It occurs when there is persistent blood flow into the aneurysm sac due to retrograde blood flow from patent lumbar arteries, inferior mesenteric artery, or other collateral vessels. Management of type II endoleaks is controversial and depends on the size of the endoleak. Most institutions favor initial conservative observation and possible intervention if the sac expands or changes on follow-up. Minimally invasive endovascular coil embolization is the treatment for type II endoleaks, either through trans-arterial approach, or direct translumbar puncture (73). Type III endoleaks is related to inadequate seals at the junction points between different graft segments, or rupture of the graft fabric. These endoleaks rapidly repressurize the aneurysm sac, causing rupture, and must be addressed urgently, usually with the placement of an additional cuff or stent at the level of the disruption or complete relining of the stent-graft with a new one. Type IV endoleak is related to the porosity of the fabric of the graft, is self-limited, and is uncommon with contemporary grafts. Type V endoleak is defined as continued growth of the aneurysm sac with no apparent endoleak, and its cause of uncertain (73).

Another complication of EVAR is stent migration, which is defined as greater than 10 mm caudal displacement of the stent (73). It occurs in 1—3% of patients after EVAR, and may be due to inadequate overlap of the aneurysm neck with the device (85), excessive graft oversizing, or progressive enlargement of the aneurysm neck after EVAR (86). Stent migration requires prompt attention to avoid limb occlusion, type I endoleak, and sac rupture (73). Treatment involves placement of extensions cuffs or additional graft limbs. Another complication of endovascular aortic aneurysm repair is stent graft-limb thrombosis, which has been reported in 6.4% of patients in the first 30 days after surgery and 0.5% to 11% in the follow-up period (87, 88). Stent kinking as a result of iliac tortuosity and small diameters of the distal aorta are the most common causes of this complication (73). Other complications of EVAR include stent graft wire fracture, stent graft stenosis, graft kinking, and graft infections. Intense research and development efforts are focusing on the design of new stent grafts to minimize these complications. Since different stent grafts have inherent design advantages and disadvantages, it is important to match these characteristics with patient and AAA anatomy (76).

In addition to stent-related complications, other non-stent-related complications can also occur, including local wound infection, hematoma, and lymphoceles, access artery injury, colonic ischemia, bleeding, and renal dysfunction, which are also known complications of open repair (89-91). Studies have shown that while renal dysfunction is more severe in patients after open repair, this is short-lived and they recover by three months post-operative. Patients who have undergone EVAR on the other hand, had worse renal function in the long term, presumably from serial contrast injections for frequent monitoring of the stent graft postoperatively (90, 91).

Many studies have examined the outcome of open versus endovascular therapy to determine if one approach has better survival than the other (75, 77, 88, 92-94). Studies have shown that while EVAR has significantly lower perioperative mortality when compared to open surgery, their long-term stent complications and need for re-intervention worsen long-term outcome (75, 77, 88, 92, 93). The Dutch Randomized Endovascular Aneurysm Management (DREAM) trial and the United Kingdom Endovascular Aneurysm Repair trial (EVAR 1) compare the two surgical modalities (75, 88, 92, 93). Both trials address AAAs that are larger than 5.5 cm. The EVAR 1 trial showed a 3% lower 30-day mortality in the endovascular repair group, with a persistent reduction in aneurysm-related death at 4 years, but no survival benefit after 4 years. Similarly, the DREAM trial observed an initial advantage in survival but the overall 1-year survival was equivalent in both groups (75, 88, 92, 93).

Several conditions preclude the use of endovascular techniques in repair of AAAs, including occlusive disease of the renal, mesenteric, or iliac arteries (3). Delivery and fixation of the endograft can also be hindered by certain tortuous anatomy. A final factor in the endovascular approach is surgeon technique, though this technique is now a major part of training for all vascular surgeons. Long-term follow-up results are necessary to select the optimal therapeutic management of patient with AAAs. Optimal therapy for patients with AAAs involves comprehensive assessment of patient risk factors, their aortic anatomy, their age, and other important components.

Medical Therapeutic Strategies

Aside from surgical therapy, medical management has been under intense investigation for the prevention of growth and rupture of AAAs. While there is currently no proven focused medical therapy to reduce aneurysm growth, emerging potential medical approaches highlight the importance of inflammation, proteolysis, vascular smooth muscle loss, and antioxidant mechanisms in aortic degeneration (1, 5, 95). Studies have focused on medications that inhibit MMPs, angiotensin II synthesis and receptors, and oxidative stress

(5). Protease inhibitors and antibiotics like tetracyclins, which inhibit MMPs, have been shown to have a protective effect on aneurysm growth (3, 96, 97). Mouse models have shown that doxycycline decreases aortic growth by 33-66%, with increased doxycycline levels corresponding to AAA growth suppression (76). However, while studies have shown that treatment with tetracycline lowers serum levels of MMP-9 and C-reactive protein, and mice models are promising, actual aneurysm size in humans showed little response over a 6-month period (96, 97). Angiotensin II blockers have been shown to reduce the production of cytokines from aortic aneurysm explants (98). Angiotensin converting enzyme inhibitors (ACEI) such as captopril, lisinopril, and enalapril have been shown to bind zinc, an important cofactor for MMP activity (99) and a large epidemiologic study has shown that ACEI reduced risk of AAA rupture, and this effect was observed apart from its blood-pressure lowering effects (100). Also, lipid-lowering agents, such as statins, have anti-inflammatory effects. It has been shown that they lower MMP-3 and MMP-9 concentrations in AAA biopsies in patients (101, 102), and reduce mortality in patients with AAAs who have undergone surgery (103). Statin use has been shown to be associated with almost 50% reduction in AAA growth (104, 105). While preliminary, small studies are promising, large-scale human trials examining anti-inflammatory medications such as cyclooxygenase inhibitors, beta blockers such as propranolol, and various antibiotics have not shown to be effective in limiting AAA growth, altering the rate of intervention, and decreasing mortality (5).

New basic science research has highlighted the importance of c-Jun N-terminal kinase (JNK) in the pathways involved in inflammation causing aortic degeneration and some studies have shown that SP600125, which inhibits JNK causes regression of AAA in the mouse model (106). Finally, smoking cessation should always be a priority to slow AAA progression.

While medical therapy specifically targeting AAA is being developed, focus needs to be placed on secondary prevention since these patients are at an increased risk of cardiovascular events, and perioperative risk needs to be minimized in patients that undergo aneurysm repair. There have been no randomized trials of cardiovascular risk reduction in patients with AAA, and current recommendations are extrapolated from risk reduction trials in patients with other cardiovascular diseases (5). Important modifiable risk factors that need to be addressed include smoking cessation (107), blood pressure control, and lipid control (108). New initiatives will need to be formed, as compliance with current recommendations is grossly insufficient: 25% of AAA patients receive platelet inhibitors, 17% statins, 24% beta-blockers, and 25% ACE inhibitors (1, 109). In addition, medical therapy is also critical around the time of operative intervention of aortic aneurysms, since the main cause of perioperative mortality are cardiac events. In these patients, beta-blockers have been shown to improve perioperative survival by ten fold in high risk patients (110). Statins have also been show to decrease the incidence of myocardial infarction or stroke within 30 days of surgery (111).

Thoracic Aortic Aneurysm

The incidence of thoracic aortic aneurysms (TAA) is also increasing, with improvements in screening and advances in imaging (112). Sixty percent of all TAA involve the aortic root or ascending aorta (or both), 40% involve the descending aorta, 10% involve the arch, and 10% involve the descending thoracic and abdominal aorta (113). TAA are more common in males and typically occur in patients between 50 and 70 years of age (114). Causes of TAA include sporadic degeneration, connective tissue disorders, and syphilitic aneurysm, which are exceeding rare today (37). Hypertension and a bicuspid aortic valve are frequently present, as is a positive family history (115, 116).

The microscopic findings in TAA are drastically different from those that characterize AAA. Elastin content in aneurismal thoracic aorta is significantly lower than normal, and there is a loss of smooth muscles in the diseased aorta (37). TAAs are frequently characterized by cystic medial degeneration and loss of elastic fibers that are replaced by a disorganized matrix lacking cellular structures, reflecting a non-inflammatory process (1, 9, 37). This is in contrary to AAA, which arises from severe intimal atherosclerosis, chronic transmural inflammation, neovascularization, and destructive remodeling of the elastic media (1). Absi *et al.* recently showed in the more than 100 genes whose expression was aberrant in aneurysm versus normal tissue, only four were concordantly different in thoracic and abdominal aortic aneurysms (117). Therefore, although some similarities between the pathogeneses of TAA and AAA exist, there are still substantial differences in these two different disease processes. A well-known cause of thoracic aortic aneurysm is the inheritable Marfan syndrome, which affects 1 in 10,000 people, and consists of a mutation of the gene for fibrillin-1, leading to disorganized elastic fibers and premature cystic medial degeneration (37).

In patients without Marfan syndrome, studies show that the thoracic aorta grows 0.07 to 0.2 cm per year, and risk factors for increased growth rate include increasing age, female gender, presence of chronic obstructive pulmonary disease (COPD), hypertension, family history, initial aortic diameter, and presence of aortic dissection (37). It has been demonstrated that the mean aortic diameter at time of rupture is 6 cm, and the mortality rate of TAA > 6 cm in diameter is 15.6% (118). While the recommendations are to intervene when TAA reach 5.5 cm, other factors such as the rate of expansion may prompt earlier intervention (37). The International Registry of Acute Aortic Dissection (IRAD) consortium demonstrate that aneurysms smaller than 5 cm can rupture, highlighting the importance of optimizing medical adjunct therapy, including blood pressure control, avoidance of strenuous exercise and adequate surveillance (37, 119). In addition, patients with known biscuspid aortic valves with TAA have higher annual expansion rates than those with tricupid aortic valves (120). The presence of aortic stenosis also increases the rate of rupture, dissection, and death in patients with TAA (37).

The definitive therapy for TAA consists solely of surgical repair. In patients with Marfan syndrome, studies show that early elective aortic root replacement is associated with 1.5% early mortality rate, as compared to 11.7% in those who undergoes emergency surgery (121). In these patients, early intervention as well as advances in imaging has improved life expectancy from 42 years to 71 years (37). Surgical intervention for patients with TAA involve adequate preoperative workup that includes coronary angiography and echocardiography to evaluate the need for concomitant cardiac procedures, as well as to assess the aortic valve and aortic root (37). Pulmonary function tests, carotid duplex, and computerized tomography to examine the remaining aorta are also performed to fully prepare the patient for the invasive operative. Operative intervention involves resection of the dilated part of the aortic root, valve, and/or arch and replacing it with a graft, with or without concomitant aortic valve replacement, and re-implantation of coronary arteries. For elective aneurysm repairs, mortality and strokes rates range from 2% to 5%, which is increased to 5% to 7% if the arch needs to be resected, and increase still if the operation is done as an emergency or if dissection is present, with mortality for repair of type A dissection exceeding 20% (37, 122). It has been demonstrated, however, that these numbers are lower for institutions that have high volume and surgical expertise (123).

Endovascular approaches are also increasingly utilized for TAA repair, though this is limited by the involvement of proximal and middle arch branches such as the left common carotid artery and the innominate arteries. However, various bypass procedures can partially solve the problem. Another limiting factor of endovascular repair of TAA involves curvature of the arch, making some aortas not amenable to this mode of therapy. Additionally, proximity of the TAA to the celiac axis can prevent endovascular repair. Long-term data for this mode of therapy continues to be gathered.

Like AAA, medical therapy as the only modality of therapy for TAA has been associated with poor prognosis. Medications that have been studied in thoracic aortic dissections and patients with Marfan syndrome include propranolol and other beta-blockers, ACEI, and angiotensin receptor blockers (ARB), which have all had promising but preliminary results (37). Lifestyle changes are also important in these patients, which include avoidance of strenuous physical activity, especially heavy weight lifting. Ultimately, however, TAA need to be diligently followed, and expansion almost always requires surgical intervention.

Conclusion

Abdominal And Thoracic Aortic Aneurysms Are Increasing, Due To Both Increased Smoking And Other Associated Risk Factors, As Well As Improved Modes Of Detection. Pathophysiology Of The Disease Processes Are Under Intense Investigation, With A Special Focus On Discovering Molecular Markers For More Reliable Methods Of Diagnosis As Well As Prediction Of Patients At Increased Risk Of Rupture. Surgical Intervention Is Being Revolutionized With Introduction And Increased Usage And Proficiency Of The Endovascular Approach. Medical Therapies Are Also Under Investigation To Prevent Progression Of Smaller Aneurysm. Medications Targeted At Reducing Inflammation And Proteolysis Will Most Likely Be Beneficial, Though There Are No Formal Guidelines For Medical Therapy To Date. In Addition To These Efforts, However, Primary Prevention Must Also Be An Important Focus. Smoking Cessation And Control Of Cholesterol And Blood Pressure Could Reduce The Number Of Patients Developing AAA. Therefore, Treatment Of This Common Illness Will Involve A Multi-Faceted Approach And Involve Both Clinicians And Clinician Scientists.

References

[1] Diehm N, Dick F, Schaffner T, Schmidli J, Kalka C, Di Santo S, et al. Novel insight into the pathobiology of abdominal aortic aneurysm and potential future treatment concepts. *Prog Cardiovasc Dis.* 2007;50(3):209-17.

[2] Pleumeekers HJ, Hoes AW, van der Does E, van Urk H, Hofman A, de Jong PT, et al. Aneurysms of the abdominal aorta in older adults. The Rotterdam Study. *Am J Epidemiol.* 1995;142(12):1291-9.

[3] Zankl AR, Schumacher H, Krumsdorf U, Katus HA, Jahn L, Tiefenbacher CP. Pathology, natural history and treatment of abdominal aortic aneurysms. *Clin Res Cardiol.* 2007;96(3):140-51.

[4] Annambhotla S, Bourgeois S, Wang X, Lin PH, Yao Q, Chen C. Recent advances in molecular mechanisms of abdominal aortic aneurysm formation. *World J Surg.* 2008;32(6):976-86.

[5] Golledge J, Muller J, Daugherty A, Norman P. Abdominal aortic aneurysm: pathogenesis and implications for management. *Arterioscler Thromb Vasc Biol.* 2006;26(12):2605-13.

[6] Singh K, BÃ¸naa KH, Jacobsen BK, BjÃ¸rk L, Solberg S. Prevalence of and risk factors for abdominal aortic aneurysms in a population-based study : The TromsÃ¸ Study. *Am J Epidemiol.* 2001;154(3):236-44.

[7] Johnston KW, Rutherford RB, Tilson MD, Shah DM, Hollier L, Stanley JC. Suggested standards for reporting on arterial aneurysms. Subcommittee on Reporting Standards for Arterial Aneurysms, Ad Hoc Committee on Reporting Standards, Society for Vascular Surgery and North American Chapter, International Society for Cardiovascular Surgery. *J Vasc Surg.* 1991;13(3):452-8.

[8] Bengtsson H, Bergqvist D. Ruptured abdominal aortic aneurysm: a population-based study. *J Vasc Surg.* 1993;18(1):74-80.

[9] Rutherford RB. *Vascular surgery. 6th ed.* Philadelphia: Saunders; 2005.

[10] Keeling WB, Armstrong PA, Stone PA, Bandyk DF, Shames ML. An overview of matrix metalloproteinases in the pathogenesis and treatment of abdominal aortic aneurysms. *Vasc Endovascular Surg.* 2005;39(6):457-64.

[11] Kuivaniemi H, Shibamura H, Arthur C, Berguer R, Cole CW, Juvonen T, et al. Familial abdominal aortic aneurysms: collection of 233 multiplex families. *J Vasc Surg.* 2003 Feb;37(2):340-5.

[12] Jamrozik K, Norman PE, Spencer CA, Parsons RW, Tuohy R, Lawrence-Brown MM, et al. Screening for abdominal aortic aneurysm: lessons from a population-based study. *Med J Aust.* 2000;173(7):345-50.

[13] Lederle FA, Johnson GR, Wilson SE, Chute EP, Littooy FN, Bandyk D, et al. Prevalence and associations of abdominal aortic aneurysm detected through screening. Aneurysm Detection and Management (ADAM) Veterans Affairs Cooperative Study Group. *Ann Intern Med.* 1997;126(6):441-9.

[14] Albornoz G, Coady MA, Roberts M, Davies RR, Tranquilli M, Rizzo JA, et al. Familial thoracic aortic aneurysms and dissections--incidence, modes of inheritance, and phenotypic patterns. *Ann Thorac Surg.* 2006 Oct;82(4):1400-5.

[15] Brady AR, Thompson SG, Fowkes FGR, Greenhalgh RM, Powell JT, Participants UKSAT. Abdominal aortic aneurysm expansion: risk factors and time intervals for surveillance. *Circulation*. 2004;110(1):16-21.
[16] Wilmink TB, Quick CR, Day NE. The association between cigarette smoking and abdominal aortic aneurysms. *J Vasc Surg*. 1999;30(6):1099-105.
[17] Shibamura H, Olson JM, van Vlijmen-Van Keulen C, Buxbaum SG, Dudek DM, Tromp G, et al. Genome scan for familial abdominal aortic aneurysm using sex and family history as covariates suggests genetic heterogeneity and identifies linkage to chromosome 19q13. *Circulation*. 2004;109(17):2103-8.
[18] Monux G, Serrano FJ, Vigil P, De la Concha EG. Role of HLA-DR in the pathogenesis of abdominal aortic aneurysm. *Eur J Vasc Endovasc Surg*. 2003;26(2):211-4.
[19] Ogata T, Gregoire L, Goddard KAB, Skunca M, Tromp G, Lancaster WD, et al. Evidence for association between the HLA-DQA locus and abdominal aortic aneurysms in the Belgian population: a case control study. *BMC Med Genet*. 2006;7:67.
[20] Brown LC, Powell JT. Risk factors for aneurysm rupture in patients kept under ultrasound surveillance. UK Small Aneurysm Trial Participants. *Ann Surg*. 1999;230(3):289-96; discussion 96-7.
[21] Lederle FA, Johnson GR, Wilson SE, Ballard DJ, Jordan WD, Blebea J, et al. Rupture rate of large abdominal aortic aneurysms in patients refusing or unfit for elective repair. *JAMA*. 2002;287(22):2968-72.
[22] Lindholt JS, Heegaard NH, Vammen S, Fasting H, Henneberg EW, Heickendorff L. Smoking, but not lipids, lipoprotein(a) and antibodies against oxidised LDL, is correlated to the expansion of abdominal aortic aneurysms. *Eur J Vasc Endovasc Surg*. 2001;21(1):51-6.
[23] Dobrin PB, Baker WH, Gley WC. Elastolytic and collagenolytic studies of arteries. Implications for the mechanical properties of aneurysms. *Arch Surg*. 1984;119(4):405-9.
[24] Dobrin PB, Mrkvicka R. Failure of elastin or collagen as possible critical connective tissue alterations underlying aneurysmal dilatation. *Cardiovasc Surg*. 1994;2(4):484-8.
[25] Cohen JR, Mandell C, Chang JB, Wise L. Elastin metabolism of the infrarenal aorta. *J Vasc Surg*. 1988;7(2):210-4.
[26] Abdul-Hussien H, Soekhoe RGV, Weber E, von der ThÃ¼sen JH, Kleemann R, Mulder A, et al. Collagen degradation in the abdominal aneurysm: a conspiracy of matrix metalloproteinase and cysteine collagenases. *Am J Pathol*. 2007;170(3):809-17.
[27] Birkedal-Hansen H, Moore WG, Bodden MK, Windsor LJ, Birkedal-Hansen B, DeCarlo A, et al. Matrix metalloproteinases: a review. *Crit Rev Oral Biol Med*. 1993;4(2):197-250.
[28] McMillan WD, Tamarina NA, Cipollone M, Johnson DA, Parker MA, Pearce WH. Size matters: the relationship between MMP-9 expression and aortic diameter. *Circulation*. 1997;96(7):2228-32.
[29] Sakalihasan N, Delvenne P, Nusgens BV, Limet R, LapiÃ¨re CM. Activated forms of MMP2 and MMP9 in abdominal aortic aneurysms. *J Vasc Surg*. 1996;24(1):127-33.

[30] Thompson RW, Parks WC. *Role of matrix metalloproteinases in abdominal aortic aneurysms.* Ann N Y Acad Sci. 1996;800:157-74.

[31] Davis V, Persidskaia R, Baca-Regen L, Itoh Y, Nagase H, Persidsky Y, et al. Matrix metalloproteinase-2 production and its binding to the matrix are increased in abdominal aortic aneurysms. *Arterioscler Thromb Vasc Biol.* 1998;18(10):1625-33.

[32] McMillan WD, Patterson BK, Keen RR, Shively VP, Cipollone M, Pearce WH. In situ localization and quantification of mRNA for 92-kD type IV collagenase and its inhibitor in aneurysmal, occlusive, and normal aorta. *Arterioscler Thromb Vasc Biol.* 1995;15(8):1139-44.

[33] Petersen E, WÃ¥gberg F, Angquist KA. Proteolysis of the abdominal aortic aneurysm wall and the association with rupture. *Eur J Vasc Endovasc Surg.* 2002;23(2):153-7.

[34] Goodall S, Crowther M, Hemingway DM, Bell PR, Thompson MM. Ubiquitous elevation of matrix metalloproteinase-2 expression in the vasculature of patients with abdominal aneurysms. *Circulation.* 2001;104(3):304-9.

[35] Freestone T, Turner RJ, Coady A, Higman DJ, Greenhalgh RM, Powell JT. Inflammation and matrix metalloproteinases in the enlarging abdominal aortic aneurysm. *Arterioscler Thromb Vasc Biol.* 1995;15(8):1145-51.

[36] Wilson WRW, Anderton M, Schwalbe EC, Jones JL, Furness PN, Bell PRF, et al. Matrix metalloproteinase-8 and -9 are increased at the site of abdominal aortic aneurysm rupture. *Circulation.* 2006;113(3):438-45.

[37] Patel MI, Melrose J, Ghosh P, Appleberg M. Increased synthesis of matrix metalloproteinases by aortic smooth muscle cells is implicated in the etiopathogenesis of abdominal aortic aneurysms. *J Vasc Surg.* 1996;24(1):82-92.

[38] Hovsepian DM, Ziporin SJ, Sakurai MK, Lee JK, Curci JA, Thompson RW. Elevated plasma levels of matrix metalloproteinase-9 in patients with abdominal aortic aneurysms: a circulating marker of degenerative aneurysm disease. *J Vasc Interv Radiol.* 2000;11(10):1345-52.

[39] McMillan WD, Pearce WH. Increased plasma levels of metalloproteinase-9 are associated with abdominal aortic aneurysms. *J Vasc Surg.* 1999;29(1):122-7; discussion 7-9.

[40] Pyo R, Lee JK, Shipley JM, Curci JA, Mao D, Ziporin SJ, et al. Targeted gene disruption of matrix metalloproteinase-9 (gelatinase B) suppresses development of experimental abdominal aortic aneurysms. *J Clin Invest.* 2000;105(11):1641-9.

[41] Lorelli DR, Jean-Claude JM, Fox CJ, Clyne J, Cambria RA, Seabrook GR, et al. Response of plasma matrix metalloproteinase-9 to conventional abdominal aortic aneurysm repair or endovascular exclusion: implications for endoleak. *J Vasc Surg.* 2002;35(5):916-22.

[42] Sangiorgi G, D'Averio R, Mauriello A, Bondio M, Pontillo M, Castelvecchio S, et al. Plasma levels of metalloproteinases-3 and -9 as markers of successful abdominal aortic aneurysm exclusion after endovascular graft treatment. *Circulation.* 2001;104(12 Suppl 1):I288-95.

[43] Knox JB, Sukhova GK, Whittemore AD, Libby P. Evidence for altered balance between matrix metalloproteinases and their inhibitors in human aortic diseases. *Circulation.* 1997;95(1):205-12.

[44] Eskandari MK, Vijungco JD, Flores A, Borensztajn J, Shively V, Pearce WH. Enhanced abdominal aortic aneurysm in TIMP-1-deficient mice. *J Surg Res.* 2005;123(2):289-93.

[45] Nishimura K, Ikebuchi M, Kanaoka Y, Ohgi S, Ueta E, Nanba E, et al. Relationships between matrix metalloproteinases and tissue inhibitor of metalloproteinases in the wall of abdominal aortic aneurysms. *Int Angiol.* 2003;22(3):229-38.

[46] Choke E, Thompson MM, Dawson J, Wilson WRW, Sayed S, Loftus IM, et al. Abdominal aortic aneurysm rupture is associated with increased medial neovascularization and overexpression of proangiogenic cytokines. *Arterioscler Thromb Vasc Biol.* 2006;26(9):2077-82.

[47] Herron GS, Unemori E, Wong M, Rapp JH, Hibbs MH, Stoney RJ. Connective tissue proteinases and inhibitors in abdominal aortic aneurysms. Involvement of the vasa vasorum in the pathogenesis of aortic aneurysms. *Arterioscler Thromb.* 1991;11(6):1667-77.

[48] Paik DC, Fu C, Bhattacharya J, Tilson MD. Ongoing angiogenesis in blood vessels of the abdominal aortic aneurysm. *Exp Mol Med.* 2004;36(6):524-33.

[49] Rundhaug JE. Matrix metalloproteinases and angiogenesis. *J Cell Mol Med.* 2005;9(2):267-85.

[50] Vorp DA, Lee PC, Wang DH, Makaroun MS, Nemoto EM, Ogawa S, et al. Association of intraluminal thrombus in abdominal aortic aneurysm with local hypoxia and wall weakening. *J Vasc Surg.* 2001;34(2):291-9.

[51] Holmes DR, Liao S, Parks WC, Thompson RW. Medial neovascularization in abdominal aortic aneurysms: a histopathologic marker of aneurysmal degeneration with pathophysiologic implications. *J Vasc Surg.* 1995;21(5):761-71; discussion 71-2.

[52] Curci JA, Liao S, Huffman MD, Shapiro SD, Thompson RW. Expression and localization of macrophage elastase (matrix metalloproteinase-12) in abdominal aortic aneurysms. *J Clin Invest.* 1998;102(11):1900-10.

[53] Jones KG, Brull DJ, Brown LC, Sian M, Greenhalgh RM, Humphries SE, et al. Interleukin-6 (IL-6) and the prognosis of abdominal aortic aneurysms. *Circulation.* 2001;103(18):2260-5.

[54] Norman P, Spencer CA, Lawrence-Brown MM, Jamrozik K. C-reactive protein levels and the expansion of screen-detected abdominal aortic aneurysms in men. *Circulation.* 2004;110(7):862-6.

[55] Rohde LE, Arroyo LH, Rifai N, Creager MA, Libby P, Ridker PM, et al. Plasma concentrations of interleukin-6 and abdominal aortic diameter among subjects without aortic dilatation. *Arterioscler Thromb Vasc Biol.* 1999;19(7):1695-9.

[56] Vainas T, Lubbers T, Stassen FRM, Herngreen SB, van Dieijen-Visser MP, Bruggeman CA, et al. Serum C-reactive protein level is associated with abdominal aortic aneurysm size and may be produced by aneurysmal tissue. *Circulation.* 2003;107(8):1103-5.

[57] Pearce WH, Sweis I, Yao JS, McCarthy WJ, Koch AE. Interleukin-1 beta and tumor necrosis factor-alpha release in normal and diseased human infrarenal aortas. *J Vasc Surg.* 1992;16(5):784-9.

[58] Juvonen J, Surcel HM, Satta J, Teppo AM, Bloigu A, SyrjÃ¤lÃ¤ H, et al. Elevated circulating levels of inflammatory cytokines in patients with abdominal aortic aneurysm. *Arterioscler Thromb Vasc Biol.* 1997;17(11):2843-7.

[59] Van den Steen PE, Proost P, Wuyts A, Van Damme J, Opdenakker G. Neutrophil gelatinase B potentiates interleukin-8 tenfold by aminoterminal processing, whereas it degrades CTAP-III, PF-4, and GRO-alpha and leaves RANTES and MCP-2 intact. *Blood.* 2000;96(8):2673-81.

[60] Tham DM, Martin-McNulty B, Wang Y-x, Wilson DW, Vergona R, Sullivan ME, et al. Angiotensin II is associated with activation of NF-kappaB-mediated genes and downregulation of PPARs. *Physiol Genomics.* 2002;11(1):21-30.

[61] Daugherty A, Manning MW, Cassis LA. Angiotensin II promotes atherosclerotic lesions and aneurysms in apolipoprotein E-deficient mice. *J Clin Invest.* 2000;105(11):1605-12.

[62] Henderson EL, Geng YJ, Sukhova GK, Whittemore AD, Knox J, Libby P. Death of smooth muscle cells and expression of mediators of apoptosis by T lymphocytes in human abdominal aortic aneurysms. *Circulation.* 1999;99(1):96-104.

[63] Rowe VL, Stevens SL, Reddick TT, Freeman MB, Donnell R, Carroll RC, et al. Vascular smooth muscle cell apoptosis in aneurysmal, occlusive, and normal human aortas. *J Vasc Surg.* 2000;31(3):567-76.

[64] Liao S, Curci JA, Kelley BJ, Sicard GA, Thompson RW. Accelerated replicative senescence of medial smooth muscle cells derived from abdominal aortic aneurysms compared to the adjacent inferior mesenteric artery. *J Surg Res.* 2000;92(1):85-95.

[65] Lindholt JS, Vammen S, Juul S, Henneberg EW, Fasting H. The validity of ultrasonographic scanning as screening method for abdominal aortic aneurysm. *Eur J Vasc Endovasc Surg.* 1999;17(6):472-5.

[66] Ashton HA, Buxton MJ, Day NE, Kim LG, Marteau TM, Scott RAP, et al. The Multicentre Aneurysm Screening Study (MASS) into the effect of abdominal aortic aneurysm screening on mortality in men: a randomised controlled trial. *Lancet.* 2002;360(9345):1531-9.

[67] Urbonavicius S, Urbonaviciene G, HonorÃ© B, Henneberg EW, Vorum H, Lindholt JS. Potential circulating biomarkers for abdominal aortic aneurysm expansion and rupture--a systematic review. *Eur J Vasc Endovasc Surg.* 2008;36(3):273-80; discussion 81-2.

[68] Ashton HA, Buxton MJ, Day NE, Kim LG, Marteau TM, Scott RA, et al. The Multicentre Aneurysm Screening Study (MASS) into the effect of abdominal aortic aneurysm screening on mortality in men: a randomised controlled trial. *Lancet.* 2002 Nov 16;360(9345):1531-9.

[69] Mortality results for randomised controlled trial of early elective surgery or ultrasonographic surveillance for small abdominal aortic aneurysms. The UK Small Aneurysm Trial Participants. *Lancet.* 1998;352(9141):1649-55.

[70] Long-term outcomes of immediate repair compared with surveillance of small abdominal aortic aneurysms. *N Engl J Med.* 2002 May 9;346(19):1445-52.

[71] Lederle FA, Wilson SE, Johnson GR, Reinke DB, Littooy FN, Acher CW, et al. Immediate repair compared with surveillance of small abdominal aortic aneurysms. *N Engl J Med.* 2002;346(19):1437-44.

[72] Parodi JC, Palmaz JC, Barone HD. Transfemoral intraluminal graft implantation for abdominal aortic aneurysms. *Ann Vasc Surg.* 1991 Nov;5(6):491-9.

[73] Liaw JV, Clark M, Gibbs R, Jenkins M, Cheshire N, Hamady M. Update: Complications and management of infrarenal EVAR. *Eur J Radiol.* 2008 Jul 8.

[74] Endovascular aneurysm repair and outcome in patients unfit for open repair of abdominal aortic aneurysm (EVAR trial 2): randomised controlled trial. *Lancet.* 2005 Jun 25-Jul 1;365(9478):2187-92.

[75] Endovascular aneurysm repair versus open repair in patients with abdominal aortic aneurysm (EVAR trial 1): randomised controlled trial. *Lancet.* 2005 Jun 25-Jul 1;365(9478):2179-86.

[76] Tan JW, Yeo KK, Laird JR. Food and Drug Administration-approved endovascular repair devices for abdominal aortic aneurysms: a review. *J Vasc Interv Radiol.* 2008 Jun;19(6 Suppl):S9-S17.

[77] Sajid MS, Desai M, Haider Z, Baker DM, Hamilton G. Endovascular aortic aneurysm repair (EVAR) has significantly lower perioperative mortality in comparison to open repair: a systematic review. *Asian J Surg.* 2008 Jul;31(3):119-23.

[78] Bernhard VM, Mitchell RS, Matsumura JS, Brewster DC, Decker M, Lamparello P, et al. Ruptured abdominal aortic aneurysm after endovascular repair. *J Vasc Surg.* 2002 Jun;35(6):1155-62.

[79] Zarins CK, Heikkinen MA, Lee ES, Alsac JM, Arko FR. Short- and long-term outcome following endovascular aneurysm repair. How does it compare to open surgery? *J Cardiovasc Surg* (Torino). 2004 Aug;45(4):321-33.

[80] Eskandari MK, Yao JS, Pearce WH, Rutherford RB, Veith FJ, Harris P, et al. Surveillance after endoluminal repair of abdominal aortic aneurysms. *Cardiovasc Surg.* 2001 Oct;9(5):469-71.

[81] Stavropoulos SW, Clark TW, Carpenter JP, Fairman RM, Litt H, Velazquez OC, et al. Use of CT angiography to classify endoleaks after endovascular repair of abdominal aortic aneurysms. *J Vasc Interv Radiol.* 2005 May;16(5):663-7.

[82] Thomas SM, Beard JD, Ireland M, Ayers S. Results from the prospective registry of endovascular treatment of abdominal aortic aneurysms (RETA): mid term results to five years. *Eur J Vasc Endovasc Surg.* 2005 Jun;29(6):563-70.

[83] Veith FJ, Baum RA, Ohki T, Amor M, Adiseshiah M, Blankensteijn JD, et al. Nature and significance of endoleaks and endotension: summary of opinions expressed at an international conference. *J Vasc Surg.* 2002 May;35(5):1029-35.

[84] White GH, May J, Waugh RC, Chaufour X, Yu W. Type III and type IV endoleak: toward a complete definition of blood flow in the sac after endoluminal AAA repair. *J Endovasc Surg.* 1998 Nov;5(4):305-9.

[85] Napoli V, Sardella SG, Bargellini I, Petruzzi P, Cioni R, Vignali C, et al. Evaluation of the proximal aortic neck enlargement following endovascular repair of abdominal aortic aneurysm: 3-years experience. *Eur Radiol.* 2003 Aug;13(8):1962-71.

[86] Sampaio SM, Panneton JM, Mozes G, Andrews JC, Noel AA, Kalra M, et al. AneuRx device migration: incidence, risk factors, and consequences. *Ann Vasc Surg.* 2005 Mar;19(2):178-85.

[87] Arko FR, Hill BB, Olcott C, Harris EJ, Jr., Fogarty TJ, Zarins CK. Endovascular repair reduces early and late morbidity compared to open surgery for abdominal aortic aneurysm. *J Endovasc Ther.* 2002 Dec;9(6):711-8.

[88] Prinssen M, Verhoeven ELG, Buth J, Cuypers PWM, van Sambeek MRHM, Balm R, et al. A randomized trial comparing conventional and endovascular repair of abdominal aortic aneurysms. *N Engl J Med.* 2004;351(16):1607-18.

[89] Becquemin JP, Majewski M, Fermani N, Marzelle J, Desgrandes P, Allaire E, et al. Colon ischemia following abdominal aortic aneurysm repair in the era of endovascular abdominal aortic repair. *J Vasc Surg.* 2008 Feb;47(2):258-63; discussion 63.

[90] Mills JL, Sr., Duong ST, Leon LR, Jr., Goshima KR, Ihnat DM, Wendel CS, et al. Comparison of the effects of open and endovascular aortic aneurysm repair on long-term renal function using chronic kidney disease staging based on glomerular filtration rate. *J Vasc Surg.* 2008 Jun;47(6):1141-9.

[91] Parmer SS, Fairman RM, Karmacharya J, Carpenter JP, Velazquez OC, Woo EY. A comparison of renal function between open and endovascular aneurysm repair in patients with baseline chronic renal insufficiency. *J Vasc Surg.* 2006 Oct;44(4):706-11.

[92] Blankensteijn JD, de Jong SECA, Prinssen M, van der Ham AC, Buth J, van Sterkenburg SMM, et al. Two-year outcomes after conventional or endovascular repair of abdominal aortic aneurysms. *N Engl J Med.* 2005;352(23):2398-405.

[93] Greenhalgh RM, Brown LC, Kwong GPS, Powell JT, Thompson SG, participants Et. Comparison of endovascular aneurysm repair with open repair in patients with abdominal aortic aneurysm (EVAR trial 1), 30-day operative mortality results: randomised controlled trial. *Lancet.* 2004;364(9437):843-8.

[94] De Rango P, Cao P, Parlani G, Verzini F, Brambilla D. Outcome after endografting in small and large abdominal aortic aneurysms: a metanalysis. *Eur J Vasc Endovasc Surg.* 2008 Feb;35(2):162-72.

[95] Golledge J, Powell JT. Medical management of abdominal aortic aneurysm. *Eur J Vasc Endovasc Surg.* 2007 Sep;34(3):267-73.

[96] Baxter BT, Pearce WH, Waltke EA, Littooy FN, Hallett JW, Kent KC, et al. Prolonged administration of doxycycline in patients with small asymptomatic abdominal aortic aneurysms: report of a prospective (Phase II) multicenter study. *J Vasc Surg.* 2002;36(1):1-12.

[97] Mosorin M, Juvonen J, Biancari F, Satta J, Surcel HM, Leinonen M, et al. Use of doxycycline to decrease the growth rate of abdominal aortic aneurysms: a randomized, double-blind, placebo-controlled pilot study. *J Vasc Surg.* 2001;34(4):606-10.

[98] CS, McCann M, Karan M, Norman P, Ketheesan N, Golledge J. Association of osteoprotegerin with human abdominal aortic aneurysm progression. *Circulation.* 2005;111(23):3119-25.

[99] da Cunha V, Tham DM, Martin-McNulty B, Deng G, Ho JJ, Wilson DW, et al. Enalapril attenuates angiotensin II-induced atherosclerosis and vascular inflammation. *Atherosclerosis.* 2005;178(1):9-17.

[100] Hackam DG, Thiruchelvam D, Redelmeier DA. Angiotensin-converting enzyme inhibitors and aortic rupture: a population-based case-control study. *Lancet.* 2006;368(9536):659-65.

[101] Evans J, Powell JT, Schwalbe E, Loftus IM, Thompson MM. Simvastatin attenuates the activity of matrix metalloprotease-9 in aneurysmal aortic tissue. *Eur J Vasc Endovasc Surg.* 2007 Sep;34(3):302-3.

[102] Wilson WRW, Evans J, Bell PRF, Thompson MM. HMG-CoA reductase inhibitors (statins) decrease MMP-3 and MMP-9 concentrations in abdominal aortic aneurysms. *Eur J Vasc Endovasc Surg.* 2005;30(3):259-62.

[103] Kertai MD, Boersma E, Westerhout CM, van Domburg R, Klein J, Bax JJ, et al. Association between long-term statin use and mortality after successful abdominal aortic aneurysm surgery. *Am J Med.* 2004;116(2):96-103.

[104] Schouten O, van Laanen JH, Boersma E, Vidakovic R, Feringa HH, Dunkelgrun M, et al. Statins are associated with a reduced infrarenal abdominal aortic aneurysm growth. *Eur J Vasc Endovasc Surg.* 2006 Jul;32(1):21-6.

[105] Sukhija R, Aronow WS, Sandhu R, Kakar P, Babu S. Mortality and size of abdominal aortic aneurysm at long-term follow-up of patients not treated surgically and treated with and without statins. *Am J Cardiol.* 2006 Jan 15;97(2):279-80.

[106] Yoshimura K, Aoki H, Ikeda Y, Fujii K, Akiyama N, Furutani A, et al. Regression of abdominal aortic aneurysm by inhibition of c-Jun N-terminal kinase. *Nat Med.* 2005;11(12):1330-8.

[107] Cornuz J, Sidoti Pinto C, Tevaearai H, Egger M. Risk factors for asymptomatic abdominal aortic aneurysm: systematic review and meta-analysis of population-based screening studies. *Eur J Public Health.* 2004 Dec;14(4):343-9.

[108] Leurs LJ, Visser P, Laheij RJ, Buth J, Harris PL, Blankensteijn JD. Statin use is associated with reduced all-cause mortality after endovascular abdominal aortic aneurysm repair. *Vascular.* 2006 Jan-Feb;14(1):1-8.

[109] Bhatt DL, Steg PG, Ohman EM, Hirsch AT, Ikeda Y, Mas JL, et al. International prevalence, recognition, and treatment of cardiovascular risk factors in outpatients with atherothrombosis. *JAMA.* 2006 Jan 11;295(2):180-9.

[110] Poldermans D, Boersma E, Bax JJ, Thomson IR, van de Ven LL, Blankensteijn JD, et al. The effect of bisoprolol on perioperative mortality and myocardial infarction in high-risk patients undergoing vascular surgery. Dutch Echocardiographic Cardiac Risk Evaluation Applying Stress Echocardiography Study Group. *N Engl J Med.* 1999 Dec 9;341(24):1789-94.

[111] Kapoor AS, Kanji H, Buckingham J, Devereaux PJ, McAlister FA. Strength of evidence for perioperative use of statins to reduce cardiovascular risk: systematic review of controlled studies. *BMJ.* 2006 Dec 2;333(7579):1149.

[112] Gillum RF. Epidemiology of aortic aneurysm in the United States. *J Clin Epidemiol.* 1995 Nov;48(11):1289-98.

[113] Isselbacher EM. Thoracic and abdominal aortic aneurysms. *Circulation.* 2005 Feb 15;111(6):816-28.

[114] Cohn LH, Edmunds LH. *Cardiac surgery in the adult.* 3rd ed. New York: McGraw-Hill Medical; 2008.

[115] Coady MA, Davies RR, Roberts M, Goldstein LJ, Rogalski MJ, Rizzo JA, et al. Familial patterns of thoracic aortic aneurysms. *Arch Surg*. 1999 Apr;134(4):361-7.

[116] Nkomo VT, Enriquez-Sarano M, Ammash NM, Melton LJ, 3rd, Bailey KR, Desjardins V, et al. Bicuspid aortic valve associated with aortic dilatation: a community-based study. *Arterioscler Thromb Vasc Biol*. 2003 Feb 1;23(2):351-6.

[117] Absi TS, Sundt TM, Tung WS, Moon M, Lee JK, Damiano RR, et al. Altered patterns of gene expression distinguishing ascending aortic aneurysms from abdominal aortic aneurysms: complementary DNA expression profiling in the molecular characterization of aortic disease. *J Thorac Cardiovasc Surg*. 2003;126(2):344-57; discission 57.

[118] Davies RR, Goldstein LJ, Coady MA, Tittle SL, Rizzo JA, Kopf GS, et al. Yearly rupture or dissection rates for thoracic aortic aneurysms: simple prediction based on size. *Ann Thorac Surg*. 2002 Jan;73(1):17-27; discussion -8.

[119] Pape LA, Tsai TT, Isselbacher EM, Oh JK, O'Gara P T, Evangelista A, et al. Aortic diameter >or = 5.5 cm is not a good predictor of type A aortic dissection: observations from the International Registry of Acute Aortic Dissection (IRAD). *Circulation*. 2007 Sep 4;116(10):1120-7.

[120] Davies RR, Kaple RK, Mandapati D, Gallo A, Botta DM, Jr., Elefteriades JA, et al. Natural history of ascending aortic aneurysms in the setting of an unreplaced bicuspid aortic valve. *Ann Thorac Surg*. 2007 Apr;83(4):1338-44.

[121] Gott VL, Greene PS, Alejo DE, Cameron DE, Naftel DC, Miller DC, et al. Replacement of the aortic root in patients with Marfan's syndrome. *N Engl J Med*. 1999 Apr 29;340(17):1307-13.

[122] Mehta RH, Suzuki T, Hagan PG, Bossone E, Gilon D, Llovet A, et al. Predicting death in patients with acute type a aortic dissection. *Circulation*. 2002 Jan 15;105(2):200-6.

[123] Knipp BS, Deeb GM, Prager RL, Williams CY, Upchurch GR, Jr., Patel HJ. A contemporary analysis of outcomes for operative repair of type A aortic dissection in the United States. *Surgery*. 2007 Oct;142(4):524-8; discussion 8 e1.

In: Aneurysms: Types, Risks, Formation and Treatment
Editors: Alain Laurent and Ethan Morel
ISBN: 978-1-60741-557-2
© 2009 Nova Science Publishers, Inc.

Chapter 5

Endovascular Repair of Abdominal Aortic Aneurysm: Biomechanical Challenges and Potential Answers

Florian Dick[1,3], Juerg Schmidli[1], Dai-Do Do[2], Thierry Carrel[1], Iris Baumgartner[2]* and Nicolas Diehm[2]

Swiss Cardiovascular Center

[1]Departments of Vascular Surgery, and

[2] Clinical and Interventional Angiology, Inselspital, University Hospital Bern, Switzerland

[3]Imperial College Vascular Surgery Research Group, Division of Surgery, Oncology, Reproductive Biology and Anaesthetics, Charing Cross Hospital, London, UK

Abstract

Endovascular repair is increasingly popular as a minimally invasive treatment option for patients with abdominal aortic aneurysms. Long-term durability and cost-effectiveness of this technology, however, are still in doubt. Essentially, the mechanical reliability of the exclusion of the aneurysm sac from blood flow and pressure depends on anatomical fit between endograft and aortic-iliac attachment zones and may be challenged over time by continuing aneurysmal degeneration. Failure of endograft seal is associated with the occurrence of endoleaks and graft migration, the need for repeated interventions and a small but continuing risk of re-pressurization of the aneurysm sac potentially leading to aortic rupture.

In this chapter we review the mechanical and biological challenges which are currently associated with endovascular abdominal aortic aneurysm repair. We discuss promising new approaches and their potential limitations. Clearly, multidisciplinary efforts will be indispensable to facilitate an integrated form of endovascular management

*Corresponding author: Prof. Dr. med. Iris Baumgartner, University Hospital Bern Inselspital, Freiburgstrasse, 3010 Bern, Switzerland, Fax Number (..41-31) 632 4397, Telephone Number (..41-31) 632 4237, iris.baumgartner@insel.ch

including improved patient selection, dedicated stent graft design, pharmacological stabilization of the attachment zones and modulation of the biological background of the disease. Based on current evidence such a strategy has the best prospect of improving long-term durability and cost-effectiveness of endovascular repair and hopefully will eventually translate into optimized safety and quality of life for patients with the disease. Maybe even more importantly, such efforts have the potential to pave future ways for dedicated proteomic and genomic interventions to prevent the genesis of the disease at all in the large population of patients at risk.

Introduction

Abdominal aortic aneurysm is a potentially fatal condition as aneurysms have a propensity to rupture with increasing diameter [1]. It was estimated that only half of all patients with ruptured aortic aneurysm reach the hospital alive [2], and those who reach the operating theatre still incur an excessive operative mortality rate [3]. Currently there is no known method to prevent aneurysm from occurring. Therefore, present-day management aims at timely elective repair which - in conjunction with population-based aneurysm screening - is thought to have the potential to prevent at least ruptures of abdominal aortic aneurysm from occurring [4].

Open aneurysm repair was the established treatment for decades, but has been challenged since the introduction of endovascular aneurysm repair (EVAR) in the early 1990ies [5]. Current evidence is persuasive that both methods have eventually become equivalent alternatives, each with distinct assets and drawbacks [6]. A hallmark of both approaches, however, is that they address a dynamic biologic process, i.e. progressive aortic expansion and increasing risk of rupture, by static mechanical means [7, 8]. The list of similar instances where pathologic *phenomena* are being tackled mechanically before actual treatment *of the disease* becomes available is long and includes indications for cardiac, orthopedic and vascular surgery, endovascular medicine, and dentistry.

The unidimensional approach to aortic aneurysm, however, might just be changing. An increasing understanding of the biologic background has recently led to the recognition of crucial pathologic pathways of aneurysmal degeneration and to the definition of potential drug targets [9-11]. The main mechanisms which are thought to control aneurysm expansion include proteolytic destruction of extracellular matrix, atrophy of smooth-muscle cells, and inflammation [12]; and various promising pharmacological approaches are being scrutinized to interfere with them [9, 11, 13, 14]. Thus, although no preventive treatment of aortic aneurysms has emerged thus far, we might be on the verge of an up-coming era of molecular aneurysm management.

The increasing awareness of the physiopathology may also have practical consequences on current management. A major difference between open and endovascular repair lies in the mode of graft fixation. Whereas in open repair the prosthetic graft can be sewed directly and stably onto the aortic wall, the fixation of the endovascular stent-graft depends essentially on a tight anatomical fit between graft and predefined aorta-iliac attachment zones [15]. Flawed anatomical appraisal at the beginning and continued aneurysmal degeneration of these zones may critically compromise sustained tightness of endovascular fit over time. Thus, endovascular repair is exposed to unique biomechanical challenges to which answers must be sought if durability and cost-effectiveness of this fascinating technology are to be improved [6]. Potential strategies include efforts towards superior patient selection using new developments of dedicated 3-dimensional imaging [15] and pharmacological stabilisation of attachment zones which might be a first practical application of the emerging molecular understanding of the disease [7].

Aim of this chapter is to highlight the biomechanical challenges of endovascular repair in depth and to review emerging concepts to answer them critically. The historical background and the current evidence for abdominal aortic aneurysm repair are given as a basis first to put clinical importance and characteristic limitations of endovascular repair into perspective.

Historical Aspects

The phenomenon of an undue arterial widening – i.e., an aneurysm – has been literally known for thousands of years and was probably first described in the Ebers papyrus 4000 years ago. Associated risks were soon recognised and, as early as 200 A.D., Antyllus observed rightly [16]: *'To decline treatment of any aneurysms is foolish, but it is also dangerous to operate on all of them.'*. This axiom still holds true although our treatment options of course are not comparable to those at that time. Modern management of aneurysm developed along intermediate steps including compressive therapy, induction of thrombotic occlusion, external wrapping or aneurysmorraphy and total extirpation with extraanatomical reconstruction. However, it was not until the early 1950-ies that operative logistics had matured enough to facilitate successful open aortic aneurysm repair by autologous inlay vein graft [17] or by homograft [16, 18]. The introduction of biocompatible synthetic fabrics such as Dacron and the production of commercially available Y-shaped prosthetic grafts established the gold standard of open aneurysm repair for many decades. Open repair can be performed with a high degree of patient safety and operative mortality rates range well below 1% in dedicated centres [3]; however, even today severity of the operative trauma must not be underestimated and average operative mortality rates may be as high as 5% [19, 20].

Around 1990 a conceptual shift occurred when endovascular aortic repair was introduced. The idea was based on experimental studies performed by Alexis Carrel who had used endovascular grafts in canine experiments already in 1912 [21]. The concept of minimally invasive access and endoluminal treatment of arterial lesions soon revolutionized management of occlusive and aneuriysmal aortic disease [22-24]. In humans, endovascular aneurysm repair was first performed by Volodos in 1986 [25] and it was first published in English by Parodi in 1991 [5].

The primary endovascular devices consisted of aorto-aortic tube grafts and were attached to a large Palmaz stent for endovascular fixation at both ends. This tube graft design, however, was only applicable to a particular aneurysm morphology; therefore tapered aorto-mono-iliac or –femoral grafts were soon developed to widen the applicability of endovascular aortic repair [26]. The unilateral approach, however, required inevitably an iatrogenic occlusion of the ipsilateral hypogastric artery and the contralateral common iliac artery, and mandated the construction of a femoro-femoral crossover bypass to revascularize the contralateral limb. Thus, most of these early, surgeon-made solutions disappeared with the advent of commercially available modular, bifurcated and fully stented endografts, because they overcame most of the initial limitations [26]. Since then, a wide array of dedicated graft designs has been developed including balloon- and self-expandable stent grafts which may partly support proximal fixation with the use of hooks or barbs and some of them are suitable for suprarenal fixation. Moreover, fenestrated and branched graft designs are being utilized increasingly for complex aneurysm morphologies [27].

Evidence for Aneurysm Repair and Screening

The evidence basis for aneurysm repair was established before endovascular repair became widely available. The UK Small Aneurysm Trial (UK SAT) [28] was the first randomised trial to challenge the empirical approach to aortic aneurysm repair. Its results terminated an era of debate, where on one end of the spectrum Jack Collin claimed in the Lancet (1987) [29]: *„It is now no longer acceptable for a patient of any age with an abdominal aortic aneurysm of more than 4 cm to be denied the life-saving routine elective operation of aneurysm replacement“*, and on the other end Alan Scott advised in the British Medical Journal (1988) [30], that watchful waiting was justified for abdominal aortic aneurysms up to a diameter of 6 cm. Both were sure they were right. Obviously there was a 'grey area of clinical uncertainty' at the time, the dimensions of which had to be defined precisely before it was known which question had to be answered by the UK SAT. A survey was performed and consensus was that there was significant uncertainty about what was the appropriate treatment for *asymptomatic aortic aneurysms between 4.0 and 5.5 cm in male patients aged 60 to 79 years* [6]. UK SAT tested the question whether it was superior for these patients (1) to undergo early surgery (within 3 months) or (2) to remain under ultrasound surveillance until the aorta reached 5.5 cm, provided that the aorta did not become symptomatic or showed evidence of rapid growth. Detection of these events was to be ascertained by periodic control visits and repeated ultrasound scans and it triggered elective open repair. Importantly, an '*early surgery* strategy for small aneurysms' was compared to a '*delayed surgery* strategy until the aneurysm satisfied defined critera', and *not* against a '*no surgery* strategy' [31].

UK SAT randomised 1090 patients and became the basis upon which it is now known that it is safe to leave an asymptomatic aneurysm to reach 5.5 cm before surgery is considered. The US Aneurysm Detection and Management (ADAM) Trial tested a nearly identical protocol in 1136 patients [32]. The findings of the trials were essentially the same and showed that the annual rupture rate of stable small aneurysms ranged between 0.6% and 1%. We know now, that approximately 75% of the patients in the surveillance arm reached the criteria for repair eventually during 12 years of follow-up [33]. Thus all the trials demonstrated was that it was safe to observe them until they do, and no clinical benefit could be claimed by an early surgery strategy whereas treatment costs were considerably increased. As abdominal aortic aneurysms are much more prevalent in men, UK SAT and ADAM both involved almost exclusively male patients. However, the risk of rupture is estimated four times as high among women as among men. The fact that aneurysms rupture at smaller diameters in women has been explained by a tendency for the normal aortic diameter to be smaller in women than in men, and that, thus, a given diameter may represent a greater relative dilatation of the original diameter. Thus for women, the threshold diameter of 5.5 cm for aneurysm repair is probably too high, but trial data do not permit the specification of a lower threshold [14].

The cost-effectiveness of population screening is closely related to the validity of the criteria that are used to trigger therapeutic consequences. The UK Multicentre Aneurysm Screening Study (MASS) was based on the above criteria and was designed to answer the question whether it made sense to screen men aged 65 years for aortic aneurysm or not. It randomised 67'800 patients to either ultrasound screening or no screening and demonstrated after 4 years of follow-up that screening reduced aneurysm-related deaths by 42% (intention to treat analysis). In those patients who had actually attended ultrasound screening (per protocol analysis) the reduction of aneurysm-related deaths was even higher at 53%. However, overall mortality was not reduced by aneurysm screening [34]. The Gloucestershire's screening project is a practical application of this and has offered a single aortic ultrasound scan to every man reaching the age of 65 years since 1990 [35]. It showed an impressive reduction of interventions for ruptured aortic aneurysm and, interestingly, a reduced elective operative mortality of screen detected aneurysms (3%) as compared to incidentally discovered aneurysms (9%). Combined, the findings suggested that a single scan could largely rule out aneurysm disease for life in 95% of men (i.e. those with aortas < 2.6 cm at the age of 65) [36] and that population aneurysm screening had every possibility of virtually eradicating ruptured aneurysm over a 20 year period [4].

Endovascular Aneurysm Repair

Endovascular aneurysm repair was introduced in the early 1990ies with the expectation that it would considerably reduce the risks associated with open aortic surgery and, thus, provide a treatment alternative for the subset of patients who were not considered suitable surgical candidates [6]. Initial reports from institutional experiences, registries, and the United States Food and Drug Administration device trials seemed to reconfirm these expectations. However, when long-term follow-up from large registries such as the EUROSTAR registry became available in the late 90ies an alarming incidence of problems, reinterventions and even late aortic ruptures became apparent [37].

The UK Endovascular Aneurysm Repair Trials (EVAR 1 [19] and 2 [38]) were the first trials to test endovascular repair properly and started in 1999. They compared endovascular repair against open repair in *surgically fit* patients (EVAR 1) and endovascular repair against best medical management in *surgically unfit* patients (EVAR 2). Of note, *surgical high risk* patients were included and analysed in EVAR 1 [31]. The Dutch Randomized Endovascular Aneurysm Management (DREAM) Trial [20] tested a very similar protocol as EVAR 1, and two further randomised trials are underway but have not reported yet [6]. The findings of EVAR 1 and DREAM were very consistent. Both trials found a threefold reduction of operative mortality in favour of endovascular repair (1.7% *versus* 4.7% for EVAR 1 and 1.2% *versus* 4.6% for DREAM). The difference was statistically significant and it was preserved during follow-up as advantage regarding *aneurysm-related* deaths. Neither trial, however, was able to establish an overall survival benefit for endovascular repair during follow-up, and graft-related complications and re-interventions occurred significantly more frequently in the endovascular groups. This contributed to significantly higher treatment costs of endovascular repair. In addition and quite unexpectedly, initial advantages of endovascular repair regarding health-related quality of life disappeared completely within the first six months [39].

The findings of EVAR 2 were completely unexpected. The trial found no benefits in favour of endovascular aortic repair as compared to best medical management for patients deemed unfit for open surgery at any stage during follow-up and in terms of analyses by intention-to-treat or per-protocol. On the contrary, complications and subsequent procedures were more frequent in the endovascular group which generated higher treatment costs. Thus, of all things, EVAR 2 showed that endovascular repair was unsuited for exactly the subgroup of patients it had originally been designed for. These findings have remained unchallenged so far. Thus, until further evidence of equal quality becomes available it must be assumed that patients with aortic aneurysms who are not eligible for open repair are just so unfit due to their co-morbidities that endovascular aneurysm repair does not alter their expected date of death but it only increases costs.

Available data of randomised controlled trials [19, 20] and observational series [40] suggested that graft-related complications occur in up to 40% of patients during the first four years of follow-up after endovascular repair, and that about 20% of patients eventually need a reintervention. Corresponding findings after open repair were considerably lower at 9% and 6%, respectively, in the randomised trials. The characteristic complications of endovascular repair include occurrence of endoleak, graft migration and limb occlusion and they may eventually lead to re-pressurisation of the aneurysm sac. Therefore a small but finite risk of aneurysm rupture persists after endovascular repair which has been estimated around 0,7% per year [41-43]; and patients who do not undergo close follow-up surveillance after endovascular repair might be at increased risk of poor outcome. Thus dedicated surveillance programmes are still considered mandatory.

Against the background of these potentially serious complications and the need of costly surveillance, it is consoling to remember that it is safe for the patient to leave an aortic aneurysm up to 5.5cm and less expensive. Again, the key to the safety is the very low spontaneous risk of rupture of small aortic aneurysm (4.0 to 5.4 cm) which ranges between 0.6% and 1% per year, and this translates into a lower mortality than any active treatment has achieved so far. Therefore, any attempts to erode the established threshold of intervention are at least dubious. For instance, it was assumed that endovascular repair could be used legitimately for smaller aneurysm based on non-randomised observations which suggested that endovascular repair might achieve better results in smaller as compared to larger abdominal aneurysms. This is a flawed assumption of course, since the proper comparison is not whether endovascular repair performs better in small than in large aneurysms, but whether it performs better than watchful waiting with a defined protocol of intervention [31]. Again, this is unlikely, since the annual rupture rate for small aneurysms is lower than the reported mortality of endovascular repair. Moreover, both the 'early intervention arm' *and* the 'surveillance according to protocol arm' would profit from the reduced perioperative mortality of endovascular repair would it be used in a trial like UK SAT. Two randomised controlled endovascular trials are currently underway to test exactly this question with a very similar design to the UK SAT: is early endovascular repair associated with additional benefits to surveillance of small aortic aneurysm? The trials are the European Comparison of surveillance vs Aortic Endografting for Small Aneurysm Repair (CAESAR) Trial and the Positive Impact of EndoVascular Options for Treating Aneurysms Early (PIVOTAL) Trial and are due to report fairly soon. Hence, until these results become available there is no evidence to support a policy of treating patients with small aortic aneurysms with endovascular repair outside randomised controlled trials. Endovascular registries which include aneurysms as small as 4.0 cm such as EUROSTAR must be regarded off any evidence base, and this has been banned by practically all published national practice guidelines and international consensus recommendations of vascular surgery societies.

In summary, current level 1 evidence only supports the notion that endovascular repair offers benefits for *surgically fit* patients during the early recovery phase and in terms of aneurysm-related mortality. Other expected advantages have not been reconfirmed in prospective trials, which have however documented a higher incidence of complications and an increased need for reinterventions and resources after endovascular repair. Long-term durability of this treatment option is therefore still in doubt. The other important conclusion is that endovascular repair does not seem to confer any additional benefit to surgically *unfit* patients when compared to best medical treatment alone and that there is no justification for its use for small aneurysms (<5.5cm).

Emerging Biomechanical Challenges

As mentioned above the clinical effectiveness of endovascular aneurysm repair depends on the initial fit of the device and the sustained exclusion of blood flow and pressure from the aneurysm sac [8]. Failure of endograft seal is one of the major reasons for the occurrence of complications. The *initial anatomical fit* of a given stent-graft relates to specific anatomical requirements, which need to be appreciated carefully. Pre-procedural assessment is usually based on computed tomography (CT) scans using intraarterial contrast. Anatomical factors which are thought to be able to predict technical success include axial length, overall shape, condition and angulation of the intended attachment zones of the stent-graft [15]. Among these, the aortic neck has been identified as one of the most important determinants of outcome; however, anatomical appraisal of the neck relates closely to the ability to know exactly where it begins and where it ends for determination of length and shape, and reproducibility of such measurements has been astonishingly disappointing in the past [44, 45]. The main reasons for this have been suspected to relate to intrinsic limitations of conventional CT angiography regarding complex anatomical measurements and to the lack of a practicable and reliable definition of where an aneurysm starts [15]. However, the reliable appraisal of anatomical suitability is increasingly recognised as an underestimated challenge which may carry great importance towards superior patient selection and improved outcome of endovascular repair.

The *sustained exclusion* of the aneurysm sac depends on the stability of the seal that is achieved by the stent-graft. The tightness of the seal is challenged by ongoing degenerative processes in the aortic wall [46]. Clinical evidence suggests that neither surgical nor endovascular aneurysm repair has the potential to prevent continuing degeneration as progressive dilatation of the aortic neck is a common finding after both treatment approaches. Up to 28% and 59% of patients were shown to have relevant aortic neck dilatation at two and four years after endovascular repair, respectively [46]. Contrary to open surgical repair, this is associated with an increased risk of adverse clinical outcome since graft migration and endoleak are likely to occur as soon as the seal becomes leaky and the diameter of the infrarenal neck exceeds the dimensions of the proximal stent-graft. It was suspected before that progressive neck dilatation represented a centrifugal perpetuation of the aneurysmal disease process, and it was shown that alternative endovascular strategies including suprarenal fixation and fixation with hooks did not prevent this from happening [46]. We have recently reconfirmed this assumption on a molecular level and showed that the seemingly non-diseased infrarenal aortic neck in patients undergoing open surgical aneurysm repair already exhibited severe destruction on a histological level as well as significant up-regulation of proteolytic enzymes [10]. Therefore, progressive aortic neck dilatation after endovascular repair does not seem to be a chance finding; on the contrary it is very likely to represent an integral part of the disease. Thus it represents a major biomechanical challenge for durable endovascular fixation, and considering the increasing demand for endovascular repair particularly among younger patients [47] investigations into possibilities how to slow down or stop ongoing aneurysmal degeneration are clearly warranted.

Potential Answers to Current Challenges

The main biological mechanisms which are currently thought to control aneurysm expansion include proteolytic destruction of extracellular matrix, atrophy of smooth-muscle cells, and inflammation [12]. Increasing understanding of these processes has led many investigators to scrutinize potential pharmacological treatment options to prevent the development or decrease the growth of aortic aneurysms [9, 11, 48, 49]. For instance, angiotensin converting enzyme (ACE) inhibitors are known to prevent a wide variety of key events in vascular inflammation, and the efficacy of these blood pressure lowering agents in prohibition of abdominal aortic aneurysm development has been proven in animal studies [50]. A recent large epidemiological study showed that intake of ACE-inhibitors significantly reduced risk of aortic aneurysm rupture and the beneficial effect seemed to be independent of blood pressure lowering properties [51]. Or statins were shown to reduce the expression of various molecules involved in vascular inflammation [11]. In a rat model of aortic aneurysm, simvastatin suppressed aneurysm growth by lowering metalloproteinase levels [52]. Moreover, Wilson and colleagues have shown that statins decreased metalloproteinase concentrations in the anterior aortic aneurysm wall in humans undergoing open surgical aneurysm repair [53]. However, since statins and ACE inhibitors are already used with high prevalence in patients with abdominal aortic aneurysm who are at substantially increased risk of cardiovascular events [11], dedicated randomized trials to formally test the hypothesized effects of these drugs in human tissue face substantial difficulties regarding a meaningful study design.

As outlined above, we reported recently the discovery of increased proteolytic activity in the seemingly non-diseased infrarenal neck of patients who were treated by open repair [10]. This aortic segment would have been used for anchorage of the stent graft had these patients undergone endovascular repair. This led to the assumption that there might be a potential benefit to the durability of endovascular repair if the disease process could be modulated within the attachment zones. The emerging concept of a durable pharmacological stabilisation of the endovascular stent-graft seal by prevention of ongoing degeneration and dilatation of the involved vascular segments is very appealing and highlights a novel adjuvant treatment approach [7]. Currently, there is no data available regarding potential effectiveness of such a dedicated drug therapy. However, there is convincing evidence to justify the formulation of such a hypothesis: in a recent landmark publication, selective pharmacological inhibition of a similar proteolytic enzyme as found in our study, JNK, prohibited the development of abdominal aortic aneurysm in a in vivo mouse model, and even caused regression of existing aneurysms [54]. Thus, given biotolerance can be proven in humans, JNK inhibitors may represent an exciting new adjuvant pharmacological approach to improve outcome of endovascular repair or even prevent progression of small aneurysms to avoid repair altogether. Certainly further scrutiny of the clinical potential of these and other promising classes of substances is warranted and may become a key to improve the durability of endovascular repair.

Another potential key technology to meet the biomechanical challenges of endovascular repair is three-dimensional imaging. This method has recently emerged as a promising modality in the superior anatomical investigation and selection for endovascular repair [55]. Although anatomical complexity may affect open and endovascular repair procedures alike, endovascular repair is unique in its dependency on precise and detailed imaging *before* the procedure and during *follow-up:* as mentioned, eligibility of patients is based on distinct anatomical criteria and stent-graft dimensions must be determined by and large prior to the procedure [8]. Reliable investigation of aortic anatomy is also crucial to reduce the patient's exposure to ionising radiation during intervention; and the detection of impending complications as suggested by endoleak or subtle stent-graft migration during follow-up depends for the most part on precise imaging as well [15]. In all these instances, the validity of conventional CT angiography is likely to be limited by its susceptibility to parallax bias. Parallax may affect accuracy and reliability of all types of measurements including lengths, areas, volumes and angulations; and flawed pre-procedural imaging might be a preventable cause of impaired outcome of endovascular repair [15].

The potential of 3-dimensional CT imaging lies in its ability to reduce parallax error and to resolve typical technical measurement restrictions which may occur when reference points cannot be brought into the same planar reconstruction. Essentially, 3-dimensional imaging software converts two-dimensionally (i.e., in slices) acquired CT information consisting of picture elements (pixel) into true spatial volumetric information (voxel). This facilitates the calculation of a central luminal line along the vessel extension and unlimited assessment of anatomical characteristics in all three dimensions [55]. Measurements which are taken relative to the central luminal line are at reduced risk of parallax error and thus are likely to be more reliable and accurate. Also, the central luminal line is independent of the patient's orientation during CT acquisition, which allows for improved comparability between follow-up studies. At least theoretically 3-dimensional imaging can be expected to facilitate superior patient selection, better pre-procedural sizing of the stent-graft and more sensitive follow-up surveillance [15].

This can be illustrated in the instance of the aortic neck, but the same principles apply equally to distal landing zones or to the assessment of tortuosity. The aortic neck expands by consensus between the lowermost renal artery and the start of the aneurysm. Although this definition seems intuitively plausible and is conceptually easy to understand, it is in actual fact very difficult to agree upon the precise extension of the aortic neck on an individual CT scan [55]. Hence, there is considerable uncertainty as to 'on which CT slide' *exactly* the aneurysmal process begins [44, 56] and this decision may be further confounded by the choice of the particular planar reconstruction. Moreover, it may even be difficult to localise the start of the neck unambiguously since a planar reconstruction must be found where the renal artery and the axis of the neck are both visible. Thus, using conventional CT imaging a valid radiological definition of where the aortic neck ends and the aneurysm begins seems unrealistic [15]. Apart from the start and endpoint of the neck, the assessment of the distance between (i.e. the precise neck length) may be flawed in conventional CT if the measured distance cannot be brought completely into the same planar reconstruction and even if it can the impact of any angulation along the way can only be estimated. It is not surprising, thus, that the mean variation of neck length measurements using conventional CT angiography was almost 7mm in a study comparing four blinded readers which corresponded to more than 30% of the mean neck length [44]. Another common problem is the assessment of the angulation of the aortic neck. This is commonly estimated on biplanar (i.e., sagittal and coronal) reconstructions and the sharper angle between the long axis of the neck and the long axis of the aneurysm is recorded. However, individual interpretation of the 'vessel axis' can be very variable and kinking aneurysms have to be taken into account [44]. Moreover, it is difficult to visualise both axes on the same planar reconstruction. Together with a systematic underestimation of the true angle, measured angles have not only proven to be very imprecise, but are also likely to be faulty [15]. Three-dimensional imaging has every possibility to improve our ability significantly to know the exact neck dimensions and to reproduce them reliably. By introduction of the central luminal line the proximal starting point of the aortic neck can be defined unambiguously as the first plane orthogonal to the central luminal line at which the lowermost renal artery is not in luminal continuity with the aorta anymore; and length measurements are taken by definition from the intersection of the central luminal line with this plane. In a similar way, other neck dimensions can be established in a reproducible fashion by progressive assessment of all orthogonal cross-sections along the central luminal line of the neck. In brief, mathematical definitions for standardised assessment of anatomical dimensions become available which is the prerequisite for prospective correlation of patient anatomy and clinical outcome.

Clinical Implications

It is important to realise that minimal length or maximum angulation of the aortic neck for safe and durable endovascular sealing has never been tested experimentally and is purely based on manufacturers' recommendations and observational studies. Anecdotal evidence suggests that shorter aortic necks and sharper angles correlate with a significant deterioration of outcome [57-59]. For instance, graft migration rates were twofold greater with a fixation length of less than 15mm as compared to more than 15mm [60], and sealing zones of more than 15 mm have been associated with low overall risk [61]. Observational data from an Australian registry indicated that neck angulation of more than 45 degrees was an independent predictor of re-interventions for failed endovascular repair [62]; however, in the EUROSTAR registry this threshold was at 60 degrees [63, 64]. Hence, 'something between 40 to 60 degrees' is regarded currently the maximum neck angulation still suitable for endovascular repair [65]. However, given the assumable degree of imprecision of current neck measurements, nobody really knows *what* was measured in such studies and consistency of findings is very likely to be flawed. Consequentially, grading of aortic neck morphology towards prediction of suitability for endovascular repair has not been an easy task so far; and current classification schemes have arguably been derived on the basis of 'best current opinion' rather than acceptable levels of evidence. The *Ad Hoc Committee for Standardized Reporting Practices in Vascular Surgery* of the Society for Vascular Surgery/American Association for Vascular Surgery proposed a detailed graduation scheme of 'anatomical risk' for endovascular repair [61] which can serve as a general orientation. However, prospective research into the correlation between aortic anatomy and outcome of endovascular repair using more precise and reliable imaging tools such as 3-dimensional CT imaging is more than likely to improve the predictive value of such recommendations in the future.

In conclusion, endovascular aneurysm repair has become a well-established mechanical treatment concept that dramatically changed the overall look of aortic aneurysm repair. Distinct feature of this novel technology, however, have brought characteristic biomechanical challenges to our attention. These involve the problem of reliable appraisal of the patients' anatomy prior to the procedure and during follow-up and the preservation of a snug fit of the stent-graft over time. Both may be compromised by ongoing degenerative processes in the aortic wall. Currently, the scientific community has gained important insights into the biologic basis of aneurysmal disease and the first potential drug targets to modulate disease progression have emerged. These are promising to herald a new era of integrated aneurysm management combining mechanical repair and molecular modulation. Improved imaging technology has the potential to contribute to endovascular repair by superior selection of patients, dedicated modifications of stent-graft designs and better prediction of risk of complications. All these efforts taken together are likely to improve safety and durability of endovascular repair which will hopefully translate eventually into better quality of life of treated patients, reduced need for intensive surveillance programmes and improved cost-effectiveness. In a further step, joined efforts may even have the potential to pave the way for dedicated proteomic and genomic techniques to predict, modulate or even prevent the natural course of the disease. However, until the emerging knowledge has evolved enough to achieve these goals, endovascular aneurysm repair remains to be considered palliative.

Disclosures

Nicolas Diehm receives an unrestricted research grant by Medtronic, Inc. Switzerland.

Florian Dick currently receives independent stipendiary support for a vascular research fellowship from the Swiss National Funds (SNF, PBBSB-120858) and the Lichtenstein Stiftung, Basel, Switzerland.

References

[1] Szilagyi, DE; Smith, RF; DeRusso, FJ; Elliott, JP; Sherrin FW. Contribution of abdominal aortic aneurysmectomy to prolongation of life. *Ann Surg.* 1966, 164, 678-699.

[2] Bengtsson H; Bergqvist D. Ruptured abdominal aortic aneurysm: a population-based study. *J Vasc Surg.,* 1993, 18, 74-80.

[3] Dick, F; Grobety, V; Immer FF; et al. Outcome and quality of life in patients treated for abdominal aortic aneurysms: a single center experience. *World J Surg.,* 2008, 32, 987-994.

[4] Greenhalgh, RM. National screening programme for aortic aneurysm. *BMJ.* 2004, 328, 1087-1088.

[5] Parodi, JC; Palmaz, JC; Barone, HD. Transfemoral intraluminal graft implantation for abdominal aortic aneurysms. *Ann Vasc Surg.,* 1991, 5, 491-499.

[6] Dick, F; Brown, LC; Powell, JT; Reise, J; Greenhalgh, RM. Appraisal Era for Endovascular Repair of Abdominal Aortic Aneurysms. *Acta Chir Belg.,* 2008, 288-291.

[7] Diehm, N; Dick, F; Katzen, B; Do, D; Baumgartner, I. Endovascular abdominal aortic aneurysm repair: Just a mechanical solution for a biological problem? *J Endovasc Ther.,* 2009, 16.

[8] Greenhalgh, RM; Powell, JT. Endovascular Repair of Abdominal Aortic Aneurysm. *N Engl J Med.,* 2008, 358, 494-501.

[9] Diehm, N; Dick, F; Schaffner, T; et al. Novel insight into the pathobiology of abdominal aortic aneurysm and potential future treatment concepts. *Prog Cardiovasc Dis.,* 2007, 50, 209-217.

[10] Diehm, N; Santo, SD; Schaffner, T; et al. Severe structural damage of the seemingly non-diseased infrarenal aortic aneurysm neck. *J Vasc Surg.,* 2008.

[11] Diehm, N; Schmidli, J; Dai-Do, D; Baumgartner, I. Current evidence and prospects for medical treatment of abdominal aortic aneurysms. *Vasa.,* 2005, 34, 217-223.

[12] Shimizu, K; Mitchell, RN; Libby, P. Inflammation and cellular immune responses in abdominal aortic aneurysms. *Arterioscler Thromb Vasc Biol.,* 2006, 26, 987-994.

[13] Powell, JT; Brady, AR. Detection, management, and prospects for the medical treatment of small abdominal aortic aneurysms. *Arterioscler Thromb Vasc Biol.,* 2004, 24, 241-245.

[14] Powell, JT; Greenhalgh, RM. Clinical practice. Small abdominal aortic aneurysms. *N Engl J Med.,* 2003, 348, 1895-1901.

[15] Dick F, Greenhalgh RM. Three-dimensional imaging for EVAR: Importance of precise neck length and angulation. In: Vascular and endovascular consensus update. Ed R M Greenhalgh, BIBA Publishing, London, UK, 2009:189-95

[16] Bergqvist, D. Historical aspects on aneurysmal disease. *Scand J Surg.,* 2008, 97, 90-99.

[17] Freeman, ME; Leeds, FH. Vein inlay graft in the treatment of aneurysms and thrombosis of the abdominal aorta; a preliminary communication with report of 3 cases. *Angiology.* 1951, 2, 579-587.

[18] Dubost, C; Allary, M; Oeconomos, N. Resection of an aneurysm of the abdominal aorta: reestablishment of the continuity by a preserved human arterial graft, with result after five months. *AMA Arch Surg.,* 1952, 64, 405-408.

[19] Endovascular aneurysm repair versus open repair in patients with abdominal aortic aneurysm (EVAR trial 1): randomised controlled trial. *Lancet.,* 2005, 365, 2179-2186.

[20] Blankensteijn, JD; De Jong, SE; Prinssen, M; et al. Two-year outcomes after conventional or endovascular repair of abdominal aortic aneurysms. *N Engl J Med.,* 2005, 352, 2398-2405.

[21] Carrel, A. Results of the permanent intubation of the thoracic aorta. *Surg Gynecol Obstet.,* 1912, 15, 245-248.

[22] Dotter, CT. Transluminally-placed coilspring endarterial tube grafts. Long-term patency in canine popliteal artery. *Invest Radiol.,* 1969, 4, 329-332.

[23] Dotter, CT; Judkins, MP. Transluminal Treatment of Arteriosclerotic Obstruction. Description of a New Technic and a Preliminary Report of Its Application. *Circulation.,* 1964, 30, 654-670.

[24] Gruntzig, A; Hopff, H. Percutaneous recanalization after chronic arterial occlusion with a new dilator-catheter (modification of the Dotter technique) (author's transl). *Dtsch Med Wochenschr.,* 1974, 99, 2502-2510, 2511.

[25] Volodos, NL; Shekhanin, VE; Karpovich, IP; Troian, VI; Gur'ev, Iu A. [A self-fixing synthetic blood vessel endoprosthesis]. *Vestn Khir Im I I Grek.,* 1986, 137, 123-125.

[26] Dick, F; Greenhalgh, RM. Potential role of balloon expandable aorto-uni-femoral endografts. *Ital J Vasc Endovasc.* 2008, 15, 121-126.

[27] Diehm, N; Baum, S; Benenati, JF. Fenestrated and branched endografts: why we need them now. *J Vasc Interv Radiol.,* 2008, 19, S63-67.

[28] Mortality results for randomised controlled trial of early elective surgery or ultrasonographic surveillance for small abdominal aortic aneurysms. The UK Small Aneurysm Trial Participants. *Lancet.,* 1998, 352, 1649-1655.

[29] Collin, J. Elective surgery for small abdominal aortic aneurysms. *Lancet.,* 1987, 1, 909.

[30] Scott, RA; Ashton, HA; Kay, DN. Routine ultrasound screening in management of abdominal aortic aneurysm. *Br Med J (Clin Res Ed).,* 1988, 296, 1709-1710.

[31] Greenhalgh, RM; Brown, LC. The most important misinterpretations of the UK randomised trials on abdominal aortic aneurysm repair. *Scand J Surg.,* 2008, 97, 116-120.

[32] Lederle, FA; Johnson, GR; Wilson, SE; et al. The aneurysm detection and management study screening program: validation cohort and final results. Aneurysm Detection and

Management Veterans Affairs Cooperative Study Investigators. *Arch Intern Med.,* 2000, 160, 1425-1430.

[33] Powell, JT. Final 12-year follow-up of Surgery versus Surveillance in the UK Small Aneurysm Trial. *British Journal of Surgery.,* 2007, 94, 702-708.

[34] Ashton, HA; Buxton, MJ; Day, NE; et al. The Multicentre Aneurysm Screening Study (MASS) into the effect of abdominal aortic aneurysm screening on mortality in men: a randomised controlled trial. *Lancet.,* 2002, 360, 1531-1539.

[35] Earnshaw, JJ; Shaw, E; Whyman, MR; Poskitt, KR; Heather, BP. Screening for abdominal aortic aneurysms in men. *Bmj.,* 2004, 328, 1122-1124.

[36] Crow, P; Shaw, E; Earnshaw, JJ; Poskitt, KR; Whyman, MR; Heather, BP. A single normal ultrasonographic scan at age 65 years rules out significant aneurysm disease for life in men. *Br J Surg.,* 2001, 88, 941-944.

[37] Rutherford, RB. Randomized EVAR Trials and Advent of Level I Evidence: A Paradigm Shift in Management of Large Abdominal Aortic Aneurysms? *Seminars in Vascular Surgery.,* 2006, 19, 69-74.

[38] Endovascular aneurysm repair and outcome in patients unfit for open repair of abdominal aortic aneurysm (EVAR trial 2): randomised controlled trial. *Lancet.,* 2005, 365, 2187-2192.

[39] Prinssen, M; Buskens, E; Blankensteijn, JD. Quality of life endovascular and open AAA repair. Results of a randomised trial. *Eur J Vasc Endovasc Surg.,* 2004, 27, 121-127.

[40] Van Marrewijk, C; Buth, J; Harris, PL; Norgren, L; Nevelsteen, A; Wyatt, MG. Significance of endoleaks after endovascular repair of abdominal aortic aneurysms: The EUROSTAR experience. *J Vasc Surg.,* 2002, 35, 461-473.

[41] Brewster, DC; Jones, JE; Chung, TK; et al. Long-term outcomes after endovascular abdominal aortic aneurysm repair: the first decade. *Ann Surg.,* 2006, 244, 426-438.

[42] Sicard, GA; Zwolak, RM; Sidawy, AN; White, RA; Siami, FS. Endovascular abdominal aortic aneurysm repair: long-term outcome measures in patients at high-risk for open surgery. *J Vasc Surg.,* 2006, 44, 229-236.

[43] Zarins, CK; Crabtree, T; Bloch, DA; Arko, FR; Ouriel, K; White, RA. Endovascular aneurysm repair at 5 years: Does aneurysm diameter predict outcome? *J Vasc Surg.,* 2006, 44, 920-929.

[44] Diehm N, Katzen BT, Samuels S, Pena C, Powell A, Dick F. 64-detector computed tomography angiography of infrarenal aortic neck length and angulation: prospective analysis of inter-observer variability. J Vasc Intervent Radiol 2008;19:1283-8

[45] Diehm, N; Kickuth, R; Gahl, B; et al. Intraobserver and interobserver variability of 64-row computed tomography abdominal aortic aneurysm neck measurements. *J Vasc Surg.,* 2007, 45, 263-268.

[46] Diehm, N; Dick, F; Katzen, BT; Schmidli, J; Kalka, C; Baumgartner, I. Aortic neck dilatation after endovascular abdominal aortic aneurysm repair: A word of caution. *J Vasc Surg.,* 2008, 47, 886-892.

[47] Diehm N, Tsoukas A.I, Katzen B.T, Baum S, Pena C, Dick F. Matched-pair analysis of endovascular versus open surgical abdominal aortic aneurysm repair in young low-risk patients. J Vasc Interv Radiol 2008 May;19:645-51

[48] Baxter, BT; Terrin, MC; Dalman, RL. Medical management of small abdominal aortic aneurysms. *Circulation.*, 2008, 117, 1883-1889.

[49] Diehm N, Becker G.J, Katzen B.T, Benenati J.F, Kovacs M.E, Dick F. Statins are associated with decreased mortality in abdominal, but not in thoracic aortic aneurysm patients: propensity score-adjusted analysis. VASA 2008;37:241-9

[50] Liao, S; Miralles, M; Kelley, BJ; Curci, JA; Borhani, M; Thompson, RW. Suppression of experimental abdominal aortic aneurysms in the rat by treatment with angiotensin-converting enzyme inhibitors. *J Vasc Surg.*, 2001, 33, 1057-1064.

[51] Hackam, DG; Thiruchelvam, D; Redelmeier, DA. Angiotensin-converting enzyme inhibitors and aortic rupture: a population-based case-control study. *Lancet.*, 2006, 368, 659-665.

[52] Kalyanasundaram, A; Elmore, JR; Manazer, JR; et al. Simvastatin suppresses experimental aortic aneurysm expansion. *J Vasc Surg.*, 2006, 43, 117-124.

[53] Wilson, WR; Evans, J; Bell, PR; Thompson, MM. HMG-CoA Reductase Inhibitors (Statins) Decrease MMP-3 and MMP-9 Concentrations in Abdominal Aortic Aneurysms. *Eur J Vasc Endovasc Surg.*, 2005, 3, 259-262.

[54] Yoshimura, K; Aoki, H; Ikeda, Y; et al. Regression of abdominal aortic aneurysm by inhibition of c-Jun N-terminal kinase. *Nat Med.*, 2005, 11, 1330-1338.

[55] Filis, KA; Arko, FR; Rubin, GD; Zarins, CK. Three-dimensional CT evaluation for endovascular abdominal aortic aneurysm repair. Quantitative assessment of the infrarenal aortic neck. *Acta Chir Belg.*, 2003, 103, 81-86.

[56] Diehm, N; Katzen, BT; Samuels, S; Pena, C; Powell, A; Dick, F. Sixty-four-detector CT angiography of infrarenal aortic neck length and angulation: prospective analysis of interobserver variability. *J Vasc Interv Radiol.*, 2008, 19, 1283-1288.

[57] Albertini, J; Kalliafas, S; Travis, S; et al. Anatomical risk factors for proximal perigraft endoleak and graft migration following endovascular repair of abdominal aortic aneurysms. *Eur J Vasc Endovasc Surg.*, 2000, 19, 308-312.

[58] Leurs, LJ; Kievit, J; Dagnelie, PC; Nelemans, PJ; Buth, J. Influence of infrarenal neck length on outcome of endovascular abdominal aortic aneurysm repair. *J Endovasc Ther.*, 2006, 13, 640-648.

[59] Sampaio, SM; Panneton, JM; Mozes, GI; et al. Proximal type I endoleak after endovascular abdominal aortic aneurysm repair: predictive factors. *Ann Vasc Surg.*, 2004, 18, 621-628.

[60] Zarins, CK; Bloch, DA; Crabtree, T; Matsumoto, AH; White, RA; Fogarty, TJ. Stent graft migration after endovascular aneurysm repair: importance of proximal fixation. *J Vasc Surg.*, 2003, 38, 1264-1272; discussion 1272.

[61] Chaikof, EL; Fillinger, MF; Matsumura, JS; et al. Identifying and grading factors that modify the outcome of endovascular aortic aneurysm repair. *J Vasc Surg.*, 2002, 35, 1061-1066.

[62] Boult, M; Babidge, W; Maddern, G; Barnes, M; Fitridge, R; On Behalf Of The Audit Reference G. Predictors of success following endovascular aneurysm repair: mid-term results. *Eur J Vasc Endovasc Surg.*, 2006, 31, 123-129.

[63] Hobo, R; Kievit, J; Leurs, LJ; Buth, J. Influence of severe infrarenal aortic neck angulation on complications at the proximal neck following endovascular AAA repair: a EUROSTAR study. *J Endovasc Ther.,* 2007, 14, 1-11.

[64] Fransen, GA; Desgranges, P; Laheij, RJ; Harris, PL; Becquemin, JP. Frequency; predictive factors, and consequences of stent-graft kink following endovascular AAA repair. *J Endovasc Ther.,* 2003, 10, 913-918.

[65] Sternbergh, WC; 3rd, Carter, G; York, JW; Yoselevitz, M; Money, SR. Aortic neck angulation predicts adverse outcome with endovascular abdominal aortic aneurysm repair. *J Vasc Surg.,* 2002, 35, 482-486.

In: Aneurysms: Types, Risks, Formation and Treatment
Editors: Alain Laurent and Ethan Morel
ISBN: 978-1-60741-557-2
© 2009 Nova Science Publishers, Inc.

Chapter 6

Inflammatory Abdominal Aortic Aneurysm from a Viewpoint of IgG4-Related Disease: Proposal of IgG4-Related Chronic Periaortitis

Yasuni Nakanuma[1*], Yoh Zen[2], Yasunori Sato[1], Kenichi Harada[2] and Satomi Kasashima[3]
[1]Department of Human Pathology and
[2]Department of Diagnostic Pathology, Kanazawa University Graduate School of Medicine, Kanazawa, and
[3]Pathology, Kanazawa Medical Center, Kanazawa, Japan

Abstract

Atherosclerosis is the most common cause of abdominal aortic aneurysm (AAA). Inflammatory abdominal aneurysm (IAAA), a variant of AAA, is characterized by dense fibrosis and extensive lymphoplasmacytic infiltration of the aortic wall, particularly its adventitia and surrounding connective tissue, and belongs to a spectrum of chronic periaortitis that includes retroperitoneal fibrosis and perianeurysmal retroperitoneal fibrosis. Recent studies disclosed that retroperitoneal fibrosis belongs to the IgG4-related diseases, characterized by numerous infiltrating IgG4-positive plasma cells and fibrosis, and high serum IgG4 concentrations. However, the relationship between IgG4-related diseases and IAAA remains unclarified. Our recent studies comparing IAAA with atherosclerotic AAA and IgG4-related diseases in other organs, showed that IAAA could be classified into 2 types: those aneurysms with IgG4-positive plasma cells (IgG4-related type), and those without (IgG4-unrelated type). All patients with atherosclerotic AAA had only a few IgG4-positive plasma cells. The IgG4-related type was characterized by

*Corresponding author: Department of Human Pathology, Kanazawa University Graduate School of Medicine, Kanazawa 920-8640, Japan, Tel: +81-76-265-2197 (Japan), Fax: +81-76-234-4229 (Japan), E-mail: pbcpsc@kenroku.kanazawa-u.ac.jp

marked lymphoplasmacytic infiltration with lymph follicle formation and inflammatory extension around nerve fibers, frequent infiltration of eosinophils, and inconspicuous infiltration of neutrophils compared with the IgG4-unrelated type. Obliterative phlebitis, which is found in patients with IgG4-related diseases in other organs, was observed in all cases of IgG4-related IAAA. These histopathological features were identical to those of IgG4-related diseases in other organs such as autoimmune pancreatitis. In addition, serum IgG4 concentrations were significantly higher in IgG4-related IAAA, suggesting it to be one of the IgG4-related diseases. Because some cases of retroperitoneal fibrosis and inflammatory IAAA belong to IgG4-related diseases, such cases are categorized as "IgG4-related chronic periaortitis".

Introduction

Abdominal aortic aneurysm (AAA) is the most common type of aneurysm, developing in people older than 60 years. Inflammatory AAA is a special and rare variant of AAA, and characterized histopathologically by dense fibrosis and lymphoplasmacytic infiltration in the aneurismal wall and surrounding tissue [1-4]. The intima is relatively spared from such inflammation. While several mechanisms have been proposed, the exact pathogenesis of IAAA remains unclear [5-8]..

Recently, much attention has been focused on IgG4-related diseases, a new clinicopathological disease entity proposed with regard to autoimmune pancreatitis (AIP) [9-11]. IgG4-related disease is a unique sclerosing disorder characterized by marked lymphocyte and plasma cell infiltration, including numerous IgG4-positive plasma cells, and obliterative phlebitis. The prototype of this lesion was first reported in the pancreas as AIP, a unique form of pancreatitis and also called lymphoplasmacytic sclerosing pancreatitis [12-14]. It soon became evident that this lesion involves not only the pancreas, but also extrapancreatic tissues, including the bile duct, salivary glands, and retroperitoneum [9,10]. It is now widely accepted that IgG4-related diseases showing histological features similar to AIP can occur in various organs. These diseases are clinically characterized by elevated serum IgG4 concentrations, a high prevalence in adults, steroid sensitivity, and a frequent association with IgG4-related lesions in other organs [10]. Most IgG4-related diseases occur in glandular or ductal tissues, with retroperitoneal or mediastinal connective tissue occasionally affected. However, IgG4-related disease has not been well documented in the cardiovascular system.

Recently, we reported for the first time that some patients with inflammatory AAA showed numerous IgG4-positive plasma cells among dense lymphoplasmacytic infiltrates in aneurismal lesions of the affected aorta and in adjacent fibrotic tissue. These patients also had high serum IgG4 concentrations [15], suggesting that a subgroup of inflammatory AAA has clinicopathological characteristics similar to IgG4-related diseases. Interestingly, there were also inflammatory AAA patients without dense IgG4-bearing plasma cells and with no elevation of the serum IgG4 level. Thereafer, additional reports from Japan supporting our theory that inflammatory AAA is a IgG4-related disease emerged [16,17].

Recently, the disease entity "chronic periaortitis" was proposed [18,19] which encompass retroperitoneal fibrosis, inflammatory AAA and perianeurysmal retroperitoneal fibrosis [18,19]. Although these disorders differ in their clinical presentation, their histopathological characteristics are identical and together they compose a spectrum of one disease. Interestingly, retroperitoneal fibrosis is also postulated to be a retroperitoneal lesion of IgG4-related diseases [20,21].

Herein, the clinicopathological features of inflammatory AAA are reviewed in comparison with those of atherosclerotic AAA, and then the pathology and etiopathogenesis of inflammatory AAA are discussed with regard to IgG4-related diseases and chronic periaortitis.

Clinical and Pathological Features

A. Clinical Features

Inflammatory AAA accounts for about 3-10% of all AAA cases, and affects middle-old aged people [1,22]. Classical symptoms include intermittent lower back/abdominal pain, fever, malaise, weight loss, general fatigue, abdominal pulsatile mass, anemia of chronic disease and raised inflammatory markers. Such features may be dependent on the extent and anatomical location of the periaortic fibrosis and aneurismal dilatation [1,2]. Aneurysms always occur within the abdominal aorta in inflammatory AAA, though occasionally the thoracic and ascending aorta and iliac artery are affected [23]. The natural course of inflammatory AAA seems to involve enlargement, while patients with inflammatory AAA seldom have a history of rupture [3]. Other autoimmune diseases are occasionally diagnosed in the cases of inflammatory AAA, including rheumatoid arthritis and polyarteritis nodosa. Patients with inflammatory AAA, particularly the IgG4-related type, have a history of IgG4-related diseases such as autoimmune pancreatitis (AIP) (see below), while such complications are not found in atherosclerotic AAA [15].

In principle, treatment for inflammatory AAA could be surgical repair [24]. Corticosteroids or immunosuppressive therapy is also effective for inflammatory AAA, particularly the IgG4-related type, and should be considered as a first line of treatment and for long-term maintenance [24]. Corticosteroid therapy for inflammatory AAA needs a lot of attention, because the aneurismal wall in cases of inflammatory AAA would become thin and fragile and might rupture. While the perioperative mortality associated with open surgical repair of inflammatory AAAs is higher than that with noninflammatory AAA due to inflammation and periaortic fibrosis [25], surgical repair could be performed after steroid therapy to reduce the periaortic inflammatory reaction. Clinical studies using many cases are mandatory to determine the effectiveness of steroid therapy in the clinical management of patients with inflammatory AAA, particularly the IgG4-related type [15].

Imagings: Abdominal ultrasonography, computed tomography (CT) and magnetic resonance imaging (MRI) can show an infrarenal inflammatory AAA and retroperitoneal soft tissue surrounding the aorta (*Figure 1*) [25]. Enhanced CT confirmed a large infrarenal AAA with enhanced delineation of the periaortic mantle and a thickened aneurysmal wall, and adhesions to adjacent abdominal organs, the findings of a thickened aneurysmal wall with rigid adherence of adjacent structures [26]. Ultrasound is also useful for the detection of ureteral strictures with hydronephrosis or aortic aneurysm [24]. To identify inflammation in the aneurismal wall, positron emission tomography and computed tomography (PET/CT) are used and inflammatory AAAs showed significantly higher F18-fluorodeoxyglucose (FDG) uptake than the normal-sized aorta in age-matched controls [27]. Irrespective of the aneurysm's diameter, asymptomatic AAAs show more FDG uptake and greater inflammatory activity in the wall than the non-dilated abdominal aorta [28]. Imaging has a major role in the diagnosis of inflammatory AAA, and FDG-PET/CT in particular is regarded as a promising technique to identify inflammation of the aneurysmal wall. 3

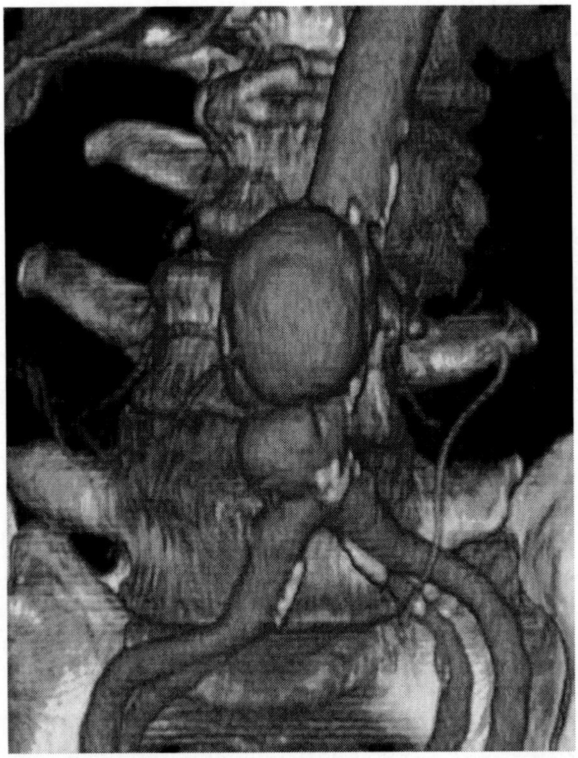

Figure 1. CT arteriography of inflammatory abdominal aortic aneurysm (an IgG4-related case). A cystic aneurysm is observed in the abdominal aorta.

Laboratory data: Levels of systemic inflammatory markers, such as the erythrocyte sedimentation rate (ESR) and C-reactive protein (CRP), are high in inflammatory AAA in comparison with atherosclerotic AAA [6,24,29]. CRP initially increases with very varying (and at times only very low) frequency [24]. The CRP level is increased mostly in patients with inflammatory AAA, but is not associated with the diameter of the periaortic mass [30]. CRP is not a reliable marker for excluding chronic periaortitis and for monitoring disease activity. Autoantibodies such as ANA and anti-smooth muscle antibody and an elevation of the serum IgG concentration are also frequently found [5,15,31]. The incidence in antinuclear antibodies (ANA) did not differ between inflammatory AAAs and atherosclerotic AAA [32]. The difference of laboratory data between IgG4-related and -unrelated types will be discussed below. There have been no specific or pathognomonic laboratory markers for the diagnosis of inflammatory AAA.

B. Pathology

Gross findings: Inflamamtory AAA is characterized by diffuse fibrous thickening of the aortic wall, particularly its adventitia, and is apparently tumorous. Fibrous adhesion between the retroperitoneum and aneurysm, especially its anterior wall, is frequently found. Dense and rigid adherence of the adjacent structures to the aneurysmal wall may cause the obstruction of adjacent abdominal organs such as ureters with hydronephrosis and the duodenum.

Microscopic findings: Inflammatory AAA is characterized by extensive fibrosis with fibroblastic proliferation and severe lymphoplasmacytic infiltration with lymph follicle formation in the media and in the adventitia of the aneurismal wall, followed by a marked thickening of the aortic wall (*Figure 2,3*) [15-17]. The infiltrating of lymphoplasmacytes are intermixed with irregular fibrotic areas. Lymphocytes are mainly composed of B cells and smaller numbers of CD4+ and CD8+ T cells. While severe infiltration of plasma cells is observed, monoclonality is not evident among the infiltrating plasma cells, which are composed of kappa- and lambda-bearing cells. Macrophages and mild eosinophilic infiltration are usually found, and conspicuous eosinophilic infiltration is occasionally encountered. Neutrophilic infiltration is not observed or minimum. Elastica van Gieson staining discloses obliterative phlebitis with the luminal occlusion of small veins with mixed inflammatory cells (*Figure 4*) [15]. In addition, similar inflammatory changes with fibrosis commonly spread into the surrounding connective tissue of the adventitia, and lymphoplasmacytic infiltration also extends along nerve fascicles. In addition, atherosclerotic changes such as fibrous thickening, cholesterol clefts, and the accumulation of foam cells and loss of elastic fibers are also observed in the intima and media of the aneurismal wall.

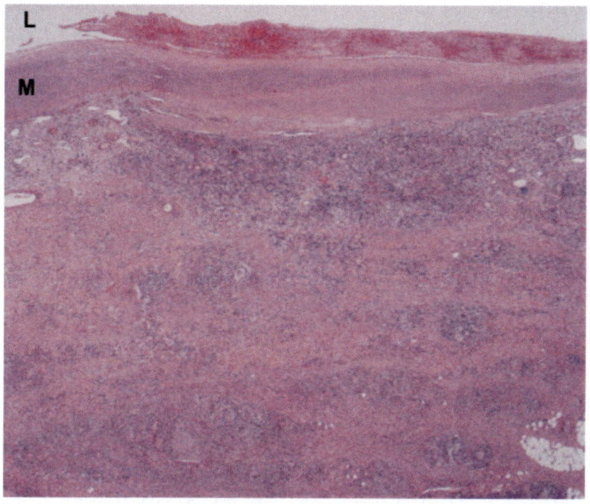

Figure 2. Histological features of IgG4-related inflammatory abdominal aortic aneurysm. The adventitia and periaortic connective tissue are severely expanded due tosclerosing inflammation. H&E, ×20. L and M: lumen and media of abdominal aorta (adapted from ref. #10)

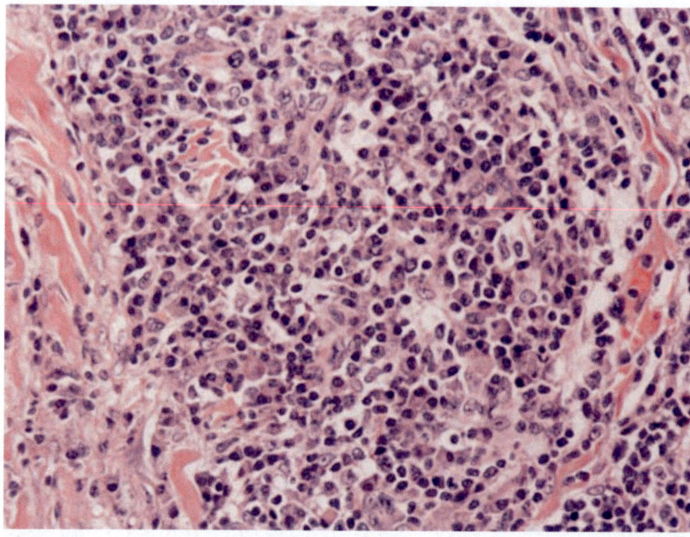

Figure 3. Histological features of IgG4-related inflammatory abdominal aortic aneurysm. Inflammatory cells consisted of many lymphocytes and plasma cells. H&E, ×200.

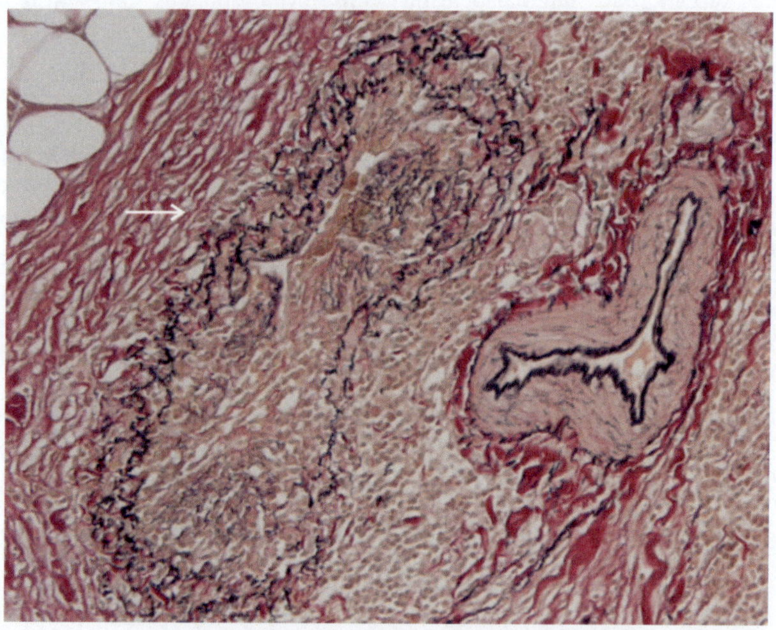

Figure 4. Elastica van Gieson staining reveals obliterative phlebitis (arrow) in the aneurysmal wall of IgG4-related inflammatory abdominal aortic aneurysm. ×200. (adapted from ref. #10)

Differences of inflammatory AAA from atherosclerotic AAA: While atherosclerotic changes are observed in both inflammatory and atherosclerotic AAAs, atherosclerotic AAA is more commonly associated with erosive and exudative changes and also has neutrophilic infiltration in the intima and media. In contrast, the adventitia was grossly significantly thicker in inflammatory AAA than atherosclerotic AAA [15,16]. Fibrosis and variable degrees of lymphoplasmacytic infiltration are seen in the media and adventitia of affected lesions in cases of both inflammatory AAA and atherosclerotic AAA, though inflammatory cell infiltrates and fibrosis are significantly more intense and extensive in the former. Inflammatory AAA is not strictly or absolutely separable from atherosclerotic AAA [2-4,32]. Numbers of IgG4-positive plasma cells were significantly larger in inflammatory AAA than in atherosclerotic AAA.

C. Subclassification of Inflammatory AAA into IgG4-Related and IgG4-Unrelated Types

Pathology: Immunohistochemically, many IgG-positive plasma cells are diffusely spread in the adventitia of all inflammatory AAAs. Interestingly, some patients with inflammatory AAA show diffuse and extensive infiltration of IgG4-positive plasma cells (*Figuge 5*). In contrast, IgG4-positive plasma cells were few or only focally accumulated in other cases of inflammatory AAA as seen in atherosclerotic AAA [15]. The ratio of IgG4/IgG-positive plasma cells is significantly higher in the former. Numbers of IgG-positive cells were not different in inflammatory AAA irrespective of IgG4-positive plasma cell infiltration. The thickness of the adventitia and degree of inflammation did not differ between them. IgG4-related inflammatory AAA was pathologically characterized by the frequent infiltration of eosinophils, lymph follicle formation, perineural inflammatory extension, and inconspicuous infiltration of neutrophils compared with IgG4-unrelated inflammatory AAA. In addition, obliterative phlebitis was more commonly observed in IgG4-related aneurysms (all cases) than in non- IgG4-related cases (50% of cases), although the difference was not significant. On the basis of the results of immunostaining of IgG and IgG4, inflammatory AAA could be classified into these cases with and those without numerous infiltrating IgG4-positive plasma cells. The former are designated IgG4-related inflammatory AAA, and the latter, IgG4-unrelated inflammatory AAA. This classification may be important therapeutically, because IgG4-related disease in other organs is known to respond favorably to corticosteroid therapy.

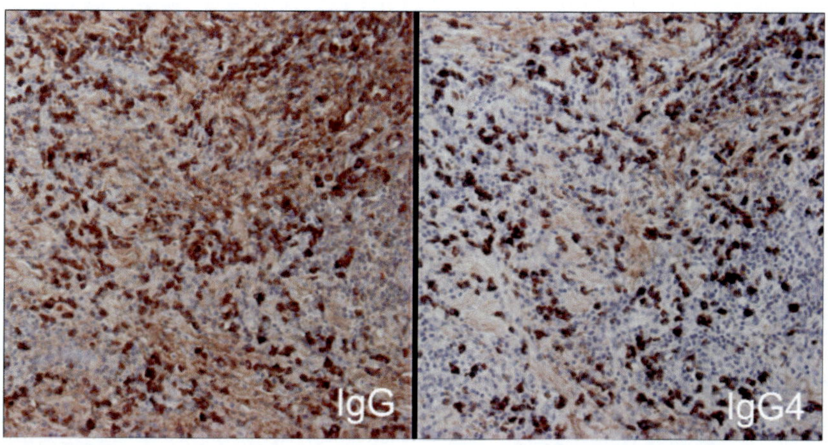

Figure 5. IgG- and IgG4-positive plasma cells in the aneurysmal wall of IgG4-related inflammatory abdominal aortic aneurysm. Immunostaining of IgG (left) reveals numerous IgG4-positive plasma cells, many of which are also positive for IgG4 (right). Both images, ×200. (adapted from ref. #10)

Laboratory and clinical data: As described above, the serum level of IgG4 and rate of association with other IgG4-related disease are high in cases of IgG4-related type. Age and sex did not differ between the IgG4-related and -unrelated type [15]. There have been no imaging data for the two types. Serum IgG4 concentrations were significantly increased in IgG4-related inflammatory AAA, though no such finding was evident in IgG4-unrelated inflammatory AAA and all atherosclerotic AAA. Serum levels of IgG, IgA, and IgM did not differ among IgG4-related inflammatory AAA, non– IgG4-related inflammatory AAA, and conventional AAA. The serum IgG4 concentration was usually elevated in IgG4-related inflammatory AAA, in some cases reaching the upper limit while in other being only slightly elevated. The incidence of ANA did not differ among IgG4-related and non-related inflammatory AAAs, and atherosclerotic AAA [15]. IgG4 is a useful marker for identifying AIP that can be effectively treated with corticosteroids, thus avoiding the need for surgery. Considering the histological similarity between IgG4-related and -unrelated inflammatory AAA, the serum IgG4 level might also be a preoperative diagnostic marker for all AAAs including inflammatory AAA.

Etiopathogenesis

Although the etiopathogenesis of inflammatory AAA may relate to inflammatory and immune response and also to fibrotic processes localized to the vessel wall of the abdominal aorta and surrounding connective tissue, the exact cause and mechanisms remain to be clarified. This disease may be a complex multifactorial disorder involving the interaction of infectious viral or bacterial agents, altered inflammatory/immune response including features of autoimmunity, and lipid oxidation [3,5,19,33]. Recent studies disclosed that inflammatory AAA could be subdivided into IgG4-related and IgG4-unrelated types, and the etiopathogenesis of the former should be discussed with respect to IgG4-related diseases. IgG4-unrelated inflammatory AAAs could be heterogeneous in their pathogenesis and some of them might correspond to atherosclerotic AAA with a relatively prominent inflammatory reaction [34].

A. Altered Immune Reactions and Autoimmune Etiology

Inflammatory AAA could be a rare disease with unusual immune and inflammatory reaction. Clinically, the presence of autoantibodies such as ANA, anti-smooth muscle antibodies, anti-thyroid microscome, and antineutrophil cytoplasmic antibodies [5,15,31,35], and an elevation of the serum IgG level are not uncommon findings in cases of chronic periaortitis including inflammatory AAA [4,15]. Histologically, the striking inflammatory reaction in the adventitia and to a lesser degree in the media involves plasma cells, lymphocytes, and macrophages [4,15,16]. Immunostaining in cases of inflammatory AAA revealed that the lymphocytes and plasma cells were polyclonal and composed of mostly B cells with lymphoid follicles and variable numbers of T cells in the aneurysmal wall [15]. On the other hand, IgA-positive or IgM-positive plasma cells were observed in either inflammatory AAA or atherosclerotic AAA.

Inflammatory AAA often affects patients with atherosclerosis, and several lines of evidence support the view that it could result from a local inflammatory reaction to antigens in the atherosclerotic plaques of the abdominal aorta such as oxidized-low density lipoproteins and ceroid. Such antigens could be related to the immune-mediated process of inflammatory AAA [4,32].

B. IgG4-Related Disease and Inflammatory AAA

Recent studies showed that in some cases, inflammatory AAA presents similar pathological and immunohistochemical features to IgG4-related diseases [11,15]. Retroperitoneal fibrosis and inflammatory AAA are related to each other, and belong to chronic periaortitis [18,19]. Interestingly, retroperitoneal fibrosis is now recognized as a IgG4-related disease and some inflammatory AAAs show a significant increase in the number of infiltrating IgG4-positive plasma cells. These findings suggest inflammatory AAA to be an aortic lesion reflecting a IgG4-related disease. [15-17,20,21]. Herein, the etiopathogenesis of inflammatory AAA will be discussed with regard to IgG4-related diseases and also chronic periaortitis.

Characteristics and spectrum of IgG4-related diseases: IgG4-related diseases are characterized histologically by a fibroproliferative change with many infiltrating lymphocytes and plasma cells and obliterative phlebitis [10,11]. Immunohistochemically, numerous IgG4-positive plasma cells are distributed diffusely within the lesions. The serum level of IgG4 is highly elevated in a majority of such patients [9]. AIP is a prototype of the IgG4-related diseases [13,36,37], and recent studies showed that such histologic and immunohistochemical features are identifiable in some cases of sclerosing cholangitis, chronic sclerosing sialadenitis, pulmonary or mammary inflammatory pseudotumor, pulmonary fibrosis, prostatitis, and mediastinal or retroperitoneal fibrosis, which are now regarded as IgG4-related diseases (*Figure 6*) [10,11]. More diseases are being nominated as candidates every year [38,39]. However, it remains to be clarified whether these diseases are variable and inconstant or protean manifestations of a single disease involving several organs or these diseases develop via common pathogenetic epiphenomena due to different etiologies.

Participation of regulatory T cell (Treg) abnormalities in the pathogenesis of IgG4-related diseases: IgG4 is the rarest of the IgG subclasses, accounting for only 3% to 6% of all the IgG in normal serum. IgG4 does not bind to complement (s) [40]. A high serum level of IgG4 is reported in a limited number of diseases including atopic dermatitis, bronchial asthma or related conditions, pemphigus vulgaris, and pemphigus foliaceus [41,42]. The pathologic significance of an elevated serum IgG4 level and numerous IgG4-positive plasma cells in the affected tissue in IgG4-related diseases has been unclear. Recently, we reported that the expression of Th2 (IL-4, IL-5, and IL-13) and regulatory cytokines (transforming growth factor-β [TGF-β] and IL-10) was increased in the affected tissue [43]. We speculated that IL-

10 is involved in increasing serum IgG4 concentrations and IgG4-positive plasma cell infiltration, because it has a major role in directing B cells to produce IgG4 [44]. TGF- β which is a powerful fibrogenic cytokine, might participate in fibroplasia. These cytokines may be related to increased number of Tregs in the affected tissues. Tregs are known to exert their functions through the modulation of both T and B cell responses, and IL-10-producing Treg can produce IL-10 [45]. We recently demonstrated that numbers of Tregs are actually increased in these lesions [43], and IL-10 and TGF- β might be released from theseTregs (*Figure 7*). The Tregs might have been generated to suppress the Th2-predominant environment in the affected tissue, though why Th2 predominates in this disease remains unclear. It is also possible that the target antigens involved in this Th2-predominant process differ among individual IgG4-related diseases in different organs. Miyoshi et al [46] also reported that increased numbers of $CD4^{+}CD25^{+}$ Tregs may influence IgG4 production in AIP, whereas decreased numbers of naïve Tregs may be involved in the pathogenesis of AIP.

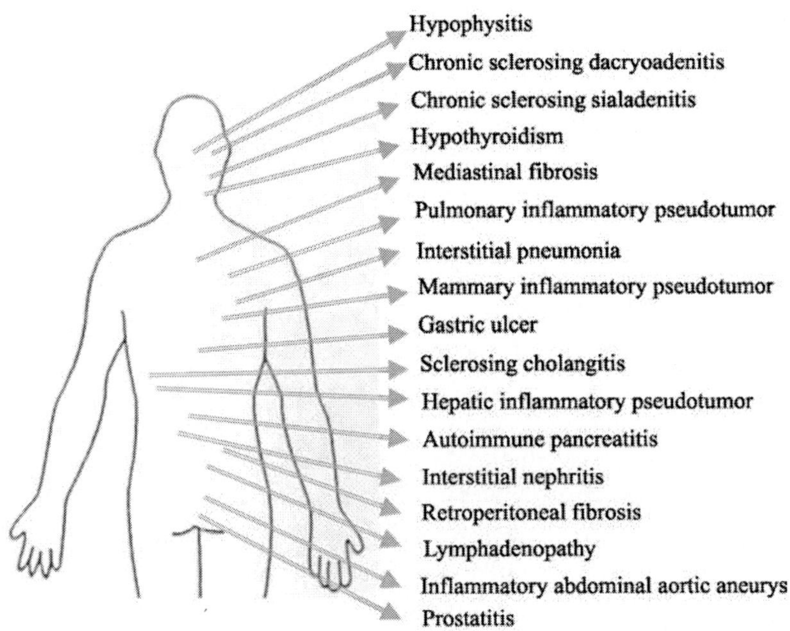

Figure 6. Systemic distribution of IgG4-related diseases.

C. Pathogenesis of IgG4-Realted Inflammatory AAA

Recently, we reported that about a half of all inflammatory AAAs belong to the spectrum of IgG4-related diseases [15]. Such patients have clinical features and histological characteristics similar to those of IgG4-related diseases. Interestingly, IgG4-related inflammatory AAA is not infrequently associated with other IgG4-related diseases such as AIP and chronic sclerosing sialadenitis, and such complications may develop simultaneously or metachronously during the course of inflammatory AAA. In contrast, such complications are not reported in IgG4-unrelated type of inflammatory AAA. This suggests IgG4-related inflammatory AAA to an abdominal aortic lesion reflecting IgG4-related disease. As for other IgG4-related diseases, the serum IgG4 level could be useful for the pre-operative differential diagnosis of inflammatory IAA.

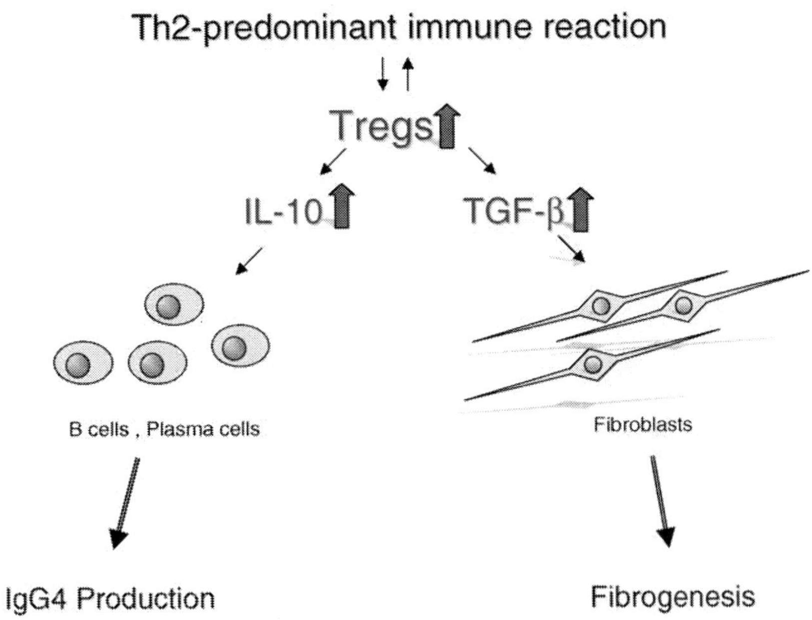

Figure 7. Hypothesis of the immunopathologenesis of IgG4-related diseases including inflammatory abdominal aortic aneurysm. Regulatory T-cells (Treg) and regulatory cytokines (IL-10 and TGF-β) might play central roles in the development of IgG4-related diseases. Tregs are induced and increased in the enviroment of a Th2-predominant reaction.

Given the Based similarity between inflammatory AAA and AIP or other IgG4-related diseases, a common pathogenetic process may be involved in these diseases. As described above, IgG4-related diseases are immunologically characterized by a Th2-dominant immune reaction and over-production of regulatory cytokines such as IL-10 and TGF-β by Tregs, resembling allergic disorders [41,43,46]. While the details of immune disturbance in inflammatory AAA remain to be clarified, an allergic hyper-immune reaction to antigen(s) in the arterial wall or peri-aorta connective tissue with a Th2-dominant reaction may result in IgG4-related inflammatory AAA probably via the proliferation of Tregs and over-secretion of Tregs-related cytokines.

Atheromatous changes found in inflammatory AAA seem to be a direct cause of inflammatory AAA. However, such changes could be an immunological trigger of inflammatory AAA or an aggravating factor for the dilatation of an aneurysm (see below). That is, inflammatory AAA may result from a local inflammatory reaction to antigen(s) in the atherosclerotic plaques of the abdominal aorta. Antibodies to atherosclerotic plaque antigens (e.g. oxidized-low density lipoproteins and ceroid) are reportedly detectable at higher titers in chronic periaortitis patients than in controls, and adventitial lipid-laden macrophages are found in aortic specimens of inflammatory AAA [4,32]. It remains, however, unclear whether such antibodies are of the IgG4 subclass or not. In addition, autoantibodies such as ANA and smooth muscle antibodies and antineutrophil cytoplasmic antibodies are detectable in inflammatory AAA patients [15,32]. It is also interesting that obliterative phlebitis is always observed in vein branches in the adventitia of the abdominal aorta [15,32]. The vasa vasorum of the aorta, which can show obliterative phlebitis, may participate in the pathogenesis of IgG4-related inflammatory AAA, though the exact contribution and significance of these vascular lesions are only unclear.

D. Pathogenesis of IgG4-Unrelated Inflammatory AAA

As described above, about a half of all patients with inflammatory AAA do not show intense IgG4-bearing plasma cells in the affected areas and do not have a high serum level of IgG4 [15]. A similar situation has been describe for chronic sclerosing cholangitis and sialadenitis [47-49]: some cases are associated with numerous IgG4-positive plasma cells and some are not, in spite of similar histopathological features in both groups. The distinction between IgG4-related and non-related types is clinically important, because the IgG4-related type could respond well to steroid therapy as reported for AIP and other IgG4-related diseases [9,36]. In contrast, the IgG4-unrelated type could be refractory to steroid therapy. The effectiveness of steroid therapy has also been reported for inflammatory AAA [3,24], and sensitivity to steroids might differ between IgG4-related and nonrelated inflammatory AAAs, though there have not been no such clinical studies using many cases. It seems necessary to classify IgG4-related inflammatory AAA using more sophisticated clinical methods or criteria [34].

The etiopathogenesis of IgG4-unrelated inflammatory AAA may be heterogeneous. That is, some IgG4-unrelated inflammatory AAAs might correspond to atherosclerotic AAA with relatively prominent chronic inflammation and adventitial fibrosis [3] or may be one phase during the natural course of IgG4-related inflammatory AAA. That is, recent evidence suggests that inflammatory AAAs arise from the same causal stimulus responsible for noninflammatory AAAs. Atherosclerosis usually occurs together with adventitial fibrosis and inflammation. Genetic and chemical factors such as smoking predispose certain individuals to noninflammatory AAAs and others to the extreme end of the inflammatory spectrum, inflammatory AAA [3]. Inflammatory AAA may develop in some individuals affected by advanced atherosclerosis of the abdominal aorta through a pathogenic B-cell response to locally presented antigens [34].

E. Relation to Chronic Periaortitis and Retroperitoneal Fibrosis

Inflammatory AAA belongs to a family of disorders often referred to as 'chronic periaortitis'. Chronic periaortitis commonly involves the infrarenal portion of the abdominal aorta. It's clinicopathological features are retroperitoneal fibrosis, inflammatory AAA and perianeurysmal retroperitoneal fibrosis, the latter being a combination of the former two [18,19,35]. Retroperitoneal fibrosis is known to cause non-specific symptoms and leads to the obstruction of the ureters and sometimes adjacent abdominal structures. When the ascending or thoracic aorta is involved, mediastinal fibrosis may develop.

Although these three disorders differ in their clinical presentation according to the degree and anatomical location of the pathological changes, their histopathological characteristics are identical: atherosclerosis of the abdominal aorta, chronic inflammatory infiltrates in the aortic adventitia, medial thinning in dilated or undilated aorta with varying degrees of periaortic fibrosis, and extension to involve adjacent structures. Altered inflammatory reactions and immunological disturbance, particularly autoimmunity, have been proposed as pathogenetic processes leading to chronic periaortitis [4,19,32], and in fact, chronic periaortitis is often associated with systemic autoimmune disorders such as rheumatoid arthritis, systemic lupus erythematosus and autoimmune thyroiditis suggesting that chronic periaortitis may be related to the autoimmune process [4-6,19]. An occasional association with HLA-DRB1*03 also supports this notion [6,49]. Interestingly, these associated conditions are different from IgG4-related diseases reported in other organs, suggesting that in some cases of inflammatory AAA, probably the IgG4-unrelated type, mechanisms common to systemic autoimmune diseases other than IgG4-related diseases may be operative.

Interestingly, retroperitoneal fibrosis was recently shown to have clinicopathological features similar to AIP and is occasionally associated with AIP and/or other IgG4-related diseases, so this disease is now recognized as an IgG4-related sclerosing disease [20,21]. IgG4-positive cells could also be identified in the retroperitoneum of those patients, suggesting that IgG4-related immune reactions occurred in the retroperitoneum. As described above, some patients with inflammatory AAA have clinicopathological features similar to IgG4-related disease. As described above, retroperitoneal fibrosis and inflammatory AAA, particularly with marked infiltration of IgG4-positive plasma cells, are forms of chronic periaortitis, so chronic periaortitis itself may belong to the same category of IgG4-related sclerosing diseases. However, there might be also inflammatory AAA and retroperitoneal fibrosis without predominant IgG4-positive plasma cells [15]. Therefore, it seems plausible that chronic periaortitis can be divided into IgG4-related and IgG4-unrelated types. The former belongs to the IgG4-related diseases, while the etiopathogenesis of the latter remains unclear.

F. Fibroplasia

Inflammatory AAA is associated with extensive fibrosis of the aneurismal wall and its surrounding tissues, and the wall is significantly thicker in cases of inflammatory AAA than atherosclerotic AAA. Increased number of myofibroblasts are important to such fibroplasia [29]. Interestingly, a significant increase in the expression of α-SMA was found in adventitial fibroblasts of inflammatory AAA compared to those of atherosclerotic AAA [29]. These results suggest that myofibroblasts are significantly involved in the development of inflammatory AAA. In fact, the cell density and MIB-1 index of adventitial myofibroblasts are significantly higher in inflammatory AAA than in atherosclerotic AAA [29]. As for the mechanisms of myofibroblastic proliferation, hypoxia-inducible factor 1alpha is reportedly involved and is actually expressed in the cytoplasm or nucleus of adventitial myofibroblasts in inflammatory AAA [29]. A recent report described that sclerosing angiomatoid nodular transformation (SANT) of the spleen is another type of IgG4-related disease, and 20-30% of the myofibroblasts were positive for Epstein-Barr-virus (EBV) [38]. This group suggested that EBV-infected myofibroblasts may be also responsible for fibroplasias of IgG4-related disease, though relevant data is not available for inflammatory AAA. Furthermore, a role for matrix metalloproteinases in the pathogenesis of abdominal aortic aneurysm is also speculated [33].

G. Infectious Etiology

Several microorganisms have been suggested as possible factors contributing to the development and/or expansion of AAAs including inflammatory AAAs, though the data are still controversial [50,51].

Chlamydia (C.) pneumoniae: Chronic C. pneumoniae infection has been suggested to contribute the development and/or expansion of AAA. Immunohistochemical staining revealed C. pneumoniae antigenic components in inflammatory cells including macrophages and T-lymphocytes in atherosclerotic plaques of patients with inflammatory AAA. Serological markers of chronic C. pneumoniae infection were more frequently found in AAA patients than in healthy controls [8]. Recently, C. pneumoniae infection was shown to be closely associated with AAA, and to be an important factor in the aneurysmal formation and dilatation in cases of AAA. These findings indicate C. pneumoniae infection to be an important mediator that accentuates the inflammatory response in the abdominal aorta leading to aneurysmal development, and to be involved in the pathogenesis of inflammatory AAA [52].

Cytomegalovirus (CMV): CMV infection is suspected of being involved in inflammatory AAAs [53-55]. Immediate early gene expression of human CMV was shown to be prevalent in IAAA by solution-phase PCR and reverse transcription PCR, respectively, suggesting that this virus plays a role in chronic inflammatory reactions in inflammatory AAA [56]. In the fibrously thickened adventitia of patients with inflammatory AAA, CMV infected cells were more frequent than in that in cases of atherosclerotic AAA or control cases. CMV-infected cells were mainly identified as macrophages, fibroblasts, endothelial cells, and lymphocytes. The expression of CMV immediate early mRNA, which suggests an active infection triggering an active inflammatory reaction, was detected in most of the macrophages, endothelial cells, and fibroblasts. These results suggest that frequent and active infections of CMV plays a significant role in the induction and acceleration of chronic inflammatory reactions in inflammatory AAA [56].

Other Vascular Lesions Related to IgG4-Related Disease

Recently, we experienced a case (67 yrs, female) of pseudotumor of the right coronary artery [57]. Echocardiography revealed a cardiac tumorous mass, and coronary arteriography revealed an almost normal flow of the right coronary artery. During surgery, an elastic hard mass was found around the mid portion of the right coronary artery, and then, the mass lesion was completely resected. The mass was found to contain diffuse lymphoplasmacytic infiltrates and fibrosis, and immunostaining of IgG showed diffusely distributed IgG-positive plasma cells, many of which were also positive for IgG4. In addition, obliterative phlebitis was observed. The intima showed mild histological changes such as fibrous thickening. Pathologically and immunopathologically, coronary arterial lesions are similar to the lesions in cases of IgG4-related disease, and can be called IgG4-related periarteritis of the right coronary artery. This case was also associated with IgG4-related inflammatory AAA, suggesting that IgG4-related disease could occur in the vascular system other than the abdominal aorta, and manifest as an aneurysm or peri-arterial mass. So, one should also be aware of whether or not IgG4-related diseases can manifest as vascular lesions other than aneurismal or tumorous lesions.

Conclusion

Inflammatory AAA is characterized by dense fibrosis and extensive lymphoplasmacytic infiltration of the aortic wall, particularly its adventitia and surrounding connective tissue. A subgroup of patients with inflammatory AAA show numerous infiltrating IgG4-positive plasma cells and high serum IgG4 concentrations. Based on these findings, inflammatory AAA could be subdivided into IgG4-related and IgG4-unrelated types. The former may be an aortic manifestation of IgG4-related sclerosing disease, and may respond well to corticosteroid therapy. The pathogenesis of the latter remains unclear, and some cases may be atherosclerotic AAA with relatively prominent inflammatory changes. It was recently reported that retroperitoneal fibrosis is related to IgG4-related diseases. Retroperitoneal fibrosis and inflammatory AAA constitute chronic periaortitis, so IgG4-related periaortitis could be proposed for these pathologic conditions. Recently, IgG4-related tumorous lesions around the coronary artery were reported, suggesting that IgG4-related diseases could occur in the vascular system, and manifest as an aneurysm or peri-arterial mass. Further clinical analysis seems mandatory to elucidate the possibility of other vascular manifestation(s) of IgG4-related disease.

References

[1] Walker, DI; Bloor, K; Williams, G; Gillie, I. Inflammatory aneurysms of the abdominal aorta. *Br J Surg*., 1972, 59, 609-14

[2] Pennell, RC; Hollier, LH; Lie, JT; Bernatz, PE; Joyce, JW; Pairolero, PC; Cherry, KJ; Hallett, JW. Inflammatory abdominal aortic aneurysms: a thirty-year review. *J Vasc Surg.*, 1985, 2, 859-69.

[3] Rasmussen, TE; Hallett, JW Jr. Inflammatory aortic aneurysms. A clinical review with new perspectives in pathogenesis. *Ann Surg.*, 1997, 225, 155-64.

[4] Parums, DV. The spectrum of chronic periaortitis. *Histopathology*, 1990, 16, 423-31.

[5] Vaglio, A; Corradi, D; Manenti L; Ferretti, S; Garini G; Buzio C. Evidence of autoimmunity in chronic periaortitis: a prospective study. *Am J Med.*, 2003, 114, 454-62.

[6] Vaglio, A; Palmisano, A; Ferretti, S; Alberici, F; Casazza, I; Salvarani, C; Buzio, C. Peripheral inflammatory arthritis in patients with chronic periaortitis: report of five cases and review of the literature. Rheumatology (Oxford). 2008, 47, 315-8.

[7] Vaglio, A; Greco, P; Corradi, D; Palmisano, A; Martorana, D; Ronda, N; Buzio, C. Autoimmune aspects of chronic periaortitis. *Autoimmun Rev.*, 2006, 5, 458-64.

[8] Mazur, E; Niedwiadek, J; Wolski, A; Siezieniewska-Skowrońska, Z; Zywick, W; Korolczuk, A; Korobowicz, E; Kozioł-Montewka, M. Chlamydia pneumoniae infection in abdominal aortic aneurysm (AAA) patients and its clinical impact. *Pol J Pathol*, 2004, 55, 155-64.

[9] Hamano, H; Kawa, S; Horiuchi, A; Unno, H; Furuya, N; Akamatsu, T; Fukushima, M; Nikaido, T; Nakayama, K; Usuda, N; Kiyosawa, K. High serum IgG4 concentrations in patients with sclerosing pancreatitis. *N Engl J Med.*, 2001, 344, 732-8.

[10] Kamisawa, T; Funata, N; Hayashi, Y; Tsuruta, K; Okamoto, A; Amemiya, K; Egawa, N; Nakajima, H. Close relationship between autoimmune pancreatitis and multifocal fibrosclerosis. *Gut.*, 2003, 52, 683-7.

[11] Nakanuma, Y; Zen, Y. Pathology and immunopathology of immunoglobulin G4-related sclerosing cholangitis: The latest addition to the sclerosing cholangitis family. *Hepatol Res.*, 2007 Oct., 37 Suppl., 3, S478-86.

[12] Kawaguchi, K; Koike, M; Tsuruta, K; Okamoto, A; Tabata, I; Fujita, N. Lymphoplasmacytic sclerosing pancreatitis with cholangitis: a variant of primary sclerosing cholangitis extensively involving pancreas. *Hum Pathol.*, 1991, 22, 387-95.

[13] Yoshida, K; Toki, F; Takeuchi, T; Watanabe, S; Shiratori, K; Hayashi, N. Chronic pancreatitis caused by an autoimmune abnormality. Proposal of the concept of autoimmune pancreatitis. *Dig Dis Sci.*, 1995, 40, 1561-8.

[14] Wakabayashi, T; Kawaura, Y; Satomura, Y; Fujii, T; Motoo, Y; Okai, T; Sawabu, N. Clinical study of chronic pancreatitis with focal irregular narrowing of the main pancreatic duct and mass formation: comparison with chronic pancreatitis showing diffuse irregular narrowing of the main pancreatic duct. *Pancreas*, 2002, 25, 283-9.

[15] Kasashima, S; Zen, Y; Kawashima, A; Konishi, K; Sasaki, H; Endo, M; Matsumoto, Y; Kawakami, K; Kasashima, F; Moriya, M; Kimura, K; Ohtake, H; Nakanuma, Y. Inflammatory abdominal aortic aneurysm: close relationship to IgG4-related periaortitis. *Am J Surg Pathol.*, 2008, 32, 197-204.

[16] Sakata, N; Tashiro, T; Uesugi, N; Kawara, T; Furuya, K; Hirata, Y; Iwasaki, H; Kojima, M. IgG4-positive plasma cells in inflammatory abdominal aortic aneurysm: the

possibility of an aortic manifestation of IgG4-related sclerosing disease. *Am J Surg Pathol*, 2008, 32, 553-9.

[17] Ito, H; Kaizaki, Y; Noda, Y; Fujii, S; Yamamoto, S. IgG4-related inflammatory abdominal aortic aneurysm associated with autoimmune pancreatitis. *Pathol Int.*, 2008, 58, 421-6.

[18] Jois, RN; Gaffney, K; Marshall, T; Scott, DG. Chronic periaortitis. *Rheumatology (Oxford)*, 2004, 43, 1441-6.

[19] Vaglio, A; Greco, P; Corradi, D; Palmisano, A; Martorana D; Ronda N; Buzio C. Autoimmune aspects of chronic periaortitis. *Autoimmun Rev.*, 2006 , 5, 458-64.

[20] Zen Y; Sawazaki A; Miyayama S; Notsumata K; Tanaka N; Nakanuma Y. A case of retroperitoneal and mediastinal fibrosis exhibiting elevated levels of IgG4 in the absence of sclerosing pancreatitis (autoimmune pancreatitis). *Hum Pathol.*, 2006, 37, 239-43.

[21] Taniguchi, T; Kobayashi, H; Fukui, S; Ogura, K; Saiga, T; Okamoto, M. A case of multifocal fibrosclerosis involving posterior mediastinal fibrosis; retroperitoneal fibrosis; and a left seminal vesicle with elevated serum IgG4. *Hum Pathol*, 2006, 37, 1237-9.

[22] Baker, LR; Mallinson, WJ; Gregory, MC; Menzies, EA; Cattell, WR; Whitfield, HN; Hendry, WF; Wickham, JE; Joekes, AM. Idiopathic retroperitoneal fibrosis. A retrospective analysis of 60 cases. *Br J Urol,* 1987, 60, 497-503.

[23] Dhareshwar, J; Estrera, AL; Covinsky, MH; Safi, HJ. Inflammatory aneurysm of the ascending aorta. *Eur J Cardiothorac Surg*., 2006, 30, 806-7.

[24] Warnatz, K; Keskin, AG; Uhl, M; Scholz, C; Katzenwadel, A; Vaith, P; Peter, HH; Walker, UA. Immunosuppressive treatment of chronic periaortitis: a retrospective study of 20 patients with chronic periaortitis and a review of the literature. *Ann Rheum Dis.,* 2005, 64, 828-33.

[25] Sueyoshi, E; Sakamoto, I; Uetani, M. Endovascular repair of inflammatory abdominal aortic aneurysm: serial changes of periaortic fibrosis demonstrated by CT. *Abdom Imaging*, 2008 (in press)

[26] Pipitone, N; Ghinoi, A; Versari, A; Vaglio, A; Palmisano, A; Salvarani, C. Images in cardiovascular medicine. *Chronic periaortitis. Circulation,* 2008, 118, 1214-6.

[27] Salvarani, C; Pipitone, N; Versari, A; Vaglio, A; Serafini, D; Bajocchi, G; Salvo, D; Buzio, C; Greco, P; Boiardi, L. Positron emission tomography (PET): evaluation of chronic periaortitis. *Arthritis Rheum*, 2005, 53, 298-303.

[28] Truijers, M; Kurvers, HA; Bredie, SJ; Oyen, WJ; Blankensteijn JD. In vivo imaging of abdominal aortic aneurysms: increased FDG uptake suggests inflammation in the aneurysm wall. *J Endovasc Ther*., 2008, 15, 462-7.

[29] Sakata, N; Nabeshima, K; Iwasaki, H; Tashiro, T; Uesugi, N; Nakashima, O; Ito H, Kawanami, T; Furuya, K; Kojima, M. Possible involvement of myofibroblast in the development of inflammatory aortic aneurysm. *Pathol Res Pract.,* 2007, 203, 21-9.

[30] Nitecki, SS; Hallett, JW, Jr; Stanson, AW; Ilstrup, DM; Bower, TC; Cherry, KJ; Jr; Gloviczki, P; Pairolero, PC. Inflammatory abdominal aortic aneurysms: a case-control study. *J Vasc Surg.,* 1996, 23, 860–8.

[31] Kaipiainen-Seppänen, O; Jantunen, E; Kuusisto, J; Marin, S. Retroperitoneal fibrosis with antineutrophil cytoplasmic antibodies. *J Rheumatol*, 1996, 23, 779-81.

[32] Parums, DV; Brown, DL; Mitchinson, MJ. Serum antibodies to oxidized low-density lipoprotein and ceroid in chronic periaortitis. *Arch Pathol Lab Med.*, 1990, 114, 383-7.

[33] Pearce, WH; Shively, VP. Abdominal aortic aneurysm as a complex multifactorial disease: interactions of polymorphisms of inflammatory genes; features of autoimmunity, and current status of MMPs. *Ann N Y Acad Sci.,* 2006, 1085, 117-32.

[34] Pasquinelli, G; Preda, P; Gargiulo, M; Vici, M; Cenacchi, G; Stella, A; D'Addato, M; Martinelli, GN; Pileri, S. An immunohistochemical study of inflammatory abdominal aortic aneurysms. *J Submicrosc Cytol Pathol.*, 1993, 25, 103-12.

[35] Moroni, G; Del Papa, N; Moronetti, LM; Vitali, C; Maglione, W; Comina, DP; Urgnani, F; Sandri, S; Ponticelli, C; Cortelezzi, A. Increased levels of circulating endothelial cells in chronic periaortitis as a marker of active disease. *Kidney Int.*, 2005, 68, 562-8.

[36] Okazaki, K. Is IgG4-associated multifocal systemic fibrosis the same disease entity as autoimmune pancreatitis? *Intern Med.*, 2007, 46, 117-8.

[37] Okazaki, K; Uchida, K; Fukui, T. Recent advances in autoimmune pancreatitis: concept, diagnosis, and pathogenesis. *J Gastroenterol.*, 2008, 43, 409-18.

[38] Kashiwagi, S; Kumasaka, T; Bunsei, N; Fukumura, Y; Yamasaki, S; Abe, K; Mitani, K; Abe, H; Matsumoto, T; Suda, K. Detection of Epstein-Barr virus-encoded small RNA-expressed myofibroblasts and IgG4-producing plasma cells in sclerosing angiomatoid nodular transformation of the spleen. *Virchows Arch.*, 2008, 453, 275-82.

[39] Chen, TS; Montgomery, EA. Are tumefactive lesions classified as sclerosing mesenteritis a subset of IgG4-related sclerosing disorders? *J Clin Pathol.,* 2008, 61, 1093-7.

[40] Oxelius, VA. Immunoglobulin constant heavy G subclass chain genes in asthma and allergy. *Immunol Res.*, 2008, 40, 179-91.

[41] Jarvis, D; Zock, JP; Heinrich, J; Svanes, C; Verlato, G; Olivieri, M; Villani, S; Ponzio, M; Leynaert, B; Sunyer, J; Dahlman-Hoglund, A; Chinn, S; Luczynska, C; Norbäck, D; Burney, P. Cat and dust mite allergen levels, specific IgG and IgG4, and respiratory symptoms in adults. *J Allergy Clin Immunol.*, 2007, 119, 697-704.

[42] Sitaru, C; Mihai, S; Zillikens, D. The relevance of the IgG subclass of autoantibodies for blister induction in autoimmune bullous skin diseases. *Arch Dermatol Res.,* 2007, 299, 1-8.

[43] Zen, Y; Fujii, T; Harada, K; Kawano, M; Yamada, K; Takahira, M; Nakanuma, Y. Th2 and regulatory immune reactions are increased in immunoglobin G4-related sclerosing pancreatitis and cholangitis. *Hepatology.* 2007, 45, 1538-46.

[44] Satoguina, JS; Weyand, E; Larbi, J; Hoerauf, A. T regulatory-1 cells induce IgG4 production by B cells: role of IL-10. *J Immunol.* 2005, 174, 4718-26.

[45] Satoguina, JS; Adjobimey, T; Arndts, K; Hoch, J; Oldenburg, J; Layland, LE; Hoerauf, A. Tr1 and naturally occurring regulatory T cells induce IgG4 in B cells through GITR/GITR-L interaction, IL-10 and TGF-beta. *Eur J Immunol,* 2008 (in press)

[46] Miyoshi, H; Uchida, K; Taniguchi, T; Yazumi, S; Matsushita, M; Takaoka, M; Okazaki, K. Circulating naïve and CD4+CD25high regulatory T cells in patients with autoimmune pancreatitis. *Pancreas*. 2008, 36, 133-40.

[47] Kitagawa, S; Zen, Y; Harada, K; Sasaki, M; Sato, Y; Minato, H; Watanabe, K; Kurumaya, H; Katayanagi, K; Masuda, S; Niwa, H; Tsuneyama, K; Saito, K; Haratake, J; Takagawa, K; Nakanuma, Y. Abundant IgG4-positive plasma cell infiltration characterizes chronic sclerosing sialadenitis (Küttner's tumor). *Am J Surg Pathol.*, 2005, 29, 783-91.

[48] Martorana, D; Vaglio, A; Greco, P; Zanetti, A; Moroni, G; Salvarani, C; Savi, M; Buzio, C; Neri, TM. Chronic periaortitis and HLA-DRB1*03: another clue to an autoimmune origin. *Arthritis Rheum*. 2006, 55, 126-30.

[49] Portman, BC; Nakanuma, Y. Diseases of bile ducts. In: Pathology of the Liver (Eds. MacSween RNM; Burt, AD; Portman, BC; Ishak, KG; Scheuer, PJ; Anthody PP) Churchill Livingstone 4th ed., London et al, 2001 pp. 435-506.

[50] Sharif, MA; Soong, CV; Lee B; McCallion K; Hannon RJ. Inflammatory infrarenal abdominal aortic aneurysm in a young woman. *J Emerg Med.*, 2008, 34, 147-50.

[51] Nyberg, A; Skagius, E; Englund, E; Nilsson, I; Ljungh, A; Henriksson, AE. Abdominal aortic aneurysm and the impact of infectious burden. *Eur J Vasc Endovasc Surg.*, 2008, 36, 292-6.

[52] Takemoto, M; Takigami, C; Sakamoto, M; Nakano, R. Inflammatory abdominal aortic aneurysm and Chlamydia pneumoniae infection. *Int J Cardiol.*, 2005, 100, 509-10.

[53] Nyberg A; Skagius E; Nilsson I; Ljungh A; Henriksson AE. Abdominal aortic aneurysm and cytomegalovirus infection. *J Med Virol.*, 2008, 80, 667-9.

[54] Nyberg, A; Skagius, E; Nilsson, I; Ljungh, A; Henriksson, AE. Abdominal aortic aneurysm and infection with CagA positive strains of Helicobacter pylori. *Scand J Infect Dis.*, 2008, 40, 204-7.

[55] Nyberg, A; Skagius, E; Nilsson, I; Ljungh, A; Henriksson, AE. Lack of association between Chlamydophila pneumoniae seropositivity and abdominal aortic aneurysm. *Vasc Endovascular Surg.*, 2007, 41, 246-8.

[56] Yonemitsu, Y; Nakagawa, K; Tanaka, S; Mori, R; Sugimachi, K; Sueishi, K. In situ detection of frequent and active infection of human cytomegalovirus in inflammatory abdominal aortic aneurysms: possible pathogenic role in sustained chronic inflammatory reaction. *Lab Invest.*, 1996, 74, 723-36.

[57] Matsumoto, Y; Kasashima, S; Kawashima, A; Sasaki, H; Endo, M; Kawakami, K; Zen, Y; Nakanuma, Y. A case of multiple immunoglobulin G4-related periarteritis: a tumorous lesion of the coronary artery and abdominal aortic aneurysm. *Hum Pathol.*, 2008, 39, 975-80.

In: Aneurysms: Types, Risks, Formation and Treatment
Editors: Alain Laurent and Ethan Morel
ISBN: 978-1-60741-557-2
© 2009 Nova Science Publishers, Inc.

Chapter 7

Rupture of Abdominal Aneurysms during Pregnancy

Mathieu Poilblanc [1*], *Loïc Sentilhes* [1], *Céline Lefèbvre-Lacoeuille* [1], *Philippe Gillard* [1], *Alain Fournié* [1], *Claude Clément* [2] *and Philippe Descamps* [1]
[1]Department of Obstetrics and Gynecology, University Hospital of Angers, 4 rue Larrey, 49033 Angers, France (Faculty of Medicine of Angers, France).
[2]Department of Vascular Surgery, University Hospital of Rheims, rue Cognacq-Jay, 51100 Rheims, France (Faculty of Medicine of Reims, France).

Summary

The rupture of an arterial aneurysm during pregnancy is a rare event and can potentially be lethal. It is a difficult clinical situation with likely consequences for the maternal and fetal prognosis and it requires immediate and multidisciplinary treatment.

This chapter describes the physiopathology, clinical features, diagnostic methods and therapeutic principles of aneurysmal ruptures of the splenic, renal and ovarian arteries during pregnancy and postpartum.

In previous studies, it has been estimated that 50% of the ruptures of arterial aneurysms in women under 40 are linked to pregnancy [1]. Many elements suggest that pregnancy is involved in the formation and rupture of aneurysms. These mechanisms are still poorly understood, but it seems that the hemodynamic and hormonal modifications caused by the gestation are preponderant factors [2].

In a pregnant women, two-thirds of the ruptures of aneurysms happen during the third trimester and the postpartum period [3,4]. In the abdomen, these ruptures most often take place on the aorta, splenic artery, renal arteries, ovarian arteries [1] and uterine arteries.

*Corresponding author: Mathieu Poilblanc, University Hospital of Angers – France; Department of Obstetrics and Gynecology, 4 rue Larrey, 49 033. Angers, France. mpoilblanc@yahoo.fr

Most of the aneurysms are asymptomatic until their rupture [5]. The clinical presentation of the rupture is nonspecific. When it happens during the third trimester of the pregnancy, the rupture of an aneurysm can be a dangerous trap and mislead the obstetrical team to a diagnosis of placental abruption or uterine rupture [2,3,6-8]. Ultrasound examination, CT scan and abdominal arteriography are the main diagnostic means to confirm the presence and the rupture of an aneurysm.

When the rupture happens at the end of the pregnancy and in the presence of signs of hemodynamic instability, resuscitation measures and the realisation of a caesarean section as a matter of urgency, together with an exploratory laparotomy, will have to be carried out without delay. As Pfannenstiel incision does not allow suitably satisfactory access to the sub-mesocolic level, a median longitudinal laparotomy will have to be realised immediately if there is an active hemorrhage causing hemodynamic instability and whose origin remains unexplained after exploring the sub-mesocolic level. The standard reference treatment remains the surgical resection of the aneurysm. Some authors report cases of selective embolisation of the sites of the ruptures, especially for aneurysms of the ovarian arteries [3,9,10]. This therapeutic option seems attractive when the symptomatology occurs during the postpartum period in a stable patient.

1. Introduction

The rupture of an aneurysm during pregnancy is a rare event marked by a high maternal and fetal mortality. The mechanism of the apparition of an aneurysm and those leading to its rupture are still poorly understood, but it seems that the hormonal and hemodynamic modifications observed in a pregnant woman are preponderant factors.

This chapter describes the physiopathology, clinical presentation, diagnostic methods and therapeutic strategies of aneurysmal ruptures of the renal, splenic and ovarian arteries during pregnancy and postpartum.

2. Epidemiology

As most aneurysms are asymptomatic, the actual incidence of the aneurysm/pregnancy association is difficult to determine [5,11,12]. It is, however, a rare clinical situation. In the general population, the prevalence of splenic artery aneurysms ranges from 0.1% [13] to 10% according to different studies [11,14].

It is very difficult to know whether or not the rupture is occurring on a vascular malformation anterior to the pregnancy. In the past, most abdominal aneurysms were discovered during their ruptures or on autopsic series [12]. At present, with the generalisation of imagery techniques such as CT scan or ultrasound examination, an increasing number of asymptomatic aneurysms are diagnosed by chance during the exploration of biliary or renal colic, for example [15,17]. Around 70% of the aneurysms of the splenic artery calcify and appear on pictures of the abdomen without preparation as a calcified ring with a central lucent area to the left of the first lumbar vertebral body [18]. Their presence can thus be detected without any rupture.

In the case of a rupture occurring during the pregnancy, the global materno-fetal mortality is estimated at around 75% on average [11] with, according to different studies, the highest rates reaching 90%, especially in the case of a rupture of the splenic artery [19].

At the abdomen, the aneurysmal ruptures associated with a pregnancy happen preferentially on the aorta, the splenic artery, the renal and the ovarian arteries [1]. In a review of the literature dated 2003, Selo and Welsh report about a hundred cases of ruptures of aneurysms situated on the splenic artery [5]. In 2006, Solimane et al. counted about 30 cases of ruptures on the renal arteries [7] and a more recent analysis, published in 2008, finds a dozen cases localised on the ovarian arteries [3].

Some rare cases of spontaneous ruptures of aneurysms involving the uterine arteries have been described in Anglo-Saxon literature [20]. At the moment, most of the published cases reports regarding the rupture of false aneurysms of the uterine arteries are of post-traumatic origin, following a vascular wound during a caesarean section.

3. Physiopathology

The etiology of the aneurysms remains unclear [6]. Yet, for all preponderant causes, the final vascular lesion is a local alteration of the connective tissue of the arterial wall [5]. The result of this is a defect in the integrity of the wounded vessel, which is the essential beginning of the formation of an aneurysm.

In the past, many abdominal aneurysms had a syphilitic or mycotic origin [12]. Nowadays, we consider the main non-traumatic risk factors to be pregnancy [11,22,23], atherosclerosis, fibromuscular dysplasia, local inflammatory conditions such as peptic ulcer disease or pancreatitis [11], angiodysplasia, diabetes, hypertension and alpha-1-antitryspine deficiency [6,24]. According to Barrett et al., around 50% of the ruptures of aneurysms in women under 40 are linked to pregnancy [1].

In 1942, Trimble and Hill mentioned the combination of two general and complementary factors at the origin of the apparition of an aneurysm: on one side the fragility of the vascular wall, and on the other side, the increase in the arterial pressure [25]. This pathophysiological model—which is still valid today—is entirely applicable to the vascular and hemodynamic modifications observed during the pregnancy.

3.1. Vascular Modifications Linked to Pregnancy

The increase in estrogen and progesterone rates during the gestation is the origin of alterations to the structure of the vascular walls. In 1967, Manalo-Estrola and Barrer proved the existence of specific alterations to the reticular substance and to the arterial elastic tissue during pregnancy [26].

Estrogen and progesterone modify the structure of the internal elastic lamina by means of hormonal receptors to steroids located on the smooth muscle structure of the arteries, and provoke a fragmentation of the elastic fibres [5]. According to some authors, the physiological secretion of relaxin observed during pregnancy may cause an increase in these effects.

Moreover, other histological abnormalities have been accounted for such as the sub-endothelial thickening, the apparition of a fibrodysplasia among the medial layer or an accumulation of the glycoaminoglycans in the arterial walls [6]. All these lesions lead to the apparition of areas of vascular fragility whose intensity becomes maximal at the third trimester [10]. During the postpartum period, these areas recede spontaneously and reappear during subsequent pregnancies. The more the parity increases, the less the restitution ad integrum occurs and the more the vascular fragility settles [5,10]. As a result, multiparity appears as a risk factor for the apparition and rupture of an aneurysm located on the ovarian or the uterine arteries.

At the same time as these histological modifications, the ovarian and uterine arteries undergo important anatomical and mechanical variations following the progressive increase in the volume of the uterus. The involution observed during the postpartum can lead to the apparition of tortuous and fragile arterial segments, as Burnett et al. suggest. These zones may be involved in the formation of aneurysms during a subsequent pregnancy which could also explain partly the increase in the occurrences of aneurismal ruptures in multiparous women, especially on ovarian arteries [2,27].

3.2. Hemodynamic Modifications Linked to the Pregnancy

In addition to these transitory alterations, there are physiological hemodynamic modifications, essential to the vascularisation, to the utero-placental perfusion and to the harmonious development of the foetus. The cardiac output increases by around 1.5L per minute from the first weeks of the pregnancy. This increase will persist until the end of the pregnancy when the debit reaches around 6L per minute on average [28].

The changes in the renal function observed in pregnant women provoke an important volumic growth. Thus the volume of plasmatic blood increases by more than 50% over the 3 trimesters.

However, the peripheral arterial resistances are considerably diminished (by around 21%) [28] because of the pergravidic production of estrogen and prostaglandin, of cardial natriuretic factors or because of the action of the relaxin secreted by the corpus luteum [30]. As a result, there is a vasodilatation (decrease in the post-charge) which balances the increase in the cardiac output and in the volume of circulating blood (increase in the pre-charge) which leads to a relative stability of the average arterial pressure. When these mechanisms of compensations are defective or unable to cope, hypertension can appear and potentially be the cause of the onset of an aneurism.

The increase in the uterine volume progressively leads to a portal hypertension which is possibly responsible for the formation of aneurysms located on the splenic artery.

4. Clinical Presentation of the Ruptures of Aneurysms during Pregnancy

4.1. Generalities

Wherever they are located, most aneurysms which are not ruptured are totally asymptomatic. However, some signs, attributed to the probable increase in the size of the aneurysm preceding its rupture, seem to be found, such as intermittent pains, bouts of nausea or even vomiting [22].

More often than not, the aneurysm only expresses itself by its rupture. This preferentially happens during the third trimester of the pregnancy (in about 70% of the cases) and brutally [31].

The clinical presentation of this rupture is non-specific [3,17]. Apart from possible bouts of nausea and vomiting, the predominant symptom remains the pain which can appear brutally or in a sporadic manner. The initial localisation of the pain will be different according to the site of the rupture [11]. Thus the rupture of an aneurysm of the splenic artery will show by the apparition of a pain in the left upper abdomen, with a possible irradiation towards the left shoulder (Sign of Kehr) [6]. A lumbar pain will guide towards a rupture located on the renal artery and a pelvic pain towards an ovarian location. In the case of a rupture of the renal artery, some authors also report the apparition of a haematuria [4].

Other signs appear more or less quickly at the same time as the pain: there are signs of hemodynamic instability, then signs of shock, linked to the apparition of a hemoperitoneal collection in the case of the rupture of the splenic artery or of a retroperitoneal hematoma following the rupture of a renal or ovarian artery. When the symptomatology occurs in peripartum, abnormalities of the fetal heart rate, in line with a secondary hypoxemia are observed. The suspicion of fetal hypoxemia often appears before the maternal shock as the mechanisms of hemodynamic adaptation reduce precociously the placental vascularisation [5, 22]. This vasoconstriction to the detriment of the foetus explains partly the difference which can be observed between the maternal and the fetal mortality. According to Hillemans, in the case of rupture of the splenic artery, these rates are respectively 75% and 95% [31].

4.2. The Double-Rupture Phenomenon in the Case of Splenic Artery Aneurysm

Around a fourth of the aneurysmal ruptures of the splenic artery occur according to this mode of rupture in *two phases* [32]. This phenomenon was initially described by Brockman [33] in 1930 and is explained by the anatomic position of the splenic artery and by its links with the peritoneal folds. When the rupture appears the effusion of blood is collected at the back of the pancreas and the stomach, at the level of the lesser sac. The formation of clots inside this cavity leads to a temporary obstruction of the foramen of Winslow confining the hematoma at the back of the pancreas. This first phase is often accompanied by abdominal pains of varying intensity: these are real signs of alarm. After a few hours, even a few days, the pressure rises in the lesser sac and clots and blood then go through the foramen of

Winslow or the pars flacida of the omentum. The rupture becomes complete and hemoperitoneal collection and signs of shock appear. When the diagnosis is made during the first phase, the chances of survival of the mother and foetus are increased, probably because the intervention can be prepared in better conditions [5].

4.3. Differential Diagnoses

The aneurysmal rupture is a real diagnostic trap, especially when it happens at the end of the pregnancy. The lack of knowledge and the rarity of this ailment often induce a delay in the care and explain the high mortality rate [22]. Indeed, even in the case of a complete symptomatology, diagnoses of placental abruption or of uterine rupture are wrongly made as they are more frequent [3,6,22]. The absence of metrorrhagia must raise suspicions, and without delaying the obstetrical care, other diagnostic hypotheses must be considered. During a caesarean section, the absence of placental abruption or of uterine rupture demands a more accurate peritoneal exploration, because if the presence of a hemoperitoneal collection is simple to objectivise, the retroperitoneal hematoma is more difficult to diagnose. In 1999, Fender et al. reported the case of an aneurysmal rupture of the splenic artery in peripartum, the clinical signs of which were initially hidden by an epidural anesthesia [32].

When it occurs outside labour or postpartum, the abdominal pain can suggest a peptic ulcer disease, a pancreatitis, a cholecystitis or an acute renal colic [34].

5. Radiological Investigations

The radiological investigations which are necessary to confirm the diagnosis and if it is the case, to locate the aneurysm must not delay its therapeutic care [6]. Whether these complementary tests will be carried out depends on the hemodynamic state to the mother and on the fetal heart rate. Schematically two situations are possible.

When the rupture occurs during pregnancy (third trimester or peripartum): abdominal ultrasound, fast and non-invasive, enables the identification of a peritoneal effusion [6,17] and the evaluation of the well-being of the foetus [35-37]. In most cases, surgical care will prevail. In the case of the absence of hemoperitoneal collection, or if there is a diagnostic doubt, a CT scan can be realised if the state of the mother and the foetus allows it [31].

When the rupture occurs postpartum: the computed tomography with contrast media, remains the gold standard to reveal a retroperitoneal hematoma or a hemoperitoneal collection. The visualisation of a leak of contrast media, showing an active hemorrhage, will make it possible to locate the site of the rupture [3]. The absence of signs of pancreatititis or peptic ulcer on CT-Scan will allow to eliminate some differential diagnoses. Normally, the visceral angiography is the standard reference test to diagnose the presence of an aneurysm [11]. This diagnostic option can only be considered in the case of a stable patient whose hemodynamic state is not preoccupying in any way [37]. However we will have to favour this examination, especially in the case of a retroperitoneal hematoma because it is very difficult to identify the origin of the bleeding during the surgical exploration, blindly, without any preliminary visual tests, and as a matter of urgency, even for an experienced vascular surgeon. Losing a small amount of time must be accepted in order to save some valuable minutes during the surgical procedure if the hemodynamic situation of the patient allows it.

6. Treatment

An aneurysmal rupture is a surgical emergency and its therapeutic care must take place without delay. In general, two procedures are possible: the exploratory laparotomy coupled with an emergency fetal extraction by caesarean section and the selective embolisation of the site of the rupture [3,9,38]. The technique to use will be chosen according to the hemodynamic state of the mother, the location of the aneurysm and the moment of the rupture. Indeed, even if there is no consensus, when the symptomatology appears at the third trimester of the pregnancy, there is not place for the selective embolisation. To our knowledge and according to recent publications [6] no case of embolisation of an abdominal aneurysm during pregnancy has ever been described in the international literature. The reported cases were realized postpartum.

6.1. Treatment of Asymptomatic Aneurysms of the Splenic Artery

The risk of rupture of an asymptomatic aneurysm of the splenic artery is estimated between around 3% and 5% in the general population and rises to 25% in a pregnant woman [31,35]. As such an event is marked by a high maternal and fetal mortality, preventive care is the rule upon unexpectedly discovering an aneurysm of the splenic artery. Normally, an aneurism with a diameter superior to 2cm will have to be treated [6,22,35,39]. However, according to some authors like Mattar and Lumsden [17], the argument of the size must not be retained for some categories of patients like pregnant women: any aneurysm discovered in a woman old enough to procreate, pregnant or aiming to be, will have to be treated [17,35,40].

The surgical treatment of the aneurysm of the splenic artery is presently well codified and depends partly on their location. The treatments by laparotomy or laparoscopy remain the main techniques. An endovascular approach is also possible out of a pregnancy [5]. Aneurysms located on the proximal and medial thirds will be treated by excision and by proximal and distal ligature of the splenic artery. The collateral vascularisation of the spleen, especially around the gastrosplenic short vessels, will make it possible to avoid a secondary splenic infarcissement. In the case of a small aneurysm located near the celiac trunk, some authors realized a resection of the aneurysm then an end-to-side or end-to-end anastomosis of the splenic artery [35,39].

Aneurysms located on the distal third and near the hile will justify in most cases a resection with splenectomy [5,6].

6.2. Treatment of Rupture

70% of ruptures in pregnant women happen during the third trimester of the pregnancy. Besides the necessary resuscitation methods and wherever the rupture is located, the emergency laparotomy with fetal extraction are the essential key elements to ensure the best chances of maternal and fetal survival. Thus the treatment will be multidisciplinary and an obstetrician, an anaesthesiologist, a vascular surgeon and a radiologist will be involved. The main difficulty remains the initial diagnostic mistake because many authors justify their decision of an emergency caesarean section by a suspected uterine rupture or placental abruption. But the Starck or Pfannenstiel incisions which are carried out in most cases do not allow an accurate exploration of the peritoneal cavity and, except in the case of the rupture of an ovarian or uterine vessel, surgical care of an aneurysm of the renal or splenic artery is therefore impossible. The presence of a hemoperitoneal collection objectivised during the caesarean section will guide the surgeon towards a possible rupture of the spleen or towards an aneurysm of the splenic artery and a median longitudinal laparotomy will then be carried out. The treatment will therefore be identical to that of aneurysms which are not ruptured.

The aneurysmal rupture of the renal artery justifies a resection followed by either an anastomisis or a nephrectomy. When conserving the kidney seems impossible, it is essential to confirm the presence of the controlateral kidney [1]. In 1966, Patterson reported the case of a maternal death after a left nephrectomy for a rupture of aneurysm in a patient with a congenital absence of right kidney [41].

In the case of an aneurysmal rupture of the ovarian artery, resection of the aneurysm associated with an ovariectomy, if need be, is the classic procedure. However, for these last two locations, the rupture takes place in the retroperitoneal area. As this space is closed and not very extensible, a kind of tamponnade appears which explains the stability of the hemodynamic state, at least during the initial phase. This phenomenon can be compared with that of the rupture in two phases described for the ruptures of the splenic artery. Several authors report cases of ruptures for which an angiography followed by an embolisation were undertaken during the latency period [3,9,10,42]. These were cases of ruptures postpartum or after the discovery of a retroperitoneal hematoma during a caesarean section. This option, both diagnostic and therapeutic, was described by King in 1990 in the case of an aneurysmal rupture of the ovarian artery four days after the delivery [9]. The vascular approach therefore makes it possible to avoid exploratory laparatomy and delicate surgery of the retroperitoneal area [3]. Yet, this technique enables the treatment of the cause but not the drainage of the hematoma. In the case of lumbar pain, drainage by lomboscopy can be proposed [3,10]. In the case of hemodynamic instability or if the embolisation procedure fails, an emergency laparotomy will have to be carried out.

As the same causes lead to the same effects, the presence of an aneurysm, ruptured or not, must be considered as a sign of alert. The presence of other locations must be mentioned and must lead to diagnostic and therapeutic treatment if need be. Diagnostic arteriography is therefore the most accurate option.

Conclusion

The rupture of an abdominal aneurysm during pregnancy is a rare event and is still not well known. Its symptomatology is non-specific, but the apparition of hemodynamic shock without metrorrhagia must raise suspicions and bring about consideration of other diagnostic hypotheses. The treatment will be multidisciplinary and will often lead to an exploratory laparotomy which will first enable fetal extraction and then the resection of the aneurysm. The presence of a retroperitoneal hematoma will actuate consideration of an arteriography in order to locate the origin of the bleeding and, if possible, to continue with embolisation. In the case of a secondary laparotomy, knowing the site of the rupture will therefore enable a direct and quick access to the wounded vessel and will limit the exploration of the retroperitoneal area. Finally, the discovery, fortuitous or not, of an aneurysm must be considered as a general pathology. The other potential sites of aneurysms will have to be explored and, if need be, treated in the case of a woman who wants to get pregnant and is old enough to procreate.

Acknowledgment

We thank Nicolas Poilblanc for his invaluable assistance.

Chapter reviewed by Claude Clément, MD, PhD, Department of Vascular Surgery, Robert Debré Hospital, University Hospital of Rheims, France

References

[1] Barrett, JM; Van, Hooydonk, JE; Boehm, FH. Pregnancy-related rupture of arterial aneurysms. *Obstet Gynecol Surv,* 1982, 37, 557-566.

[2] Blachar, A; Bloom, AI; Golan, G; Venturero, M; Bar-Ziv J. Case reports. Spiral ct imaging of a ruptured post-partum ovarian artery aneurysm. *Clin Radiol,* 2000, 55, 718-720.

[3] Poilblanc, M; Winer, N; Bouvier, A; Gillard, P; Boussion, F; Aube, C; Descamps, P. Rupture of an aneurysm of the ovarian artery following delivery and endovascular treatment. *Am J Obstet Gynecol,* 2008. 199(4):e7-8.

[4] Popham, P; Buettner, A. Arterial aneurysms of the lienorenal axis during pregnancy. *Int J Obstet Anesth,* 2003, 12, 117-119.

[5] Selo-Ojeme, DO; Welch, CC. Review: Spontaneous rupture of splenic artery aneurysm in pregnancy. *Eur J Obstet Gynecol Reprod Biol,* 2003, 109, 124-127.

[6] Sadat, U; Dar, O; Walsh, S; Varty, K. Splenic artery aneurysms in pregnancy--a systematic review. *Int J Surg.,* 2008, 6, 261-265.

[7] Soliman, KB; Shawky, Y; Abbas, MM; Ammary, M; Shaaban, A. Ruptured renal artery aneurysm during pregnancy, a clinical dilemma. *BMC Urol.,* 2006, 6, 22.

[8] Raft, J; Lalot, JM; Meistelman, C; Longrois, D. Influence of pregnancy on renal angiomyolipoma. *Gynecol Obstet Fertil,* 2005, 33, 898-906.

[9] King,WL. Ruptured ovarian artery aneurysm: A case report. *J Vasc Surg.,* 1990, 12, 190-193.

[10] Guillem, P; Bondue, X; Chambon, JP; Lemaitre, L; Bounoua, F. Spontaneous retroperitoneal hematoma from rupture of an aneurysm of the ovarian artery following delivery. *Ann Vasc Surg.,* 1999, 13, 445-448.

[11] Wagner, WH; Allins, AD; Treiman, RL; Cohen, JL; Foran, RF; Levin, PM; Cossman DV. Ruptured visceral artery aneurysms. *Ann Vasc Surg.,* 1997, 11, 342-347.

[12] Carr, SC; Pearce, WH; Vogelzang, RL; McCarthy, WJ; Nemcek, AA; Jr.; Yao JS. Current management of visceral artery aneurysms. *Surgery,* 1996, 120, 627-633.

[13] Babb, RR. Aneurysm of the splenic artery. *Arch Surg.,* 1976, 111, 924-925.

[14] Bedford, PD; Lodge, B. Aneurysm of the splenic artery. *Gut.,* 1960, 1, 312-320.

[15] Warshauer, DM; Keefe, B; Mauro, MA. Intrahepatic hepatic artery aneurysm: Computed tomography and color-flow doppler ultrasound findings. *Gastrointest Radiol,* 1991, 16, 175-177.

[16] Bret, PM; Bretagnolle, M; Enoch, G; Partensky, C; Valette, PJ; Celles, M. Ultrasonic features of aneurysms of splanchnic arteries. *J Can Assoc Radiol,* 1985, 36, 226-229.

[17] Mattar, SG; Lumsden, AB. The management of splenic artery aneurysms: Experience with 23 cases. *Am J Surg.,* 1995, 169, 580-584.

[18] Messina, LM; Shanley, CJ. Visceral artery aneurysms. *Surg Clin North Am.,* 1997, 77, 425-442.

[19] Caillouette, JC; Merchant, EB. Ruptured splenic artery aneurysm in pregnancy. Twelfth reported case with maternal and fetal survival. *Am J Obstet Gynecol,* 1993, 168, 1810-1811; discussion 1811-1813.

[20] Steinberg, LH; Goodfellow, C; Rankin, L. Spontaneous rupture of the uterine artery in pregnancy. *Br J Obstet Gynaecol,* 1993, 100, 184.

[21] Descargues, G; Douvrin, F; Gravier, A; Lemoine, JP; Marpeau, L; Clavier, E. False aneurysm of the uterine pedicle: An uncommon cause of post-partum haemorrhage after caesarean section treated with selective arterial embolization. *Eur J Obstet Gynecol Reprod Biol.,* 2001, 97, 26-29.

[22] Gallot, D; Bournazeau, JA; Amblard, J; Pouly, JL; Lemery, D. Rupture of a splenic artery aneurysm during pregnancy. Report of a case. *J Gynecol Obstet Biol Reprod,* (Paris) 1999, 28, 168-170.

[23] Yang, JC; Hye, RJ. Ruptured renal artery aneurysm during pregnancy. *Ann Vasc Surg.,* 1996, 10, 370-372.

[24] Gaglio, PJ; Regenstein, F; Slakey, D; Cheng, S; Takiff, H; Rinker, R; Dick, D; Thung, SN. Alpha-1 antitrypsin deficiency and splenic artery aneurysm rupture: An association? *Am J Gastroenterol,* 2000, 95, 1531-1534.

[25] Trimble, WK; Hill, J. Congestive splenomegaly (banti's disease) due to portal stenosis without hepatic cirrhosis; aneurysms of the splenic artery. *Arch Pathol Lab Med.,* 1942, 34, 423.

[26] Manalo-Estrella, PBA. Histopathologic findings in human aortic media associated with pregnancy. *Arch Pathol Lab Med.,* 1967, 83, 336-341.

[27] Burnett, RA. Cafrae, DC. Spontaneous rupture of ovarian artery aneurysm in the puerperium: Two case reports and review of literature. *Br J Obstet Gynaecol,* 1976, 83, 744-750.

[28] Robson, SC; Hunter, S; Moore, M; Dunlop, W. Haemodynamic changes during the puerperium: A doppler and m-mode echocardiographic study. *Br J Obstet Gynaecol,* 1987, 94, 1028-1039.

[29] Cabanes, L. Coeur et grossesse in *Traité d'obstétrique* Cabrol D; Pons JC; Goffinet F, Médecine-Sciences Flammarion, 2003, 585 p.

[30] Novak, J; Parry, LJ; Matthews, JE; Kerchner, LJ; Indovina, K; Hanley-Yanez, K; Doty, KD; Debrah, DO; Shroff, SG; Conrad, KP. Evidence for local relaxin ligand-receptor expression and function in arteries. *Faseb J.,* 2006, 20, 2352-2362.

[31] Hillemanns, P; Knitza, R; Muller-Hocker, J. Rupture of splenic artery aneurysm in a pregnant patient with portal hypertension. *Am J Obstet Gynecol,* 1996, 174, 1665-1666.

[32] Fender, GR; Haslett, E; Leary, T; Bland, E; Hackett, G. Management of splenic artery aneurysm rupture during trial of scar with epidural analgesia. *Am J Obstet Gynecol,* 1999, 180, 1038-1039.

[33] Brockman, R. Aneurysm of splenic artery. *Br J Surgery,* 1929-1930, 17, 692-693.

[34] Mines, D. Splenic artery aneurysm rupture. *Am J Emerg Med.,* 1991, 9, 74-76.

[35] Lang, W; Strobel, D; Beinder, E; Raab, M. Surgery of a splenic artery aneurysm during pregnancy. *Eur J Obstet Gynecol Reprod Biol.,* 2002, 102, 215-216.

[36] Derchi, LE; Biggi, E; Cicio, GR; Bertoglio, C; Neumaier, CE. Aneurysms of the splenic artery: Noninvasive diagnosis by pulsed doppler sonography. *J Ultrasound Med.,* 1984, 3, 41-44.

[37] D'Ambrosio, R; Ricciardelli, L; Lanni, GL; Iarrobino, GF; Moggio, G; Casale, LS; Pagano, G; Borsi, E. Intraperitoneal hemorrhage from rupture of an aneurysm of splenic artery: Case report and literature review. *Ann Ital Chir.,* 2003, 74, 97-101.

[38] Rathod, KR; Deshmukh, HL; Asrani, A; Salvi, VS; Prabhu, S. Successful embolization of an ovarian artery pseudoaneurysm complicating obstetric hysterectomy. *Cardiovasc Intervent Radiol.,* 2005, 28, 113-116.

[39] Herbeck, M; Horbach, T; Putzenlechner, C; Klein, P; Lang, W. Ruptured splenic artery aneurysm during pregnancy: A rare case with both maternal and fetal survival. *Am J Obstet Gynecol,* 1999, 181, 763-764.

[40] Collin, J. Visceral arteries; in *Oxford textbook of surgery.* Morris PJ; Wood CW; Oxford University Press, 2000.

[41] Patterson, W. Maternal death due to undiagnosed left renal artery aneurysm associated with an absent right kidney. *Proc R Soc Med.,* 1973, 66, 761.

[42] Prabulos, AM; Chen, HH; Rodis, JF; Ruby, S; Campbell, WA. Angiographic embolization of a ruptured renal artery aneurysm during pregnancy. *Obstet Gynecol,* 1997, 90, 663-665.

In: Aneurysms: Types, Risks, Formation and Treatment ISBN: 978-1-60741-557-2
Editors: Alain Laurent and Ethan Morel © 2009 Nova Science Publishers, Inc.

Chapter 8

Endovascular Treatment of Intracranial Aneurysms

Boris Lubicz*

Interventional neuroradiology, Erasme University Hospital, 808 route de Lennik, 1070 Brussels, Belgium

This review presents the current state and advances in endovascular embolization for the treatment of intracranial aneurysms (IA), including embolic materials, therapeutic and assisting techniques, long-term effectiveness, and limitations.

Over the last decade, endovascular treatment (EVT) of IA has made remarkable progress and has become widely used. EVT by means of detachable coils has been accepted as an alternative to surgical clipping for the treatment of unruptured and ruptured IA. Until recently, EVT was mostly applied in patients with small aneurysms with a small neck. Indeed, these aneurysms have a favorable anatomical configuration that prevents coil protrusion within the parent vessel as well as stable long-term anatomical results. In this particular subgroup of patients, EVT has the same efficacy as surgical clipping and it is associated with lower morbidity and mortality rates. Therefore, EVT is now considered as the first therapeutic option in these patients.

Thanks to the recent development of new endovascular techniques and tools, more and more IA are amenable to EVT. New coils, remodeling balloons, and self-expandable stents allow to treat complex IA including wide-necked aneurysms, fusiform aneurysms, and aneurysms with a branch arising from the neck or the sac. These new techniques have thus enlarged EVT indications but the question remains as to whether these techniques justify EVT as first-intention treatment in all IA. On a technical point of view, most IA are treatable by endovascular approach and EVT is no more limited to small aneurysms with a small neck. It also appears obvious that these techniques require a long learning curve and this may explain contradictory information within the literature about their associated complication rate. On a clinical point of view, EVT as first-line treatment seems a reasonable strategy that is associated with good clinical results. However, these new developments fail to circumvent the major limitation of EVT that remains the anatomical results stability. Among new techniques, intracranial stenting seems the most promising one because stents may induce intra-aneurysmal flow reduction and parent artery healing that might lead to aneurysm thrombosis without even "touching" the sac. For the first time in the history of IA treatment, a causal therapeutic approach – that is focused on the vessel wall defect – seems thus feasible. Therefore, stenting might be the next revolution of IA treatment, 15 years after the advent of detachable coils.

ENDOVASCULAR TREATMENT OF INTRACRANIAL ANEURYSMS

The development and release of the first detachable coil [1, 2], the Guglielmi Detachable Coil (GDC), in the early nineties have revolutionized the treatment of IA. The endovascular procedure of IA coiling is performed via a microcatheter that is introduced via the femoral artery and then navigated with a guidewire within cerebral vessels. After being properly positioned within the aneurysmal sac, detachable coils are delivered through the catheter to occlude the aneurysm and to exclude it from the circulation.

Over the last decade, EVT by means of detachable coils has made remarkable progress and has become widely used. EVT has also been accepted as an alternative to surgical clipping for the treatment of unruptured and ruptured IA. Moreover, in selected cases, EVT is associated with lower morbidity/mortality rates than surgical clipping [3, 4]. These latter aneurysms are those with a favorable neck/sac ratio because this anatomical configuration prevents coil protrusion within the parent vessel and it is associated with stable long-term anatomical results (Figures 1A, B). In this subgroup of IA, EVT is now considered as the first therapeutic option [3-6].

Thanks to these very good results obtained in this particular group of IA, many technological advances have recently been made to enlarge EVT indications. These innovations include new coils, liquid embolic agent, remodeling balloons, and intracranial stents.

New Endovascular Techniques and Tools

New Coils

The main disadvantage of EVT compared to surgery is aneurysm recurrence [7], especially in case of large aneurysmal sac or wide-necked aneurysm. To circumvent this potential limitation, many investigations are currently evaluating new coils including biologically active coils [8], radioactive coils [9], and coated-coils with a swelling hydrogel [10]. The aim of these innovations is to promote intra-aneurysmal clot organization and

*Corresponding author: Tel: +3225553998, Fax: +3225556670, blubicz@ulb.ac.be

fibrosis [8, 9] or to increase packing density [10] that is associated with higher long-term occlusion rate [11]. Among these new coils, Matrix coils (Boston Scientific), Cerecyte coils (Micrus) and Hydrocoils (Microvention) are those mostly used and they have recently been evaluated in several series.

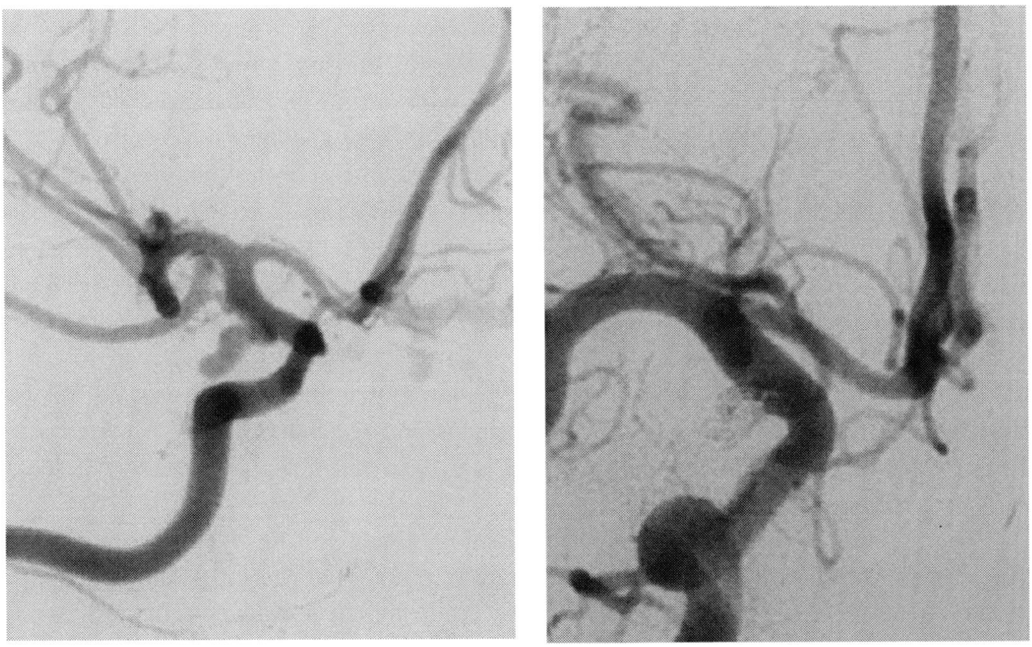

A. Small aneurysms with a small neck.

B. EVT by selective coiling with complete aneurysm occlusion.

Figure 1. Ruptured posterior communicating artery aneurysm

Matrix detachable coils were the first available coated coils with an outer coating of a bioabsorbable polymeric material (polyglycolic acid/lactide) that has been shown in swine aneurysm models to accelerate aneurysm fibrosis and neointima formation with increased neck tissue thickness but no parent artery stenosis [8]. The coil consists of 70% of polymer and 30% of platinum. Lubicz et al. [12] were the first to report the use of these coated coils for EVT of IA. They showed that the use of Matrix coils was limited by their stiffness that did not allow a complete treatment of small aneurysms with these coils alone. Indeed, Matrix coils have a tendency to compartimentalize into the aneurysmal sac and it may require to reposition the catheter to complete aneurysm occlusion. This increases the duration and the risks of the procedure. Moreover, the packing density associated with these coils is inferior when compared to bare coils because of their stiffness. These findings were confirmed by many authors who showed that EVT with Matrix coils are not associated with better aneurysm occlusion stability [13-16]. These authors showed that the recanalization rate with Matrix coils may even be higher when compared with bare coils because of the difficulty to densely pack the aneurysm.

The Cerecyte coil uses a similar polyglycolic acid material, but as an inner coating of a platinum coil to circumvent the limitation of Matrix coils. Several authors have published feasibility studies that demonstrated the safety and efficacy of Cerecyte coils for EVT of IA [17-19]. Thanks to its concept of inner coating, less limitation were encountered with these coils. However, long-term clinical efficacy of Cerecyte coils remains to be proved.

A different bioactive coil technology, the Hydrocoil, consists of a platinum coil coated with a polymer that swells on contact with blood, increasing coil volume by threefold to nine fold [20-22]. The Hydrocoil for Endovascular Aneurysm Occlusion (HEAL) study had enrolled 184 patients with 191 cerebral aneurysms as of February 2004 [20]. The preliminary data showed that the initial occlusion and complication rates were not significantly different from aneurysms treated with bare platinum coils. Follow-up angiography is currently being collected to determine whether Hydrocoil can reduce the rate of aneurysmal recanalization in their patient population. Recently, Gaba et al. [21] reviewed the outcomes of 50 aneurysms embolized primarily using Hydrocoil and compared them with aneurysms embolized with bare platinum coils. Embolization with Hydrocoil yielded a significantly greater volumetric percentage sac occlusion (84.8% versus 29.8%; $P<0.001$). Follow-up angiography showed that recurrence rates were significantly decreased in small aneurysms in the Hydrocoil cohort (5% versus 17%; $P=0.013$). Finally, one must be aware that the use of Hydrocoils has been associated with the development of hydrocephalus and meningitis [23]. Therefore, larger series with long-term follow-up are mandatory to evaluate the potential benefit of these coils as well as their limiting characteristics.

The future of bioactive endovascular technology likely will involve delivery of growth factors (vascular endothelial growth factor, transforming growth factor β, fibroblast growth factor), gene therapies, or cellular substrates within the aneurysm that will regenerate an endothelial wall layer across the aneurysm neck [24-29].

2. Liquid Embolic Agent

Liquid agents have long been considered for use in endosaccular aneurysm occlusion, despite that control of their deposition can hardly be presumed [30]. Platinum coils used for EVT only occlude a small portion of the volume of the aneurysm with significant residual dead space. Therefore, the use of liquid embolic agents is a possible alternative as filling material for the treatment of some IA and it might decrease the rate of recanalization [30]. Onyx is the first liquid embolic agent available for EVT of IA (Figures 2A-C) and it has been mostly evaluated for the treatment of large or giant IA that are more prone to recanalize [31-34].

Mawad et al. [31] reported the first series of 11 giant aneurysms successfully treated by selective obliteration of the sac with Onyx. Nine of the 11 patients showed an excellent outcome and the absence of aneurysm recanalization at 6 months. More recently, the CAMEO trial [32] and Lubicz et al. [33] reported encouraging results in case of giant IA treated with Onyx. The CAMEO study [32] reported an overall 90% of good or excellent outcomes in a series of mostly (79%) large and giant aneurysms. Procedure- or device-related permanent neurological morbidity and mortality rates were of 8% and 2% respectively. These findings were confirmed by Lubicz et al. [33] who reported good or excellent outcomes in 26 of 29 patients (90%) and procedure-related morbidity/mortality rates of 7% and 3%

respectively. Anatomical results were also encouraging with an overall 79% of complete occlusion at 12 months in the CAMEO trial [32] and a recanalization rate of 32% for giant IA in the series of Lubicz et al. [33]. These results are of course insufficient but compare favorably with those previously reported by coil occlusion in the same group of aneurysms [9, 35-38].

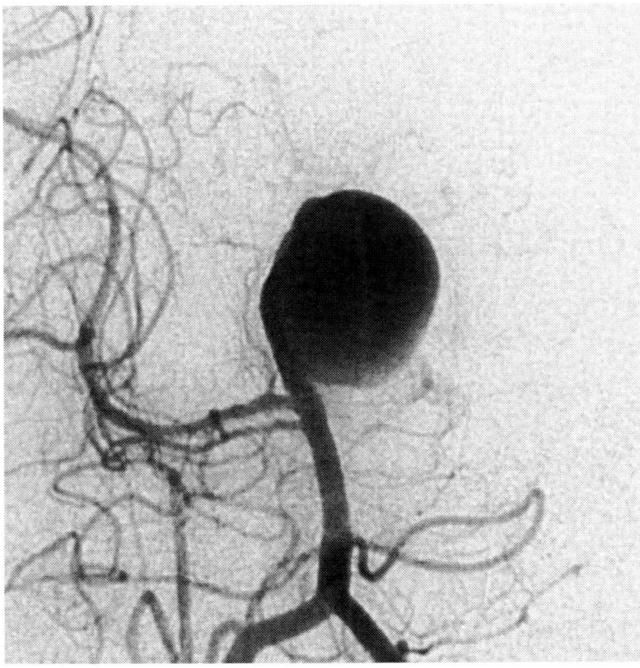

A. Giant basilar tip aneurysm.

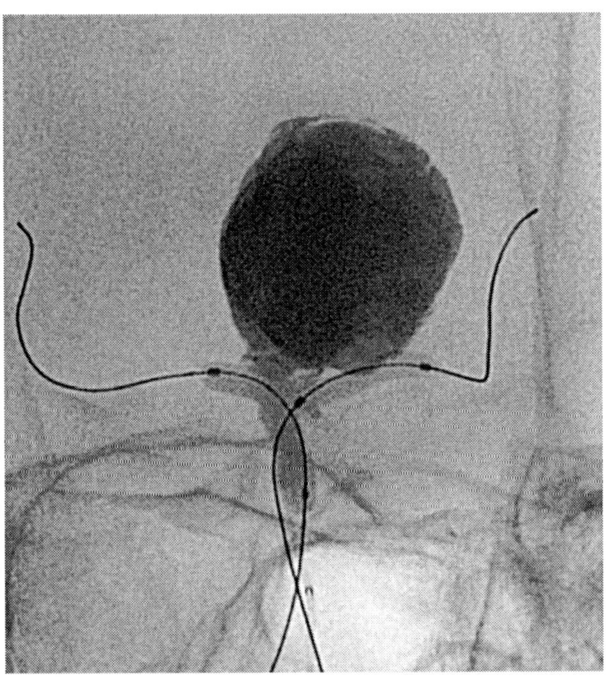

B. EVT by selective Onyx injection under balloon protection.

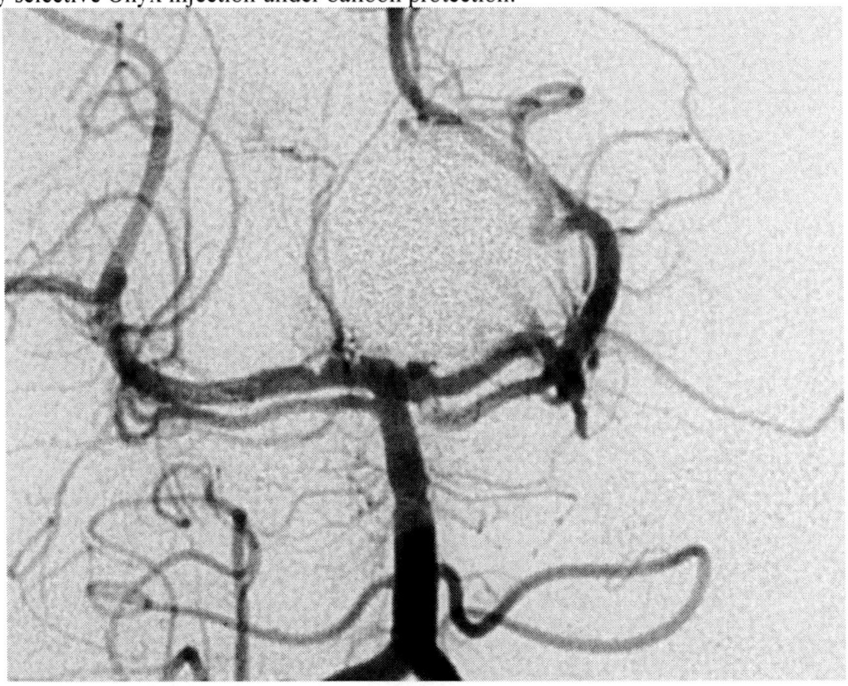

C. Complete aneurysm occlusion at the end of EVT.

Figure 2. Unruptured giant basilar tip aneurysm

The aims of treatment in patients with large or giant aneurysms, are to protect from SAH, cure symptoms, and eliminate mass effect. The goals of treatment were achieved in most patients in both series, suggesting that selective embolization with Onyx is an alternative option in case of difficult large and giant aneurysms. Nevertheless, additional technical innovations are necessary to improve the way to deliver Onyx and its combination with protecting devices (balloon, stent) in order to decrease potential complications. On the other hand, most authors agree that Onyx is not indicated for small IA for which EVT with coils remains the first option because it has proved its safety and efficacy for many years [31-34].

3. Balloon-Assisted Coiling

Balloon-assisted coiling (BAC), the so-called "remodeling technique" was first described by Jacques Moret in 1994 [39]. A small balloon-occlusion microcatheter is positioned across the aneurysm neck and a second microcatheter is placed within the aneurysmal sac. The balloon is temporarily inflated during coil deployment within the aneurysmal sac to protect the parent artery lumen. The first remodeling balloons were used to treat sidewall aneurysms [39] whereas a new one (HyperForm/EV3), more compliant, allows EVT of bifurcation aneurysms or small arteries aneurysms [40]. Many authors have shown the feasibility and the safety of the remodeling technique [39-50] and it has been accepted as an adjunctive technique for EVT of complex IA such as wide-necked aneurysms [39-49] or aneurysms with a branch arising from the neck or the sac [50].

a) BAC indications

1. Wide-necked IA (Figures 3A-C)
2. Aneurysms with a branch arising from the neck or the sac (Figures 4A-C)
3. Assistance in case of aneurysm rupture (bleb at the base of the sac, ...)
4. Assistance in case of coiling catheter instability

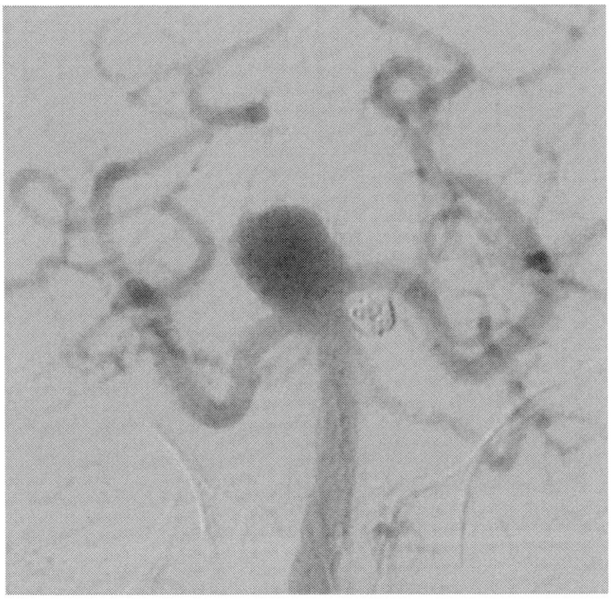

A. Very wide-necked basilar tip aneurysm.

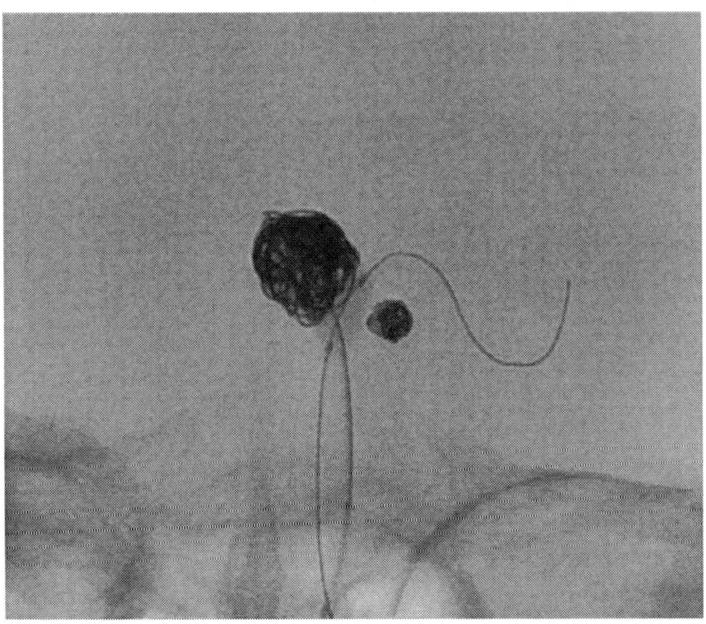

B. EVT by balloon-assisted coiling.

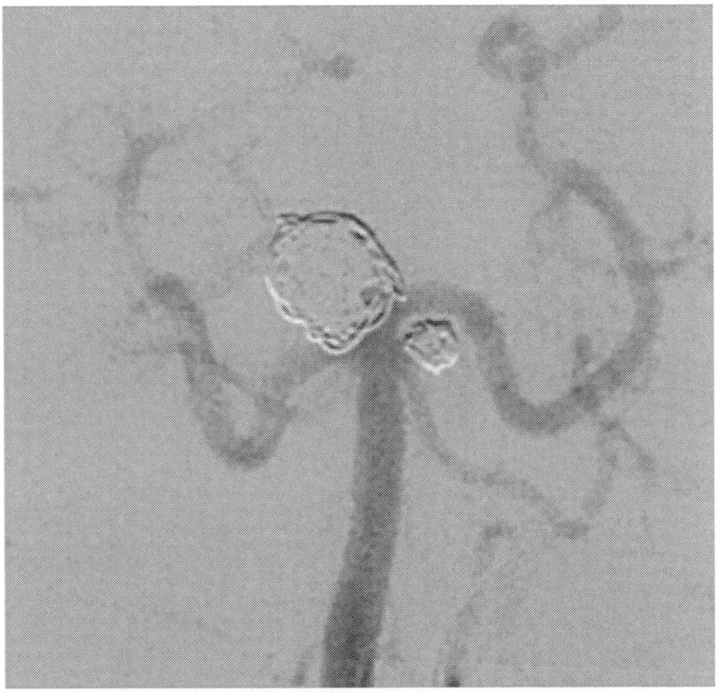

C. Complete aneurysm occlusion at the end of EVT.

Figure 3. Ruptured basilar tip aneurysm

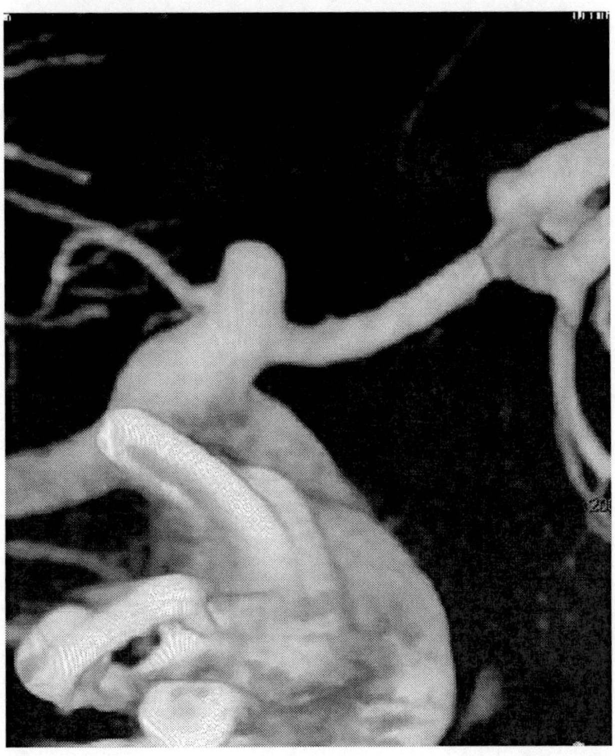

A. Wide-necked aneurysm with a branch arising from the sac.

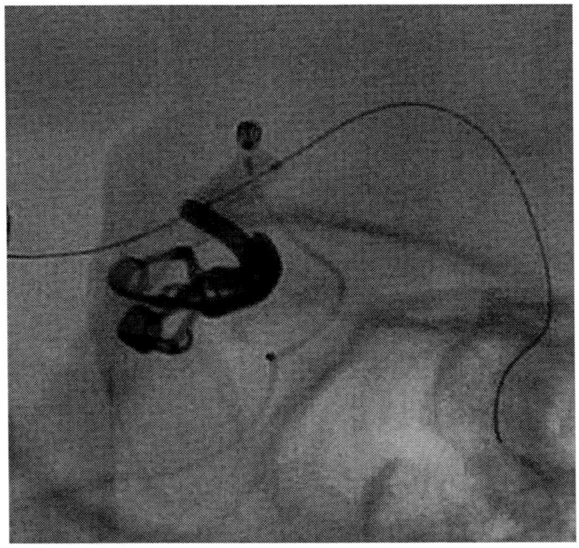

B. Balloon assisted coiling with the over-inflation technique to protect the arterial branch arising from the sac. The remodeling balloon is placed via a retrograde approach though the anterior communicating artery in order to cover the aneurysm neck.

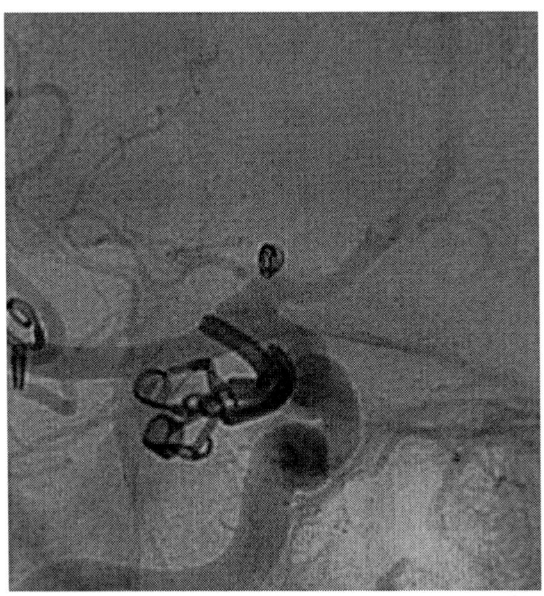

C. Satisfying aneurysm occlusion with preservation of the branch.

Figure 4. Unruptured proximal anterior cerebral artery aneurysm

Indeed, the balloon assistance is not only useful for EVT of wide-necked aneurysms, it may also be used to protect a branch arising from the aneurysm neck or from the sac [50]. Furthermore, BAC is really helpful in 2 difficult situations that may be encountered during EVT: 1) when an aneurysm perforation occurs, the balloon may be inflated to quickly stop the bleeding while coils are delivered; 2) when the coiling catheter is kicking back out of the aneurysmal sac, the balloon increases its stability.

In case of aneurysms with a branch at the neck, a remodeling balloon may be used to protect the branch. The balloon must be positioned within the origin of the artery and inflated during coils delivery. When the arterial branch emerges from the sac, a remodeling balloon can be over-inflated at the neck to bulge within the aneurysm to protect the arterial branch. Lubicz et al. [50] were the first to describe this over-inflation technique in a small series published in 2006. They showed the feasibility and safety of this technique because there was no clinical complication and the branch could be preserved in all cases when it was needed. On a technical point of view, the use of the HyperForm balloon (EV3) is mandatory because it is very compliant and it may be over-inflated to bulge within the aneurysm. The biggest available HyperForm balloon (7x7 mm) must be used because of the need of an over-inflation. Finally, one must be aware that aneurysms with a branch arising from the sac remain technically challenging to treat by endovascular approach. It requires a great amount of experience in EVT of IA especially with the use of the remodeling technique.

b) BAC complications

There is a current debate in the literature whether or not BAC might increase complication rate when compared to conventional coiling. Indeed, few authors have shown that BAC might be associated with a higher rate of thromboembolic events because of successive balloon occlusion of the parent artery [51, 52]. On the other hand, several authors have reported complication rate similar to those associated with conventional coiling [39-50]. There are only few large series that have evaluated the feasibility and the results of BAC of IA. In these series, the combined morbidity/mortality rate associated with BAC was between 0% and 7% [39-50]. Thus, most authors reported no significant increased complication rate with BAC. These good results were recently confirmed in an oral communication from a French prospective multicentre trial (Pierot et al., WIN meeting, Val d'Isère, France 2008) that reported comparable morbidity and mortality rates between conventional coiling and BAC. These findings were also confirmed by Lubicz et al. [53] in a large prospective series and in a recent meta-analysis by Shapiro et al. [54]. These latter 2 studies showed that BAC was not associated with higher complication rate than conventional coiling.

However, Sluzewski et al. [52] are the only one who reported a very high complication rate of BAC that is not in accordance with all these data. The study from Lubicz et al. [53] suggested that this difference might be related to author's experience with BAC, the rate of BAC use in daily practice, and the type of remodeling balloons used. Indeed, BAC – like conventional coiling [55] – requires a learning curve and is mostly operators' dependant [39-50, 53]. In a French prospective multicentre trial (Pierot et al., WIN meeting, Val d'Isère, France 2008) and in Lubicz et al. study [53], BAC was used in more than 20% of embolized aneurysms whereas it was used in only 8.6% of aneurysms treated by Sluzewski et al. [52]. On the other hand, the remodeling balloons that were used by Sluzewski et al. [52] are older balloons that are known to be less compliant and more traumatic than recently developed balloons (HyperForm/HyperGlide balloons, EV3). Therefore, the lesser use of BAC and the lesser quality of endovascular tools have probably influenced their complication rate. In conclusion, BAC is not associated with higher complication rate than conventional coiling when it is frequently and routinely used.

c) Anatomical outcome and re-treatment

BAC is not associated with better anatomical results stability because it is mostly used in complex IA [39-50, 53]. These findings are consistent with previously published papers showing that wide-necked aneurysms are associated with higher rate of recanalization [7, 36, 37]. However, it is now admitted that a re-treatment will be necessary in 10% of embolized IA – including mostly ruptured lesions – and that EVT should therefore be considered as a staged treatment for a certain percentage of patients. Fortunately re-treatment by endovascular approach is associated with very low complication rate [56, 57].

4. Stenting

In case of wide-necked IA, selective embolization remains difficult because of the risk of coil protrusion into the parent vessel. Several authors reported successful treatment of these aneurysms by the use of the remodeling technique [39-50]. However, this technique may fail to retain coils within the sac in aneurysms with a very large neck and it may also be technically challenging in aneurysms smaller than 3mm. Moreover, some authors have reported higher rate of thromboembolic events because of successive balloon occlusion of the parent artery [51].

The concept of stent-assisted coiling (SAC) is to bridge the aneurysm neck with the stent that will support coils that are subsequently delivered via a microcatheter through the stent struts. The idea of SAC has been reported for the first time 14 years ago. Indeed, Turjman et al. [58] and Szikora et al. [59] were the first to publish experimental studies about this technique. They showed the feasibility of SAC in an experimental swine model of wide-necked aneurysm. Then, several years later, few authors [60-62] reported the feasibility and efficacy of SAC in clinical practice for patients with wide-necked IA. However, their series concerned the use of balloon-expandable coronary stents that were the only one available at that time. These stents were not optimized for intracranial use and carried relatively high risk of dissection and/or rupture of the parent artery [60-62]. Moreover, the large profile and relative stiffness of the delivery systems were limiting locations that were safely accessible.

A few years ago, the first self-expandable intracranial stent (Neuroform stent/Boston Scientific) specifically designed for EVT of IA has been made available. This new device started a new era for EVT of IA: for the first time, a stent could be delivered via a conventional microcatheter and its placement did not require balloon inflation. The Neuroform stent has been evaluated for EVT of wide-necked IA in several series [63-69]. It has proved its efficacy and safety as procedure-related morbidity-mortality rates were low in these studies. However, the Neuroform stent presents some limiting characteristics including the impossibility to reposition it when it is partially delivered, a low radial force, and some deployment difficulties [63-69]. In one of the largest reported series of 48 aneurysms treated in 46 patients, Lylyk et al. [69] encountered difficulties in placing the Neuroform stent in up to 31% of the cases. Therefore, new stents have recently been developed to circumvent these limitations.

The first retractable stent to be released was the Leo stent. Kis et al. [70] and Lubicz et al. [71] showed that this stent may be repositioned even if a part of the stent is already delivered. This can simply be done by pulling back the stent within the delivery catheter and this may prevent from stent misplacement. Moreover, of 36 aneurysms treated in these 2 series, there was only one stent placement failure and these authors reported very good clinical and anatomical outcomes in almost all patients. Last but not least, the Leo stent has 2 radiopaques markers along its total length that makes it very visible during deployment. Nevertheless, the Leo stent presents a limiting characteristic that is the need for progressively larger and stiffer delivery catheters to place larger stents.

The second retractable and recently released stent is the Enterprise stent that has only been evaluated in few series that confirmed its efficacy and safety for EVT of complex IA [72-74]. In particular, Lubicz et al. [73] showed that this stent has two major advantages: 1) the delivery catheter that allows an easy navigation even within very tortuous arteries; 2) the possibility to reposition the stent whenever necessary. However, the current available stent has 2 limiting characteristics: 1) it must be used for aneurysms located on parent artery with a maximal diameter of 4 mm to avoid stent dislodgement or coils protrusion; 2) except from its proximal and distal markers, the stent is invisible.

a) Stenting indications

1. Wide-necked IA (Figures 5A-C)
2. Circumferential and fusiform IA (Figs 6A-D).
3. Dissecting IA

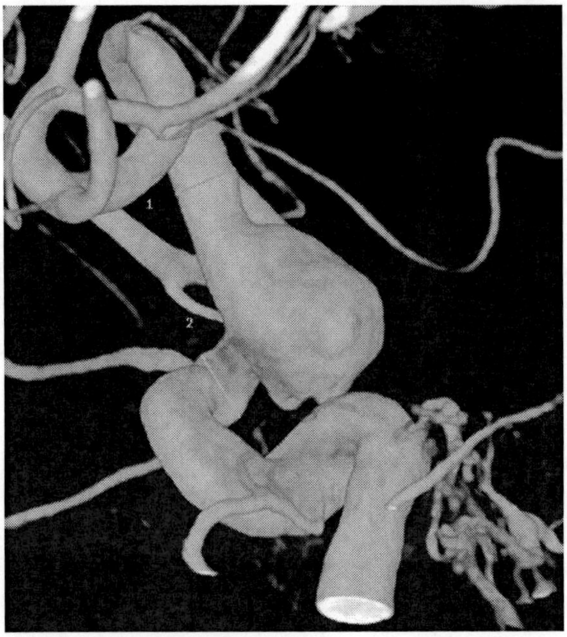

A. Very wide-necked supraclinoidal aneurysm.

Figure 5 (Continued)

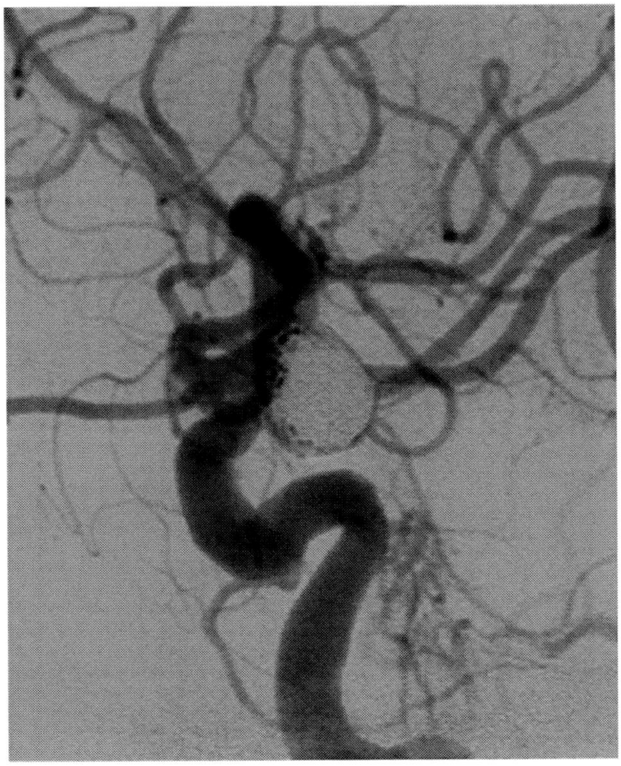

B. EVT by stent-assisted coiling with an incomplete aneurysm occlusion.

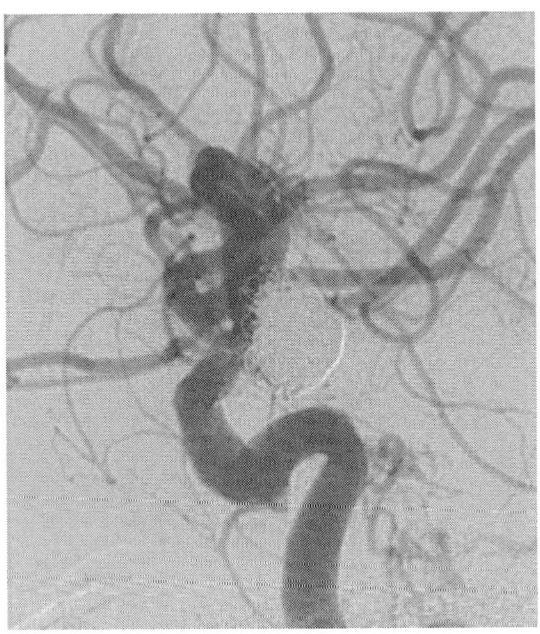

C. Angiographic control at 6 months shows a further thrombosis with a complete aneurysm occlusion.

Figure 5. Unruptured internal carotid artery aneurysm

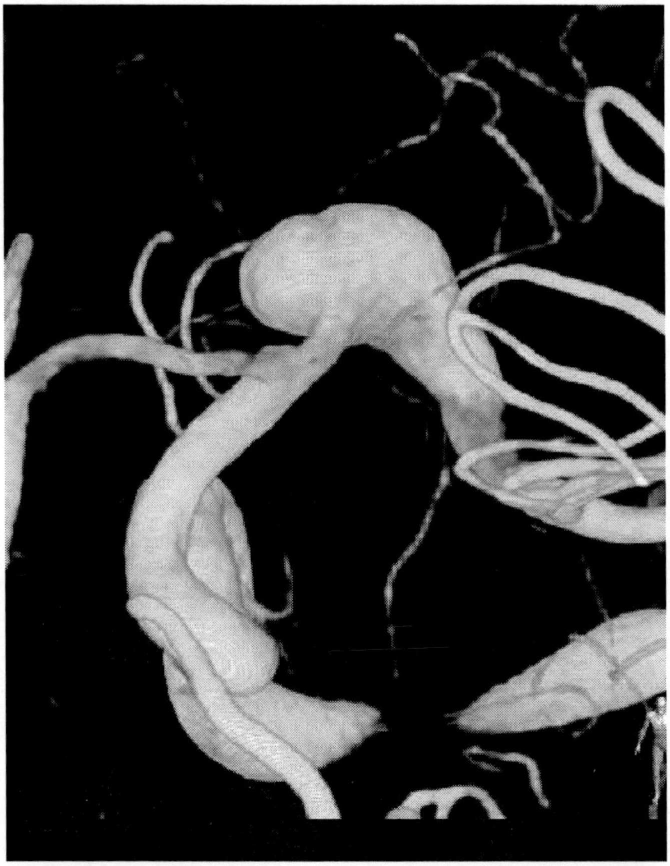

A. Large fusiform aneurysm.

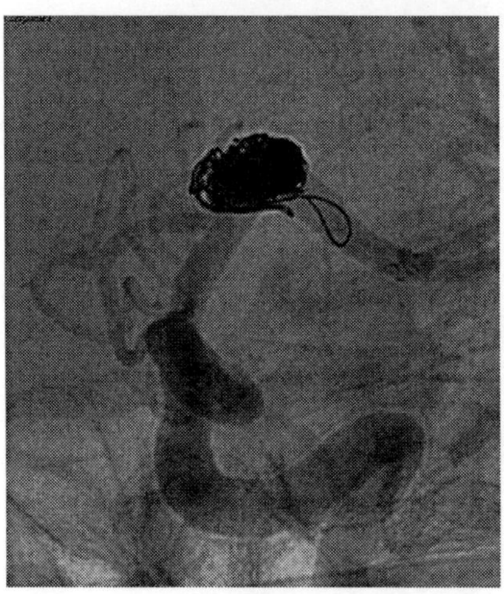

(B)

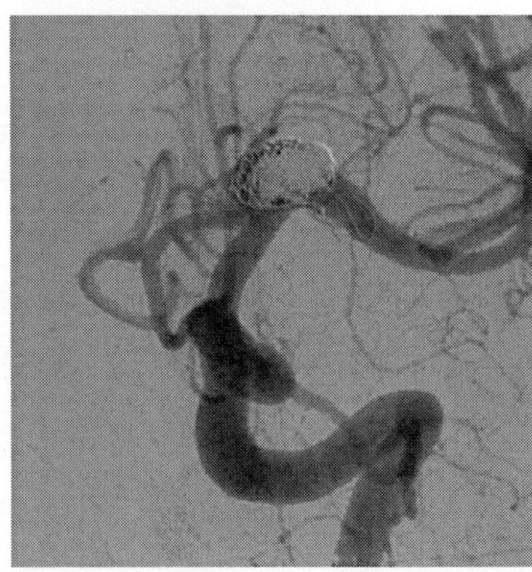

(C)

B, C. EVT by stent-assisted-coiling with incomplete aneurysm occlusion.

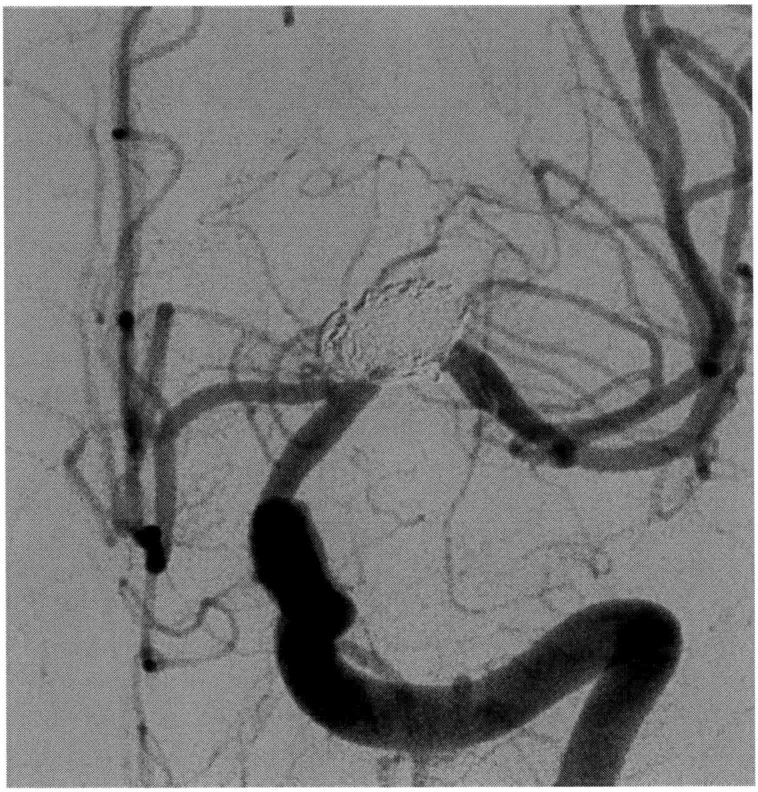

D. Angiographic control at 6 months shows a further thrombosis with a complete aneurysm occlusion.

Figure 6. Unruptured middle cerebral artery aneurysm

Among these indications, fusiform/dissecting IA are a remarkable and challenging subgroup of IA. Indeed, fusiform, circumferential aneurysms are rare and they have remained a technical challenge for both neurointerventionalists and neurosurgeons. Moreover, these aneurysms are associated with a poor natural history if left untreated. In cases in which a deconstructive treatment is possible, the affected segment of the parent vessel may be sacrificed along with the aneurysm. Parent artery occlusion provides immediate protection from subarachnoid hemorrhage (SAH), is often effective in relieving symptoms attributable to mass effect, typically results in a durable cure of the lesion, and is technically relatively uncomplicated to perform [75-78]. However, when these aneurysms arise from a vessel that is not amenable to deconstructive treatment, their management becomes much more difficult. In these cases, relatively new therapies such as the use of intracranial stents seem to be a promising technique. Only few studies have addressed this problem and were recently published [79, 80]. Fiorella et al. [79] were the first to report a small series of 7 patients treated with self-expandable stents and coils for circumferential aneurysms. They showed that this technique was safe and effective for the management of circumferential aneurysms that are not amenable to deconstructive embolization. Lubicz et al. [80] confirmed these findings because 11 of their 13 patients were treated according to this therapeutic strategy and showed an excellent clinical outcome. Both studies concluded that circumferential and fusiform IA may be treated by a reconstructive endovascular approach with self-expandable stents with or without subsequent coiling. These authors reported a therapeutic protocol which included the use of a stent within stent technique without coiling in case of aneurysms ≤ 2 mm and a combined approach of stenting and coiling for larger aneurysms. In case of a combined approach, a remodeling balloon may be temporarily inflated within the stent to ensure a safe coil delivery and the stability of the coiling catheter. Indeed, the challenging part of EVT of such complex IA is to avoid coil protrusion within the parent artery. Therefore, large 3D coils should be used to be sure that they will remain within the aneurysm. Furthermore, a remodeling balloon may be used and inflated at the stent size to assist coil delivery. Unfortunately, there is no way to be 100% sure that all coils will remain within the sac. That might explain why these aneurysms are often difficult to completely occlude because of the fear of coil protrusion at the end of EVT. Practically, and if anatomically feasible, the neuroradiologist should attempt to obtain a down-the-barrel view by manipulating the image intensifiers with the balloon inflated. If it cannot be achieved, a view that projects most of the aneurysm off of the parent vessel should be obtained. After the working angle is determined, the microcatheter can be introduced into the aneurysm and embolization initiated with balloon protection. Any shifting of the coils during balloon deflation should be interpreted as an indication of coil impingement on the parent vessel. Therefore, Fiorella et al. [79] suggested to place a second stent at the end of EVT. Because Lubicz et al. [80] felt very confident with the use of the remodeling balloon alone to prevent coil protrusion, they did not place a second stent at the end of EVT. Their therapeutic approach seemed also safe because no significant coil protrusion and/or thromboembolic complication occurred. Depending on the size of the treated aneurysm, the combined approach of stenting plus coiling is not always feasible or safe. Indeed, in aneurysms ≤ 2 mm in diameter, the risk of catheterization through the stent struts and/or coil delivery might be too dangerous [81]. Therefore, intracranial stenting alone may be an alternative therapeutic option in such cases (Figs 7A-C). Benndorf et al. [82] were the first to report spontaneous IA thrombosis by stent placement alone. Then, few authors reported the feasibility of this approach and showed good clinical and anatomical results [81-86]. This therapeutic strategy consists of an endovascular reconstruction of the diseased vascular segment with one or more self-expandable stents. Indeed, several authors [86-89] have shown that stent placement induces significant intra-aneurysmal flow modifications that may lead to spontaneous thrombosis. These findings were also confirmed by Lubicz et al. [80] because 2/13 patients were treated by this endovascular approach and showed excellent clinical and anatomical results. It is yet unknown if one or multiple stents are needed to ensure a spontaneous complete aneurysm occlusion. However, the use of 2 or more stents allows for reducing the effective size of the stent cells while maintaining the patency of the adjacent arteries. Therefore, it is associated with increased modifications of the intra-aneurysmal flow that may lead to spontaneous thrombosis of the sac. Finally, it is important to pinpoint that some patients in Fiorella et al. [79, 81] and Lubicz et al. [80] series were treated by stenting alone for a ruptured IA and it highlights the utility of this approach even in case of SAH.

However and despite these promising preliminary results, long-term follow-up is mandatory to establish the true efficacy of stenting in order to assess for the potential sequels of stenting, namely aneurysm recurrence and in-stent stenosis or thrombosis. Indeed, stenting is generally used in wide-necked, fusiform, and/or large IA that are prone to coil compaction and recanalization; on the other hand, the long-term impact of a foreign body within cerebral vessels is still unknown. Concerning in-stent re-stenosis that represents an anticipated complication of stent placement in the peripheral vasculature, it would not intuitively follow that this experience would translate to self-expandable intracranial stent deployed in a non-stenotic vessel for aneurysm treatment. This is particularly true in view of the very low radial forces of the available self-expandable stents and correspondingly low likelihood of significant vessel wall trauma during and after deployment. In large series with mid-term follow-up, the percentage of in-stent stenosis is low, around 5%, in the vast majority without clinical symptoms [63-74].

In most departments, and although this technique is very promising, patient selection for EVT with self-expandable stents mostly includes unruptured intracranial aneurysms that can not be safely treated by surgical clipping or by the use of the remodeling technique. Indeed, even if the balloon remodeling technique increases the risk of thromboembolic events [51], it avoids a permanent intravascular implant and long-term antiplatelet medication. Future larger series with long-term follow-up are required to determine the exact role of this technique for the treatment of intracranial aneurysms.

EVT Perspectives

Our paper highlights what could be expected from the development of new endovascular techniques and tools. On a technical point of view, most IA are now treatable by endovascular approach and EVT is no more limited to aneurysms with a favorable neck/sac ratio. It also appears obvious that these techniques require a learning curve that may explain contradictory information within the literature about their associated complication rate.

Among new techniques, intracranial stenting seems the most promising one because stents may induce intra-aneurysmal flow reduction and parent artery healing that might lead to aneurysm thrombosis without even "touching" the sac. Ahlhelm et al. [90] have recently confirmed this hypothesis by developing a novel highly flexible stent with a central tightly braided mesh. They have shown, in a rabbit aneurysm model, that wide-necked aneurysms may completely be treated by intracranial stenting alone. This new concept of EVT might represent a future therapeutic option for IA. However, long-term data are still missing to draw final conclusions. Nevertheless, for the first time in the history of IA treatment, a causal therapeutic approach – that is focused on the vessel wall defect – seems thus feasible. The adjunctive effect of stenting on IA occlusion has been suggested for years in experimental and early clinical studies [63-74, 81-92]. Indeed, stents have a larger potential than simple mechanical protection against coil protrusion by reducing the intra-aneurysmal flow, facilitating endothelialization at the neck, and healing the diseased vessel segment (Figures 7A-C). Stents should now be considered as mechanical, hemodynamical, and biological active devices that may help prevent aneurysm recanalization and contribute to vessel wall healing.

Currently, the industry is working to develop intracranial stent technology that will allow for safe navigation through the intracranial vasculature that will not lose its flexibility when coated with occlusive materials. Coating stents with bioactive substances that can induce collagen/fibrin formation and subsequent endothelialization are being explored. By coating alloy or biodegradable stents with compounds that can induce controlled smooth muscle proliferation, the aneurysm orifice would undergo a remodeling that would effectively reconstruct the intima and media. Therefore, stenting might be the next revolution of IA treatment, 15 years after the advent of detachable coils.

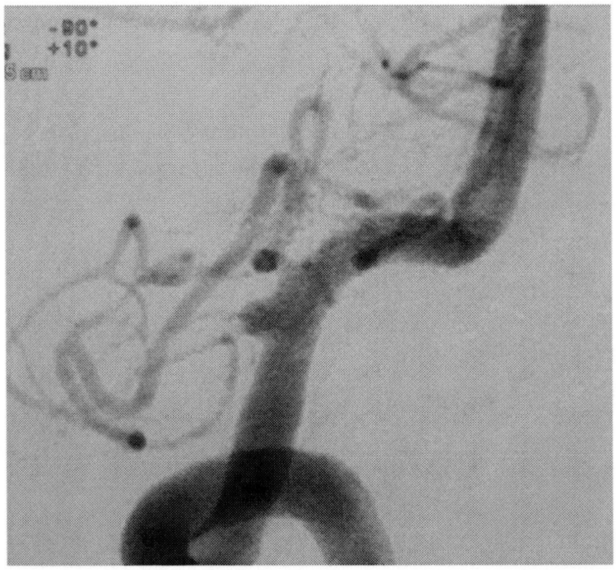

A. Very small (< 2 mm) wide-necked and circumferential aneurysm located on a unique vertebral artery close to the PICA origin.

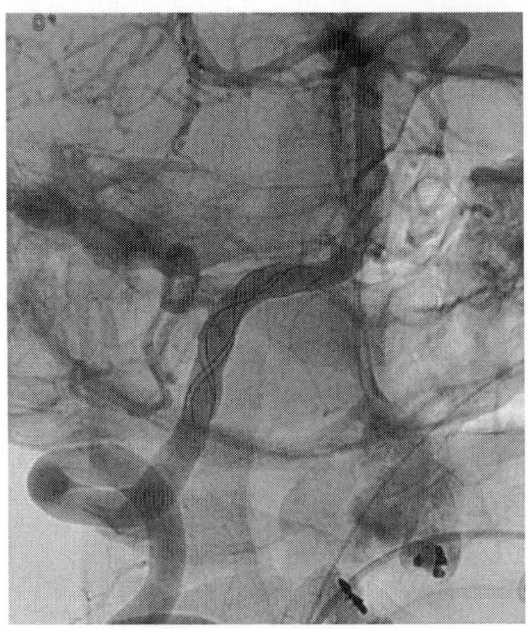

B. EVT by placement of 2 self-expandable stents to promote aneurysm thrombosis while maintaining the PICA patency.

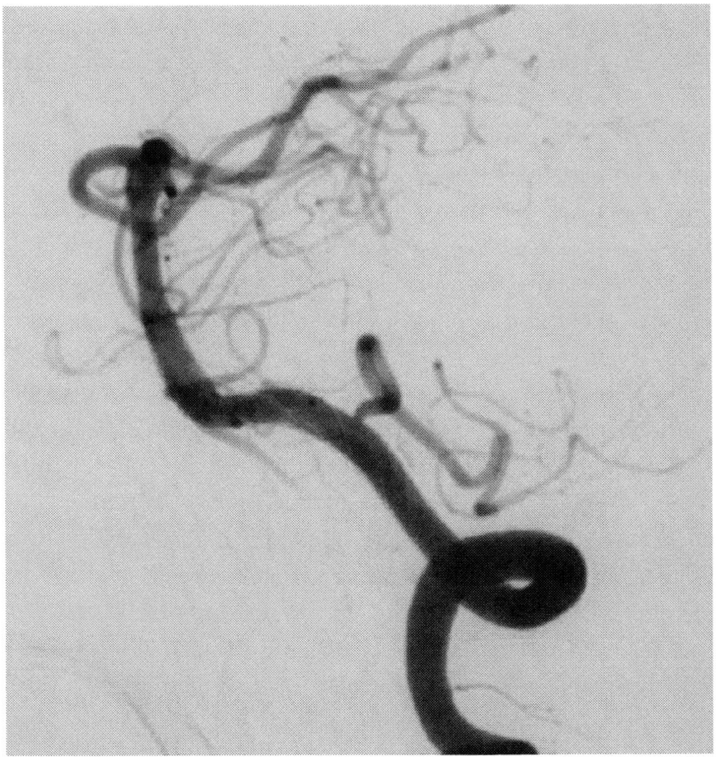

C. Angiographic control at 6 months shows a further thrombosis with a complete aneurysm occlusion.

Figure 7. Ruptured vertebral artery aneurysm

References

[1] Gulielmi, G; Vinuela, F; Dion, J; Duckwiler, G. Electrothrombosis of saccular aneurysms via endovascular approach- Part 2: Preliminary clinical experience. *J Neurosurg*, 1991, 75, 8-14.

[2] Guglielmi, G; Vinuela, F; Duckwiler, G; et al. Endovascular treatment of posterior circulation aneurysms by electrothrombosis using electrically detachable coils. *J Neurosurg,* 1992, 77, 515-524.

[3] International Subarachnoid Aneurysm Trial (ISAT) Collaborative Group. ISAT of neurosurgical clipping versus endovascular coiling in 2143 patients with ruptured intracranial aneurysms: a randomized comparison of effects on survival, dependency, seizures, rebleeding, subgroups, and aneurysm occlusion. *Lancet,* 2005, 366, 809-817.

[4] International Study of Unruptured Intracranial Aneurysms Investigators. Unruptured intracranial aneurysms: natural history, clinical outcome, and risks of surgical and endovascular treatment. *Lancet,* 2003, 362, 103-110.

[5] Mejdoubi, M; Gigaud, M; Tremoulet, M; Albucher, JF; Cognard, C. Initial primary endovascular treatment in the management of ruptured intracranial aneurysms: a prospective consecutive series. *Neuroradiology,* 2006, 48, 899-905.

[6] Lubicz, B; Balériaux, D; Lefranc, F; Brotchi, J; Bruneau, M; Levivier, M. Endovascular treatment of intracranial aneurysms as the first therapeutic option: a prospective study over 30 months in a single-centre. *J of Neuroradiol,* 2007, 34, 250-259.

[7] Raymond, J; Guilbert, F; Weill, A; et al. Long-term angiographic recurrences after selective endovascular treatment of aneurysms with detachable coils. *Stroke,* 2003, 34, 1398-1403.

[8] Murayama, Y; Tateshima, S; Gonzalez, NR; Vinuela, F. Matrix and bioabsorbable polymeric coils accelerate healing intracranial aneurysms : long-term experimental study. *Stroke,* 2003, 34, 2031-2037.

[9] Raymond, J; Leblanc, P; Desfaits, AC; et al. In situ beta radiation to prevent recanalization after coil embolization of cerebral aneurysms. *Stroke,* 2002, 33, 421-427.

[10] Cloft, HJ; Kallmes, DF. Aneurysm packing with Hydrocoil Embolic System versus platinum coils: initial clinical experience. *AJNR Am J Neuroradiol*, 2004, 25, 60-62.

[11] Tamatani, S; Ito, Y; Abe, H; et al. Evaluation of the stability of aneurysms after embolization using detachable coils: correlation between stability of aneurysms and embolized volume of aneurysms. *AJNR Am J Neuroradiol*, 2002, 23, 762-767.

[12] Lubicz, B; Leclerc, X; Gauvrit, JY; Lejeune, JP; Pruvo, JP. Endovascular treatment of intracranial aneurysms with matrix coils: a preliminary study of immediate post-treatment results. *AJNR Am J Neuroradiol*, 2005, 26, 373-375.

[13] Niimi, Y; Song, J; Madrid, M; Berenstein, A. Endovascular treatment of intracranial aneurysms using Matrix coils: early experience and mid-term follow-up. *Stroke,* 2006, 37, 028-1032.

[14] Rivet, DJ; Moran, CJ; Mazumdar, A., et al. Single-institution experience with matrix coils in the treatment of intracranial aneurysms: comparison with same-center outcomes with the use of platinum coils. *AJNR Am J Neuroradiol*, 2007, 28, 1736-1742.

[15] Piotin, M; Spelle, L; Mounayer, C; et al. Intracranial Aneurysms Coiling With Matrix. Immediate Results in 152 Patients and Midterm Anatomic Follow-Up From 115 Patients. *Stroke,* 2008, Nov 6. [Epub ahead of print]

[16] Pierot, L; Leclerc, X; Bonafe, A; et al. Endovascular treatment of intracranial aneurysms using Matrix coils: short- and mid-term results in ruptured and unruptured aneurysms. *Neurosurgery,* 2008, 63, 850-857.

[17] Bendszus, M; Bartsch, AJ; Solymosi, L. Endovascular occlusion of aneurysms using a new bioactive coil: a matched pair analysis with bare platinum coils. *Stroke,* 2007, 38, 2855-2857.

[18] Geyik, S; Yavuz, K; Ergun, O; et al. Endovascular treatment of intracranial aneurysms with bioactive Cerecyte coils: effects on treatment stability. *Neuroradiology,* 2008, 50, 787-793.

[19] Veznedaroglu, E; Koebbe, CJ; Siddiqui, A; Rosenwasser, RH. Initial experience with bioactive cerecyte detachable coils: impact on reducing recurrence rates. *Neurosurgery,* 2008, 62, 799-805.

[20] Cloft, HJ. HydroCoil for Endovascular Aneurysm Occlusion (HEAL) study: periprocedural results. *AJNR Am J Neuroradiol*, 2006, 27, 289-292.

[21] Gaba, RC; Ansari, SA; Roy, SS. Embolization of intracranial aneurysms with hydrogel-coated coils versus inert platinum coils: effects on packing density, coil length and quantity, procedure performance, cost, length of hospital stay, and durability of therapy. *Stroke,* 2006, 37, 1443-1450.

[22] Fanning, NF; Berentei, Z; Brennan, PR; THorton, J. HydroCoil as an adjuvant to bare platinum coil treatment of 100 cerebral aneurysms. *Neuroradiology,* 2007, 49, 139-148.

[23] Fanning, NF; Willinsky, RA; Ter Brugge, KG. Wall enhancement, edema, and hydrocephalus after endovascular coil occlusion of intradural cerebral aneurysms. *J Neurosurg*, 2008, 108, 1074-1086.

[24] Abrahams, JM; Diamond, SL; Hurst, RW; Zager, EL; Grady, MS. Topic review: Surface modifications enhancing biological activity of Guglielmi detachable coils in treating intracranial aneurysms. *Surg Neurol*, 2000, 54, 34–41.

[25] Abrahams, JM; Forman, MS; Grady, MS; Diamond, SL. Delivery of human vascular endothelial growth factor with platinum coils enhances wall thickening and coil impregnation in a rat aneurysm model. *AJNR Am J Neuroradiol*, 2001, 22, 1410–1417.

[26] Abrahams, JM; Song, C; DeFelice, S; Grady, MS; Diamond, SL; Levy, RJ. Endovascular microcoil gene delivery using immobilized anti-adenovirus antibody for vector tethering. *Stroke,* 2002, 33, 1376–1382.

[27] De Gast, AN; Altes, TA; Marx, WF; Do, HM; Helm, GA; Kallmes, DF. Transforming growth factor beta-coated platinum coils for endovascular treatment of aneurysms: An animal study. *Neurosurgery,* 2001, 49, 690–696.

[28] Kawakami, O; Miyamoto, S; Hatano, T; Yamada, K; Hashimoto, N; Tabata, Y. Accelerated embolization healing of aneurysms by polyethylene terephthalate coils seeded with autologous fibroblasts. *Neurosurgery,* 2005, 56, 1075–1081.

[29] Matsumoto, H; Terada, T; Tsuura, M; Itakura, T; Ogawa, A. Basic fibroblast growth factor released from a platinum coil with a polyvinyl alcohol core enhances cellular proliferation and vascular wall thickness: An in vitro and in vivo study. *Neurosurgery,* 2003, 53, 402–408.

[30] Murayama, Y; Vinuela, F; Tateshima, S; Vinuela, F: Jr, Akiba, Y. Endovascular treatment of experimental aneurysms by use of a combination of liquid embolic agents and protective devices. *AJNR Am J Neuroradiol*, 2000, 21, 1726-1735.

[31] Mawad, ME; Cekirge, S; Ciceri, E; Saatci, I. Endovascular treatment of giant and large intracranial aneurysms by using a combination of stent placement and liquid polymer injection. *J Neurosurg*, 2002, 96, 474-482.

[32] Molyneux, AJ; Cekirge, S; Saatci, I; Gal, G. Cerebral Aneurysm Multicenter European Onyx (CAMEO) Trial: results of a prospective observational study in 20 european centers. *AJNR Am J Neuroradiol*, 2004, 25, 39-51

[33] Lubicz, B; Piotin, M; Mounayer, C; Spelle, L; Moret, J. Selective endovascular treatment of intracranial aneurysms with a liquid embolic: a single-center experience in 39 patients with 41 aneurysms. *AJNR Am J Neuroradiol*, 2005, 26, 885-893.

[34] Cekirge, HS; Saatci, I; Ozturk, MH; et al. Late angiographic and clinical follow-up results of 100 consecutive aneurysms treated with Onyx reconstruction: largest single-center experience. *Neuroradiology,* 2006, 48, 113-126.

[35] Gruber, A; Killer, M; Bavinzski, G; Richling, B. Clinical and angiographic results of endosaccular coiling treatment of giant and very large intracranial aneurysms: A 7-year, single-center experience. *Neurosurgery,* 1999, 45, 793-800.

[36] Mericle, RA; Wakhloo, AK; Lopes, DK; Lanzino, G; Guterman, LR; Hopkins, LN. Delayed aneurysm regrowth and recanalization after Guglielmi detachable coil treatment. *J Neurosurg*, 1998, 89, 142-145.

[37] Murayama, Y; Nien, YL; Duckwiller, G ; et al. Guglielmi detachable coils embolization of cerebral aneurysms : 11 years experience. *J Neurosurg*, 2003, 98, 959-966.

[38] Sluzewski, M; Menovsky, T; Van Rooij, WJ; Wijnada, D. Coiling of very large and giant aneurysm: long-term clinical and serial angiographic results. *AJNR Am J Neuroradiol*, 2003, 24, 257-262.

[39] Moret, J; Pierot, L; Boulin, A; et al. "Remodelling" of the arterial wall of the parent vessel in the endovascular treatment of intracranial aneurysms. *Neuroradiology,* 1994, 36, Suppl 1:S83.

[40] Lubicz, B; Leclerc, X; Gauvrit, JY; Lejeune, JP; Pruvo, JP. HyperForm remodeling-balloon for endovascular treatment of wide-neck intracranial aneurysms. *AJNR Am J Neuroradiol*, 2004, 25, 1381-1383.

[41] Moret, J; Cognard, C; Weill, A; Castaings, L; Rey, A. The reconstruction technique in the treatment of wide-neck intracranial aneurysms: long-term angiographic and clinical results. *J Neuroradiol*, 1997, 24, 30-44.

[42] Lefkowitz, MA; Gobin, YP; Akiba, Y; et al. Balloon-assisted Guglielmi detachable coiling of wide-necked aneurysms: Part II - clinical results. *Neurosurgery,* 1999, 45, 531-536

[43] Aletich, VA; Debrun, GM; Misra, M; Charbel, F; Ausman, JI. The remodeling technique of balloon-assisted Guglielmi detachable coil placement in wide-necked aneurysms: experience at the university of Illinois at Chicago. *J Neurosurg*, 2000, 93, 388-396.

[44] Nelson, PK, Levy, DI. Balloon-assisted coil embolization of wide-necked aneurysms of the internal carotid artery: medium-term angiographic and clinical follow-up in 22 patients. *AJNR Am J Neuroradiol*, 2001, 22, 19-26.

[45] Cottier, JP; Pasco, A; Gallas S; et al. Utility of balloon-assisted Guglielmi Detachable Coiling in the treatment of 49 cerebral aneurysms : a retrospective, multicenter study. *AJNR Am J Neuroradiol*, 2001, 22, 345-351.

[46] Lubicz, B; Leclerc, X; Gauvrit, JY; Lejeune, JP; Pruvo, JP. Hyperform remodelling-balloon for endovascular treatment of wide-neck intracranial aneurysms. *AJNR Am J of Neuroradiol,* 2004, 25, 1381-1383.

[47] White, JB; Layton, KF; Kallmes, DF; Cloft, HJ. Balloon-assisted coiling through a 5-French system. *Neuroradiology,* 2006, 49, 157-159.

[48] Ross, IB; Dhillon, GS. Balloon assistance as a routine adjunct to the endovascular treatment of cerebral aneurysms. *Surg Neurol*, 2006, 66, 593-601.

[49] Layton, KF; Cloft, HJ; Gray, LA; Lewis, DA; Kallmes DF. Balloon-assisted coiling of intracranial aneurysms: evaluation of local thrombus formation and symptomatic thromboembolic complications. *AJNR Am J Neuroradiol,* 2007, 28, 1172-1175.

[50] Lubicz, B; Lefranc, F; Levivier, M; et al. Endovascular treatment of intracranial aneurysms with a branch arising from the sac. *Am J of Neuroradiol AJNR,* 2006, 27, 142-147.

[51] Soeda, A; Sakai, N; Sakai, H., et al. Thromboembolic events associated with Guglielmi Detachable Coil embolization of asymptmatic cerebral aneurysms: evaluation of 66 consecutive cases with use of Diffusion-weighted MR imaging. *AJNR Am J Neuroradiol,* 2003, 24, 127-132.

[52] Sluzewski, M; Van, Rooij, WJ; Beute, GN; Nijssen, PC. Balloon-assisted coil embolization of intracranial aneurysms: incidence, complications, and angiography results. *J Neurosurg,* 2006, 105, 396-399.

[53] Lubicz, B; Lefranc, F; Bruneau, M; Balériaux, D; De Witte, O. Balloon-assisted coiling of intracranial aneurysms is not associated with a higher complication rate. *Neuroradiology,* 2008, 50, 769-776.

[54] Shapiro, M; Babb, J; Becske, T; Nelson, PK. Safety and efficacy of adjunctive balloon remodeling during endovascular treatment of intracranial aneurysms: a literature review. *AJNR Am J Neuroradiol,* 2008, 29, 1777-1781.

[55] Singh, V; Gress, DR; Higashida, RT; Dowd, CF; Van Halbach, V; Johnston, SC. The learning curve for coil embolization of unruptured intracranial aneurysms. *AJNR Am J Neuroradiol,* 2002, 23, 768-771.

[56] Henkes, H; Fischer, S; Liebig, T; et al. Repeated endovascular coil occlusion in 350 of 2759 intracranial aneurysms: safety and effectiveness aspects. *Neurosurgery,* 2006, 58, 224-32.

[57] Slob, MJ; Sluzewski, M; Van Rooij, WJ; Roks, G; Rinkel, GJ. Additional coiling of previously coiled cerebral aneurysms: clinical and angiographic results. *AJNR Am J Neuroradiol,* 2004, 25, 1373-1376.

[58] Turjman, F; Massoud, TF; Ji C; Guglielmi, G; Vinuela, F; Robert, J. Combined stent implantation and endosaccular coil placement for treatment of experimental wide-necked aneurysms: a feasibility study in swine. *AJNR Am J Neuroradiol,* 1994, 15, 1087-1090

[59] Szikora, I; Guterman, LR; Wells, KM; Hopkins, LN. Combined use of stents and coils to treat experimental wide-necked carotid aneurysms: preliminary results. *AJNR Am J Neuroradiol,* 1994, 15, 1091-1102

[60] Phatouros, CC; Sasaki, TY; Higashida, RT; et al. Stent-supported coil embolization: The treatment of fusiform and wide-neck aneurysms and pseudoaneurysms. *Neurosurgery,* 2000, 47, 107-113

[61] Lylyk, P; Cohen, JE; Ceratto, R; Ferrario, A; Miranda, C. Endovascular reconstruction of intracranial arteries by stent placement and combined techniques. *J Neurosurg,* 2002, 97, 1306-1313

[62] Kessler, I; Mounayer, C; Piotin, M; Spelle, L; Vanzin, JR; Moret, J. The use of balloon-expandable stents in the management of intracranial arterial diseases: a 5-year single-center experience. *AJNR Am J of Neuroradiol,* 2005, 26, 2342-2348

[63] Wanke, I; Doerfler, A; Schoch, B; Stolke, D; Forsting, M. Treatment of wide-necked intracranial aneurysms with a self-expandanding stent system: initial clinical experience. *AJNR Am J Neuroradiol,* 2003, 24, 1192-1199.

[64] Alfke, K; Straube, T; Dörner, L; Mehdorn, HM; Jansen, O. Treatment of intracranial broad-neck aneurysms with a new self-expanding stent and coil embolization. *AJNR Am J Neuroradiol*, 2004, 25, 584-591.

[65] Benitez, RP; Silva, MT; Klem, J; Veznedaroglu, E; Rosenwasser, RH: Endovascular occlusion of wide-necked aneurysms with a new intracranial microstent (Neuroform) and detachable coils. *Neurosurgery,* 2004, 54, 359-1367.

[66] Broadbent, L; Moran, C; Cross, D; Derdeyn, C. Management of Neuroform stent dislodgement and misplacement. *AJNR Am J Neuroradiol*, 2003, 24, 1819-1822.

[67] Fiorella, D; Albuquerque, F; Han, P; MacDougall, C. Preliminary experience using the Neuroform stent for the treatment of cerebral aneurysms. *J Neurosurg*, 2004, 54, 6-16.

[68] Henkes, H; Bose, A; Felber, S; Miloslavski, E; Berg-Dammer, E; Kühne, D. Endovascular coil occlusion of intracranial aneurysms assisted by a novel self-expandable nitinol microstent (Neuroform). *Intervent Neuroradiol*, 2002, 8, 107-119.

[69] Lylyk, P; Ferrario, A; Pasbon, B; Miranda, C; Doroszuk, G. Buenos Aires experience with the Neuroform self-expanding stent for the treatment of intracranial aneurysms. *J Neurosurg*, 2005, 102, 235-241.

[70] Kis, B; Weber, W; Berlit, P; Kuhne, D: Elective treatment of saccular and broad-necked intracranial aneurysms using a closed-cell nitinol stent (Leo). *Neurosurgery,* 2006, 58, 443-50.

[71] Lubicz, B; Leclerc, X; Levivier, M; Brotchi, J; Pruvo, JP; Lejeune, JP; Balériaux, D. Retractable self-expandable stent for endovascular treatment of wide-necked intracranial aneurysms: preliminary experience. *Neurosurgery,* 2006, 58, 451-457.

[72] Weber, W; Bendszus, M; Kis, B; Boulanger, T; Solymosi, L; Kuhne, D. A new self-expanding nitinol stent (Enterprise) for the treatment of wide-necked intracranial aneurysms: initial clinical and angiographic results in 31 aneurysms. *Neuroradiology,* 2007, 49, 555-561.

[73] Lubicz, B; François, O; Levivier, M; Brotchi, J; Balériaux, D. Preliminary experience with the enterprise stent for endovascular treatment of complex intracranial aneurysms: potential advantages and limiting characteristics. *Neurosurgery,* 2008, 62, 1063-1069.

[74] Mocco, J; Snyder, KV; Albuquerque, FC., et al. Treatment of intracranial aneurysms with the Enterprise stent: a multicenter registry. *J Neurosurg*, 2008, Oct 31. [Epub ahead of print]

[75] Debrun, G; Fox, AJ; Drake, CG; Peerless, S; Girvin, J; Ferguson, G. Giant unclippable aneurysms: treatment with detachable balloons. *AJNR Am J Neuroradiol*, 1981, 2, 167-173.

[76] Drake, C; Peerless, S. Giant fusiform intracranial aneurysms: review of 120 patients treated surgically from 1965-1992. *J Neurosurg*, 1997, 87, 141-162.

[77] Gobin, PY; Vinuela, F; Gurian, JH; et al. Treatment of large and giant fusiform intracranial aneurysms with Guglielmi detachable coils. *J Neurosurg*, 1996, 84, 55-62.

[78] Anson, JA. Treatment strategies for intracranial fusiform aneurysms. *Neurosurg Clin N Am*, 1998, 9, 743.

[79] Fiorella, D; Albuquerque, FC; Masaryk, TJ; Rasmussen, PA; McDougall, CG. Balloon-in-stent technique for the constructive endovascular treatment of "ultra-wide necked" circumferential aneurysms. *Neurosurgery,* 2005, 57, 1218-1227.

[80] Lubicz, B; Collignon, L; Lefranc, F; et al. Circumferential and fusiform intracranial aneurysms: reconstructive endovascular treatment with self-expandable stents. *Neuroradiology,* 2008, 50, 499-507.
[81] Fiorella, D; Albuquerque, FC; Deshmukh, VR; et al. Endovascular reconstruction with the Neuroform stent as monotherapy for the treatment of uncoilable intradural pseudoaneurysms. *Neurosurgery,* 2006, 59, 291-300.
[82] Benndorf, G; Herbon, U; Sollmann, WP; Campi, A. Treatment of a ruptured dissecting vertebral artery aneurysm with double stent placement: case report. *AJNR Am J Neuroradiol*, 2001, 22, 1844-1848.
[83] Vanninen, R; Mannine, H; Ronkainen, A. Broad-based intracranial aneurysms: thrombosis induced by stent placement. *AJNR Am J Neuroradiol*, 2003, 24, 263-266.
[84] Doerfler, A; Wanke, I; Egelhof, T; Stolke, D; Forsting, M. Double-stent method: therapeutic alternative for small wide-necked aneurysms. Technical note. *J Neurosurg*, 2004, 100, 150-154.
[85] Zenteno, M; Modenesi Freitas, JM; Aburto-Murrieta, Y; Koppe, G; Machado, E; Lee, A. Balloon-expandable stenting with and without coiling for wide-neck and complex aneurysms. *Surg Neurol*, 2006, 66, 603-610.
[86] Wakhloo, AK; Schellhammer, F; De Vries, J; Haberstroh, J; Schumacher, M. Self-expanding and balloon-expandable stents in the treatment of carotid aneurysms: an experimental study in a canine model. *AJNR Am J Neuroradiol*, 1994, 15, 493-502.
[87] Ansari, SA; Lassig, JP; Nicol, E; Thompson, BG; Gemmette, JJ; Ghandi, D. Thrombosis of a fusiform intracranial aneurysm induced by overlapping neuroform stents: case report. *Neurosurgery,* 2007, 60, E950-951.
[88] Lieber, BB; Stancampiano, AP; Wakhloo, AK. Alteration of hemodynamics in aneurysm models by stenting: influence of stent porosity. *Annals of Biomedical Engineering,* 1997, 25, 460-469.
[89] Hirabayashi, M; Ohta, M; Rüfenacht, DA; Chopard, B. Characterization of flow reduction properties in an aneurysm due to a stent. *Phys Rev E Stat Nonlin Soft Matter Phys.*, 2003, 68, 02191.
[90] Ahlhelm, F; Roth, C; Kaufmann, R; Schulte-Altedorneburg, G; Romeike, BF; Reith, W. Treatment of wide-necked intracranial aneurysms with a novel self-expanding two-zonal endovascular stent device. *Neuroradiology,* 2007, 49, 1023-1028.
[91] Barath, K; Cassot, F; Fasel, JH; Ohta, M; Rüfenacht, DA. Influence of stent properties on the alteration of cerebral intra-aneurysmal haemodynamics : flow quantification in elastic sidewall aneurysm models. *Neurol Res.*, 2005, 27, S120-128.
[92] Wanke, I; Forsting, M. Stents for intracranial wide-necked aneurysms: more than mechanical protection. *Neuroradiology,* 2008, 50, 991-998.

In: Aneurysms: Types, Risks, Formation and Treatment
Editors: Alain Laurent and Ethan Morel
ISBN: 978-1-60741-557-2
© 2009 Nova Science Publishers, Inc.

Chapter 9

Diagnosis of Coronary Artery Aneurysms/Ectasia by Multidetector Row Computed Tomography, Intravascular Ultrasound, and Angioscopy

Sei Komatsu[1*], Teruaki Kamata[2], Kazuaki Miyaji[2], Yoshinobu Shimizu[2], Sachio Kuribayashi[3], Atsushi Hirayama[4] and Kazuhisa Kodama[1]

[1]Department of Cardiology, Amagasaki Central Hospital, Hyogo, Japan
[2]Department of Radiological Technology, Amagasaki Central Hospital, Hyogo, Japan
[3]Department of Diagnostic Radiology, Keio University School of Medicine, Tokyo, Japan
[4]Department of Cardiology, Nihon University School of Medicine, Tokyo, Japan

Summary

Coronary artery aneurysm/ectasia is rare, reported less than 5 % of coronary angiography. That might cause death because of thrombotic occlusion or rupture. The main cause of adult coronary aneurysm is atherosclerosis. Other cause may include Kawasaki disease, inflammatory and infectious arteritis, connective tissue disease, aortic dissection, congenital disease, and diagnostic or interventional coronary angiography. To estimate the etiology of the aneurysm, evaluating plaque component in the aneurysm is essential besides patients' history. Atherosclerotic coronary aneurysm contains yellow plaque by angioscopy and low density eccentric plaque by intravascular ultrasound (IVUS). Coronary artery aneurysms in patients with Kawasaki disease tend to have predominant egg-shell calcification. Recently, Multidetector row computed tomography (MDCT) is an excellent modality for detecting coronary artery disease with high

*Corresponding author: Department of Cardiology, Amagasaki Central Hospital. 1-12-1 Shio-e, Amagasaki, Hyogo, 661-0976 Japan. Phone +81 6 6944 3045, Fax +81 6 6499-3113 E-mail: plaquemap@yahoo.co.jp

accuracy compared to invasive coronary artery. Many previous reports mentioned that MDCT also can detect coronary anomalous condition. Also, coronary plaque is distinguishable by CT number. We developed color-coded analysis based on CT number, Plaque Map for tissue and plaque characterization. Using MDCT with Plaque Map, some kinds of aneurysm may be distinguished by their features, such as calcification and atherosclerotic plaque. We present a review of diagnostic imaging of coronary artery aneurysm by MDCT with Plaque Map and invasive plaque imaging, such as IVUS and angioscopy.

Keywords: coronary artery aneurysm, multidetector row computed tomography, angioscopy, intravascular ultrasound, Kawasaki disease

1. Introduction

Coronary artery aneurysm is rare and incidentally found in diagnostic coronary angiography (CAG), however, it might cause death because of thrombotic occlusion, arrhythmia or rupture. Coronary artery aneurysm is found both in adults and children. Main causes of coronary artery aneurysm are atherosclerosis and Kawasaki disease, however, etiology of all coronary artery aneurysm is not always conclusive when the patients' history is not clear. To detect the plaque of the aneurysm may be the key to differentiate the etiology of the coronary artery aneurysm. CAG demonstrates coronary stenosis or occlusion, but the limitation is that it is not able to demonstrate coronary plaque. Especially for detecting vulnerable plaque in patients with acute coronary syndrome, invasive coronary plaque imaging devices, such as intravascular ultrasound (IVUS) [1], angioscopy [2], and new ultrasound imaging technique such as VH (virtual histology)-IVUS [3] and IB (integrated backscatter)-IVUS [4], and optical coherence tomography (OCT) [5] have been developed. IVUS [6,7] and coronary angioscopy [7,8] have been developed. They enabled us to illustrate inside in coronary arteries and aneurysms. IVUS overview the cross-section of the vessel and angioscopy demonstrates the surface of the vessel. Atherosclerotic plaque tends to have yellow plaque by angioscopy and show dominantly lipid-rich plaque by IVUS. However, when aneurysm is occluded, composition of coronary artery aneurysm cannot be analyzed unless extracted by surgical operation.

As recent progress of multi-detector row computed tomography (MDCT) [8,9], coronary artery stenosis and occlusion has been diagnosed noninvasively with high accuracy by MDCT compared to CAG [10]. Especially, negative predictive value for detecting coronary stenosis is about 99% [10]. As the improvement of special and temporal resolution, MDCT can demonstrate morphological abnormality, such as coronary artery anomaly [11] and aneurysm. As coronary CT angiography (CTCA) becomes common, coronary aneurysm has come to be primarily diagnosed by CTCA prior to CAG. Reports about detection of coronary artery aneurysms by CTCA are increasing recently [7,12,13]. Not only detecting coronary anomaly, MDCT can demonstrate coronary plaque with high accuracy compared to IVUS and angioscopy [7]. MDCT may play a role for recognizing their etiology by analyzing inside the aneurysm.

Schroeder et al. [14] first reported that coronary plaque could be distinguished using CT number. CT number is defined as 0 HU (Hunsfield unit) for water and -1000 HU for air. A range of 2000 HU represents densities of all hard or soft tissue within the body. Using MDCT, soft plaques had a density of 14 +/- 26 HU (range -42 to +47 HU), intermediate plaques of 91 +/- 21 HU (61 to 112 HU) and calcified plaques of 419 +/- 194 HU (126 to 736 HU). To analyze the gray-scale CT images, ROI (region of interest) and profile curve are common, however, these two methods does not fit the shape of artery or plaque.

Later, color map analysis based on CT number, Plaque Map, has been developed for the analysis of CT images of short-axis view, i.e., IVUS view [8,9]. Using Plaque Map, both plaque and structure of coronary artery aneurysm can be analyzed noninvasively [7].

2. Definition and Incidence

Coronary artery aneurysm is abnormal dilatation of the coronary artery [15], first described in the 18th century [16]. Coronary artery aneurysm is defined as coronary dilatation >=1.5 times the diameter of normal adjacent segment or the diameter of the largest coronary vessel according to the Coronary Artery Surgery Study (CASS) registry [17]. Coronary artery aneurysms are classified with morphology, such as saccular and fusiform. Fusiform coronary artery aneurysm is classified four types [18]: (1) diffuse ectasia with aneurysmal lesions in two vessels (type I), (2) diffuse ectasia in one vessel and discrete ectasia in another (type II), (3) diffuse ectasia in one vessel (type III), and (4) discrete ectasia in one vessel (type IV) . These are angiographic definition, and it has been used in the majority of case reports and reviews.

Incidence of coronary aneurysm or ectasia is 1.4 % of post mortem examination [19] and 0.3-4.9 % of diagnostic invasive coronary angiography (CAG) [20]. Male predominantly affect coronary artery aneurysm three times compared with female [21]. Incidence of location of aneurysm on right coronary artery, left anterior descending coronary artery, left circumflex coronary artery, and left main trunk are 40.4%, 32.3%, 23.4%, and 3.5%, respectively [22]. Coronary artery aneurysm associated with significant obstructive coronary artery disease was found in 3.1 %, and 1.3 % was isolated coronary aneurysm [23]. Coronary artery aneurysms are commonly associated with atherosclerotic and Kawasaki disease. Other causes are arteritis (polyarteritis nodosa, syphilis, systemic lupus erythematosis, Takayasu's arteritis), mycoses, trauma, cocaine abuse, connective tissues disorders (Marfan syndrome and Ehlers-Danlos syndrome), metastic tumors, polycystic kidney disease, and percutaneous coronary interventions.

3. Symptoms and Prognosis

The symptoms in patients with coronary artery aneurysms do not correlate with the degree of coronary stenosis. It is postulated that coronary artery aneurysm renders patients to higher risk of myocardial ischemia irrespective extent of stenosis [24]. Patients with coronary artery aneurysm had significantly abnormal treadmill tests even without coronary stenosis, suggesting decrease in coronary flow reserve and microvascular dysfunction as a possible contributing factor for myocardial ischemia. Angina is most common symptom of coronary artery aneurysm [21]. Myocardial infarction, arrhythmias, and sudden cardiac death have been reported [25-27]. Coronary artery aneurysm may also break through to the right atrium, right ventricle, or coronary sinus, resulting in left-to-right shunts [15].

Prognosis of coronary artery aneurysm is unknown. In the CASS registry, no difference in survival was observed between patients with or without coronary artery ectasia [17]. In various study, elevated risk for myocardial infarction of coronary artery aneurysm has not been confirmed [17,21]. A mortality rate is reported to be 15 % at 2 years in patients with coronary artery aneurysm [18]. 5-year survival rate of coronary artery aneurysm is 71 % [28].

4. Imaging of Atherosclerotic Coronary Artery Aneurysm

The frequency of atherosclerotic coronary artery aneurysm is approximately 50 % [29]. Coronary artery aneurysm appears when the atherosclerotic process affects both the intima, forming luminal stenosis or occlusions, and the media and adventitial parts of the vessel wall resulting in arterial remodeling and dilatation [30]. The histological feature of the wall of an ectasic artery reveals grossly thickened and fibrotic intima with extensive lipid deposition and marked thinning of the media [31]. Inflammatory markers, such as interleukin-6 and C-reactive protein levels were elevated in patients with coronary artery aneurysm compared with those with normal coronary arteries [32]. Recently, significant positive correlation between the total length of ectasic segments and the levels of plasma soluble intercellular adhesion molecule-1 (ICAM-I), vascular cell adhesion molecule-1 (VCAM-I), and E-selectin has been reported [33].

When plaque is rich enough to narrowing the lumen diameter, CAG might miss coronary aneurismal formation (Figure 1). MDCT can detect coronary artery aneurysm and plaque noninvasively. In case of atherosclerotic coronary artery aneurysm, noncalcified plaque is found by MDCT (Figure 1) [7]. Curved multiplanar reformation (MPR) with Plaque Map is excellent to analyze the plaque composition of aneurysm and measure the diameter of the aneurysm. Short-axial image of the aneurysm showed CT-low-dense eccentric plaque, suggesting soft plaque [7].

IVUS study for 14 atherosclerotic coronary artery aneurysms revealed dissection and ulcer by plaque rupture and atherosclerotic plaque at both of proximal and distal edge of aneurysms [34]. IVUS allows for distinguishing true from false aneurysms. In the true aneurysm, the aneurismal wall contains the medial tissue that shows continuity with the media of the adjacent normal coronary segment; in the false aneurysm, the aneurysm is limited only by adventitial tissue or even just by the visceral pericardium [29,35].

Angioscopy is an effective modality to evaluate coronary luminal wall. Angioscopy visualizes fatty streak and thin-cap fibroatheroma as yellow plaque *in vivo*. The yellow color intensity of plaques is classified into 4 grades: Grade 0 (white), Grade 1 (light yellow), Grade 2 (yellow), and Grade 3 (intensive yellow) [9]. Kashiwase et al [7] reported that intensive yellow plaque was seen inside atherosclerotic plaque.

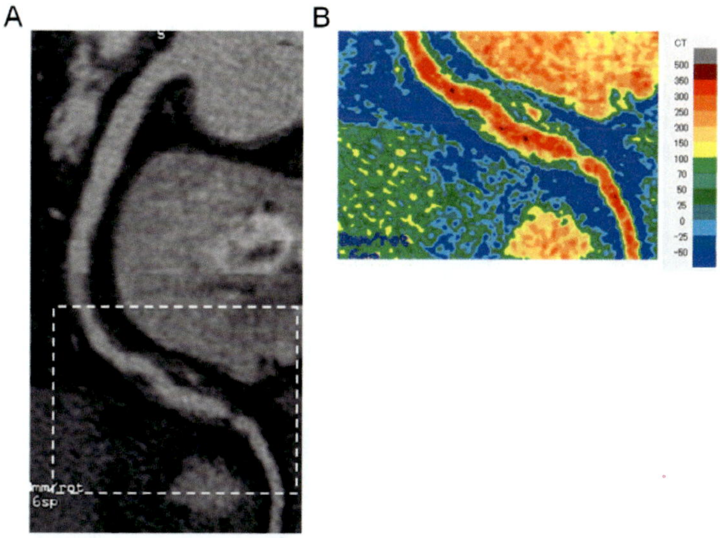

Figure 1. An example of atherosclerotic coronary artery aneurysm in right coronary artery. A. Curved multiplanar reformation image of 64-MDCT. Positive remodeling and predominant non-calcified plaque is detented. B. Plaque Map of the aneurysm. Low-CT-density plaque is seen. Lumen diameter at the aneurysm is almost same as that at normal portion.

5. Imagings of Coronary Artery Aneurysm Due to Kawasaki Disease

The second major cause of coronary artery aneurysm is Kawasaki disease, which is an acute febrile illness that arises from systemic vasculitis [36]. Kawasaki disease has been recognized in children of all racial groups, but more prevalent in Japanese [37]. The annual incidences of Japanese [38], Asians, black, Caucasians [39] were reported to be 90, 33, 23, and 12, per 100,000 the children under 5 years of age, respectively. Studies of Kawasaki disease in twins and in siblings of index cases suggested a possible role for genetic disposition that interacts with exposure to the agent or agents in the environment [37,40,41].

Kawasaki disease is characterized by 3 clinical phases [36]. The acute phase is marked by fever and symptoms of acute inflammation and lasts 1-2 weeks. The subacute phase occurs 2-4 weeks after the onset of symptoms and it is characterized periungual desquamation with accompanying thrombosis and development of coronary artery aneurysms. Approximately 25 % of patients complicated with coronary aneurysm and 3 % may progress in coronary heart disease [42]. Even if asymptomatic, large coronary aneurysm is frequently associated with coronary artery disease [43]. The convalescent phase occurs 6-8 weeks after the onset and all symptoms resolve [36].

Half of coronary artery aneurysm during acute phase of Kawasaki disease may normalize by CAG 1-2 years later [44]. Smaller aneurysms tend to regress more than large aneurysms [45]. Unresolved coronary artery aneurysms persist and developed stenotic lesion and/or thrombus [36]. The risk of myocardial infarction is highest during the first year after the onset. The most important predictor of myocardial infarction and other chronic sequelae is aneurismal size [45]. Giant coronary artery aneurysms have poor prognosis. Risk stratification of Kawasaki disease is classified 5 risk levels according to the existence and the size of the coronary artery aneurysms [46].

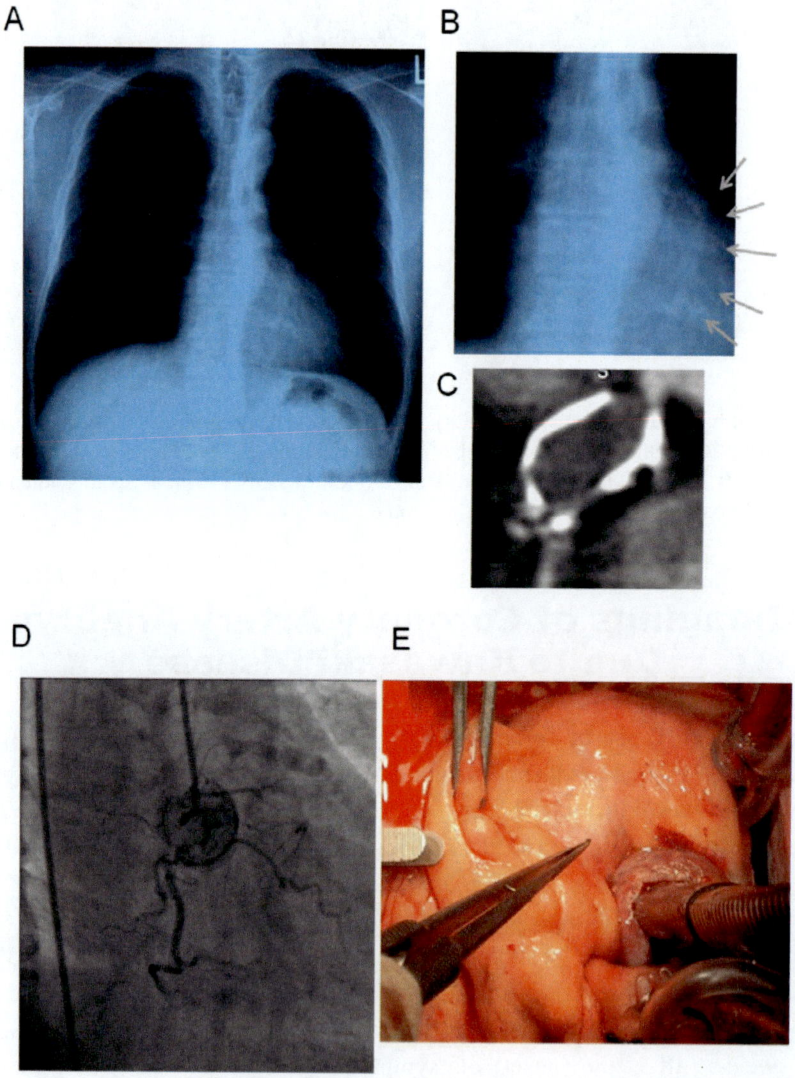

Figure. 2 An example of coronary artery aneurysm in a patient with Kawasaki disease. A Chest X-ray (PA) image. B Augmented image of Figure 2A. Calcification of coronary artery aneurysm is seen. C . Curved multiplanar reformation image of 64-MDCT. Egg-shell calcification is seen. D Coronary angiography of right coronary artery. Occluded aneurysm with collateral vessels are demonstrated at the proximal portion of right coronary artery. E Macroscopic image of coronary artery aneurysm.

Coronary artery aneurysm of Kawasaki disease is characterized with severe calcification [47,48, 49]. Large and calcified coronary aneurysm may be detected by chest X-ray (Figure 2A,B). Large aneurysm with severe calcification (Figure 2C,D) is variously named [47,48,49]. Ino et al [48]. reported that 8 of the 9 calcified lesions showed a circular or ring-shape configuration. Detection of Coronary artery aneurysm of Kawasaki disease by CTCA is increasing [7,49]. Kashiwase et al.[7] also reported egg-shell calcification in a patient with coronary artery aneurysm due to Kawasaki disease by CTCA. Calcified aneurysm is thought to be larger than non-calcified aneurysm [47]. Echocardiography is the first choice for fast and accurate diagnosis and follow-up of aneurysm in children [36]. However, the reliability of examination is strongly depending on the cardiologist experience on echocardiography. When the aneurysm is occluded (Figure 2D), invasive devices, such as IVUS and angioscopy is not available. Occluded aneurysms are often accompanied with collateral vessels. Localized and segmental stenosis for coronary artery aneurysms occurred significantly more often in the left anterior descending and the right coronary artery than in other vessels [50]. For such coronary artery aneurysm, CTCA is effective way to estimate the etiology by demonstrating the morphology and plaque composition.

6. Conclusions

CAG has been gold standard for coronary morphology for long period. CAG has potentially some non-fatal and fatal complications, such as thrombosis, rupture, and death. As the progress of MDCT, CTCA is also able to detect coronary artery aneurysm safer than CAG. By detecting coronary artery aneurysm and plaque composition by CTCA with Plaque Map combined with invasive devices, such as IVUS and angioscopy, etiology of coronary artery aneurysm may be conclusive. Main limitation of CTCA is the radiation dose. Recently, radiation dose of MDCT is decreasing using prospective ECG-gating [51]. Using this technology, MDCT may play a role for safe and rapid diagnosis of coronary artery aneurysms for adults and children.

References

[1] Nissen, SE. Who is, at risk for atherosclerotic disease? *Lessons from intravascular ultrasound, Am J Med.*, 2002, 112, 27S–33S.

[2] Asakura, M; Ueda, Y; Yamaguchi, O; et al. Extensive development of vulnerable plaques as a pan-coronary process in patients with myocardial infarction: an angioscopic study. *J Am Coll Cardiol,* 2001, 37,1284-8.

[3] Rodriguez-Granillo, GA; Aoki, J; Ong, AT; et al. Methodological considerations and approach to cross-technique comparisons using in vivo coronary plaque characterization based on intravascular ultrasound radiofrequency data analysis: insights from the Integrated Biomarker and Imaging Study (IBIS). *Int J Cardiovasc Intervent,* 2005, 7, 52-8.

[4] Komiyama, N; Berry, GJ; Kolz, ML; et al. Tissue characterization of atherosclerotic plaques by intravascular ultrasound radiofrequency signal analysis: an in vitro study of human coronary arteries. *Am Heart*, 2000, J. 140, 565-74.

[5] Huang, D; Swanson, EA; Lin, CP; et al. Optical coherence tomography. *Science*, 1991, 254, 1178-81.

[6] Gerrand, TG; Mintz, GS., et al. Intravascular ultrasound diagnosis of a coronary psudoaneurysm following percutaneous transluminal coronary angioplasty. *Am Heart J*, 1993, 125, 880-2.

[7] Kashiwase, K; Oyabu, J; Komatsu, S; et al. MDCT detection of an atherosclerotic coronary artery aneurysm: Evaluation by Plaque Map. *Int J Cardiol*, 2007, 118, 113-5.

[8] Komatsu, S; Hirayama, A; Omori, Y; et al. Detection of Coronary Plaque by Computed Tomography with the Novel Plaque Analysis System "Plaque Map" and Comparison with Intravascular Ultrasound and Angioscopy, *Circ J*, 2005, 69, 72-77.

[9] Komatsu, S; Ueda, Y; Omori, Y; et al. Diagnosis of Vulnerable Plaque and Vulnerable Patient by Coronary Angioscopy and Multi-detector Row Computed Tomography — From Invasive to Non-invasive Plaque Imaging. *Vascular Disease Prevention,* 2006, 3, 319-325.

[10] Budoff, MJ; Achenbach, S; Blumenthal, RS; et al; American Heart Association Committee on Cardiovascular Imaging and Intervention; American Heart Association Council on Cardiovascular Radiology and Intervention; American Heart Association Committee on Cardiac Imaging, Council on Clinical Cardiology. Assessment of coronary artery disease by cardiac computed tomography: a scientific statement from the American Heart Association Committee on Cardiovascular Imaging and Intervention, Council on Cardiovascular Radiology and Intervention, and Committee on Cardiac Imaging, Council on Clinical Cardiology. *Circulation*, 2006, 114, 1761-91.

[11] Komatsu, S; Sato, Y; Ichikawa, M., et al. Anomalous coronary arteries in adults detected by multislice computed tomography: presentation of cases from multi-center registry and review of the literature. *Heart and Vessels*, 2008, 23,26-34.

[12] Sato, Y; Tani, S; Kunimasa, T; Komatsu, S; et al. Multidetector-row computed tomography diagnosis of coronary artery aneurysms and collateral vessel after Kawasaki disease in an adult. *Cardiovasc Revasc Med.*, 2006, 7, 243-5.

[13] Komatsu, S; Achenbach, S; Ropers, D; et al. Occlusion of coronary aneurysms demonstrated by multidetector-row computed tomography. *Clin Res Cardiol,* 2007, 96, 575-8.

[14] Schroeder, S; Kopp, AF; Baumbach, A., et al. Noninvasive detection and evaluation of atherosclerotic coronary plaques with multislice computed tomography. *J Am Coll Cardiol*, 2001, 37; 1430-5.

[15] Chia, HM; et al. Non-atherosclerotic coronary artery aneurysm: two case reports. *Heart*, 1997, 78, 613-6.

[16] Morgagni, JB. De sedibus et causis morborum per anatomen indagatis. *Tomus primus*, Liber II, 1761, Epist 27, Article 28, Venetiis.

[17] Swaye, PS; Fisher, LD; Litwin, P; et al. Aneurysmal coronary artery disease. *Circulation*, 1983, 67, 134-8.

[18] Markis, JE; Joffe, CD; et al. Clinical significance of coronary artery ectasia. *Am J Cardiol*, 1976, 37, 217-222.

[19] Badmanaban, B; et al. Repair of left coronary artery aneurysm, recurrent ascending aortic aneurysm, and mitral valve prolapse 19 years after Bentall's procedure in a patient with Marfan syndrome. *J Card Surg*, 2004, 19, 59-61.

[20] Briguori, C; et al. Polytetrafluoroethylene-covered stent and coronary artery aneurysms. *Catheter Cardiovasc Interv*, 2002, 55, 326-330.

[21] Hartnell, GG; et al. Coronary artery ectasia. Its prevalence and clinical significance in 4993 patients. *Br Heart J.*, 1985, 54, 392-5.

[22] Syed, M; Lesch, M. Coronary artery aneurysm: a review. *Prog Cardiovasc Dis.*, 1997, 40, 77-84.

[23] Gulec, S; Aras, O; et al. Deletion polymorphism of the angiotensin I converting enzyme gene is a potent risk factor for coronary artery ectasia. *Heart*, 2003, 89, 213-214.

[24] Sayin, T; Doven, O; et al. Exercise-induced myocardial ischemia in patients with coronary artery ectasia without obstructive coronary artery disease. *Int J Cardiol,* 2001, 78, 143-149.

[25] Mrdvic, I; Jozic, T, et al. Myocardial reinfarction in a patient with coronary ectasia. *Cardiology*, 2004, 102, 32-34.

[26] Rosenberg, VD; Nepomnyashchikh, LM. Pathomorphological peculiarities of coronary artery ectasia and their role in the pathogenesis of sudden cardiac death. Bull *Exp Biol Med.*, 2004, 138, 515-521.

[27] Huikuri, HV; Mallon, SM; et al. Cardiac arrest due to spontaneous coronary artery dissection in a patient with coronary ectasia- a case report. *Angiology*, 1991, 42, 148-151.

[28] Baman, TS; Cole, JH; et al. Risk factors and outcomes in patients with coronary artery aneurysms. *Am J Cardiol*, 2004, 93, 1549-1551.

[29] Pahlavan, PS, Niroomand, F. Coronary aneurysm: A review. *Clin Cardiol,* 2006, 29, 439-443.

[30] Anfinsen, OG; Aaberge, L; et al. Coronary artery aneurysm mimicking cardiac tumor, Eur *J Echocardiogr*, 2004, 5, 308-312.

[31] Ramappa, P; Kottam, A; et al. Coronary artery ectasia-is it time for a reappraisal? *Clin Cardiol*, 2007, 30, 214-7.

[32] Tokgozoglu, L; Ergene, O; et al. Plasma interleukin-6 levels are increased in coronary artery ectasia. *Acta Cardiol*, 2004, 59, 515-519.

[33] Turhan, H; Erbay, AR; et al. Plasmal soluble adhesion moleculaes;intercellular adhesion molecule-1,vascular cell adhesion molecule-1 and E-selectin levels in patients with isolated coronary artery ectasia. *Coron Artery Dis.*, 2005, 16, 45-50.

[34] Ge, J; et al. Intravascula ultrasound approach to the diagnosis of coronary artery aneurysms. *Am Heart J,* 1995, 130, 765 71.

[35] Rubartelli, P; Terti, G; et al. Coronary artery aneurysm after stent implanatation. Acute and long-term results after percutaneous treatment with a stent graft. *Ital Heart J*, 2003, 3, 202-205.

[36] Marvrogeni, S; Papadopoulos, G; Karanasios, E; Cokkinos, D. How to image Kawasaki disease:a validation of different imaging techniques. *Int J Cardiol*, 2008, 124, 27-33.

[37] Newburger, JW; Burns, JC. Kawasaki disease. *Vascular Medicine*, 1999, 4, 187-202.

[38] Yanagawa, H; Yashiro, M; Nakamura, Y; Kawasaki, T; et al. Epidemologic pictures of Kawasaki disease in Japan: from the nationwide incidence survey in 1991 and 1992. *Pediatrics*, 1995, 95, 475-79.

[39] Davis, RL; Waller, PL; Mueller, BA; et al. Kawasaki disease in Washington state. Race-specific incidence rates and residential proximity of water. *Arch Pediatr Adolesc Med.*, 1995, 149, 66-69.

[40] Fujita, Y; Nakamura, Y; Sakata, K; et al. Kawasaki disease in families. *Pediatrics*, 1989, 84, 666-69.

[41] Harada, F; Sada, M; Kamiya, T; et al. Genetic Analysis of Kawasaki syndrome. *Am J Human Genet*, 1986, 39, 537-39.

[42] Kato, H; et al. Long-term consequences of Kawasaki disease; a 10- to 21- year follow-up study of 594 patients. *Circulation*, 1996, 94, 1379-85.

[43] Abbate, P; Patti, G; et al. Left main coronary artery aneurysms: a case report and review of the literatures. *Ital Heart J*, 2001, 2, 711-4.

[44] Akagi, T; Rose, V; et al. Outcome of coronary artery aneurysms after Kawasaki disease. *J Pediatr*, 1992, 121, 689-94.28.

[45] Suzuki, A; Kamiya, T. Visualization of coronary artery lesions in Kawasaki disease by angiography. *Cardiol Young*, 1991, 1, 225-33.

[46] Newburger, JW; Takahashi, M; et al. A statement for health professionals from the committee on rheumatic fever, endocarditis, and Kawasaki disease, council on cardiovascular disease in the young, American Heart Association. *Pediatrics*, 2004, 114, 1708-33.

[47] Nakada, T; Yonesaka, S; Sunagawa, Y; Tomimoto, K; Takahashi, T; Matsubara, T; Furukawa, H; Kamimura, K; Naka, S. Coronary arterial calcification in Kawasaki disease. *Acta Paediatr Jpn.*, 1991, 33, 443-9.

[48] Ino, T; Shimazaki, S; Akimoto, K; Park, I, Nishimoto, K; Yabuta, K; Tanaka, A. Coronary artery calcification in Kawasaki disease. *Pediatr Radiol*, 1990, 20, 520-3.

[49] Kim, YJ; Lee, HJ; Hur, J; Nam, JE; Choe, KO: Jang, Y, Choi, BW. Braid-like appearance of the coronary artery in Kawasaki disease: typical computed tomography and angiography findings. *Eur Heart J*. 2008 Nov; 29(22), 279,1.

[50] Onouchi, Z, Hamaoka, K; Kamiya, Y; et al. Transformation of coronary artery aneurysm to obstructive lesion and the role of collateral vessels in myocardial perfusion in patients with Kawasaki disease. *J Am Coll Cardiol,* 1993, 21, 158-62.

[51] Stolzmann, P; Leschka, S; Scheffel, H; et al. Dual-source CT in step-and-shoot mode: noninvasive coronary angiography with low radiation dose. *Radiology*, 2008, 249, 71-80.

In: Aneurysms: Types, Risks, Formation and Treatment
Editors: Alain Laurent and Ethan Morel
ISBN: 978-1-60741-557-2
© 2009 Nova Science Publishers, Inc.

Chapter 10

The Pathophysiology and Management of Coronary Artery Aneurysm

Masashi Ohtsuka[1*], Hiroshi Akazawa[2], Hiroyuki Takano[2], Haruaki Nakaya[3] and Issei Komuro[2]

[1]Department of Cardiology, Seirei Yokohama General Hospital, 215 Iwai-cho, Hodogaya-ku, Yokohama 240-8521, Japan

[2]Department of Cardiovascular Science and Medicine, Chiba University Graduate School of Medicine, 1-8-1 Inohana, Chuo-ku, Chiba 260-8670, Japan

[3]Department of Pharmacology, Chiba University Graduate School of Medicine, 1-8-1 Inohana, Chuo-ku, Chiba 260-8670, Japan

Abstract

Coronary aneurysm is uncommon, but occasionally encountered in patients undergoing coronary angiography. Most coronary aneurysms are caused secondarily by atherosclerosis, Kawasaki disease and infectious emboli. Whereas the pathogenesis has not been entirely clarified, an inflammatory process is crucially involved. One of the earliest histopathological changes include granulomatous inflammation within the adventia and outer layers of the affected arteries, and gradual progression to a panarteritis with inflammatory mononuclear cell infiltration. Advential inflammation and subsequent neointimal proliferation promotes the destruction of the elastic lamina and tunica muscularis, leading to formation of aneurysms. At molecular levels, matrix metalloproteinases (MMPs) are up-regulated by chronic inflammation, and promote aneurysm formation through excessive proteolysis of extracellular matrix proteins. Recently, endothelial MMP-9 emerged as a coronary flow-sensitive effector for aneurysm formation. In this section, we will summarize the current view of the pathophysiology and management of coronary aneurysms.

*Corresponding author: Department of Cardiology, Seirei Yokohama General Hospital 215 Iwai-cho, Hodogaya-ku, Yokohama 240-8521, Japan TEL: +81-45-715-3111 FAX: +81-45-715-3387 , E-mail: masaootsuka-circ@umin.ac.jp

Introduction

Coronary artery aneurysm, also termed coronary ectasia, is characterized by a pathological dilatation of a localized or diffuse segment of the coronary arteries [1,2]. According to the Coronary Artery Surgery Study (CASS) registry, coronary artery aneurysm is diagnosed when the diameter of a lesion exceeds those of normal adjacent segments or the patient's largest coronary vessel by 1.5 times [1]. Morphologically, coronary artery aneurysm is divided into two types; one is a fusiform type when the transverse diameter is smaller than the longitudinal dimension is greater, and the other is a saccular type when it is larger than the longitudinal dimension [2]. In most cases, patients with coronary artery aneurysms are asymptomatic, and the prognosis is generally favorable [1,2]. Latent coronary aneurysms are found incidentally in patients who undergo coronary angiography, and the incidence ranges from 1.2-4.9 % [3].

Although the pathogenesis remains to be fully elucidated, the most common cause of coronary artery aneurysms is atherosclerosis. Atherosclerotic process affects not only intima but also media and adventitia to cause arterial remodeling and dilatation [1,2,3]. In addition, Kawasaki disease is an important disease underlying coronary artery aneurysm, which usually affects children [4]. Besides atherosclerosis and Kawasaki disease, diverse pathological conditions underlie coronary aneurysms, as listed in Table 1 [5]. Although atherosclerosis contributes to development of coronary artery aneurysm in up to 50 % of patients [5], it is hypothesized that inflammation links atherosclerosis or other underlying conditions to destructive processes of arterial architecture. Especially, increased proteolysis of extracellular matrix (ECM) by matrix metalloproteinases (MMPs) emerges as a key mechanism of aneurysmal formation. In this section, we will review the current understanding of clinical features and pathophysiology of coronary artery aneurysm.

Table 1. Cause for coronary artery aneurysm

Coronary atherosclerosis
Kawasaki disease
Congenital abnormalities
Infections
Trauma
Coronary angioplasty
Collagen vascular disease
Ehler-Danlos syndrome
Systemic Lupus erythematousus
Polyarteritis Nodosa
Sclerodema
Juvenile idiopathic arteritis
Takayasu's disease

Clinical Featufres of Coronary Artery Aneurysm

Coronary artery aneurysms are found in 1.2-4.9 % of patients with obstructive coronary artery disease at angiography [3]. Anatomically, the proximal and middle segments of right coronary artery (RCA) are the most commonly affected sites by aneurysmal dilatation [3], and left anterior descending artery (32.3 %) and left circumflex artery (23.4 %) are less frequently involved [5]. Aneurysms in the left anterior ascending coronary artery are associated with severe stenotic lesions in most cases [6]. There is a preponderance of male over female in patients with coronary artery aneurysm [1]. Patients with coronary artery aneurysm often have no apparent symptoms, but complications such as thrombus formation, distal embolization, shunt formation, and rupture can occur [1, 2, 3].

Coronary artery aneurysm has been observed in association with diverse pathological conditions, as listed in Table 1, but more than half are caused by coronary atherosclerosis [2]. Some reports suggest that patients with coronary artery aneurysms have an increased risk of aortic aneurysm [7]. According to the CASS registry, no significant differences between aneurysmal and non-aneurysmal coronary disease patients were observed with regard to coronary risk factors such as hypertension, diabetes mellitus, hyperlipidemia, and smoking [1]. However, some papers demonstrated that there was a negative correlation between diabetes and coronary artery aneurysm [8], and that hypertension occurred more frequently in aneurysmal patients [9]. Currently, risk factors specific to coronary artery aneurysm have not been proven [10].

Pathogenesis of Coronary Artery Aneurysm

The pathogenic mechanism of coronary artery aneurysm has not been entirely clarified. Atherosclerosis participates in the pathogensis of the majority of coronary aneurysms, and it is assumed that coronary artery aneurysm and coronary artery disease are two different manifestations of atherosclerosis, especially when they coexist [2, 3, 5]. Histopathologically, the wall of an ecstatic artery is characterized by thickened and fibrotic intima with extensive lipid deposition and marked thinning of the media [2, 3]. In patients with coronary artery aneurysm, the plasma levels of inflammatory markers such as interleukin-6 and C-reactive protein are elevated, as compared with patients with normal coronary arteries [11]. In addition, plasma soluble adhesion molecules such as intercellular adhesion molecule (ICAM)-1, vascular cell adhesion molecule (VCAM)-1 and E-selectin are higher in patients with coronary artery aneurysm [12]. These findings suggest that inflammatory process is crucially involved in the pathogenesis of aneurysmal formation.

Kawasaki disease is the most common cause of coronary artery aneurysm in children and the second most common cause in adults [13]. Kawasaki disease is a systemic inflammatory syndrome affecting arteries of small and medium sizes. It has been reported that 15~25 % of patients with Kawasaki disease develop coronary artery aneurysm [14, 15], but half of the coronary aneurysms of small or medium sizes undergo spontaneous regression [16]. Immunohistochemical studies revealed that coronary artery wall was infiltrated primarily by $CD8^{+}$ cytotoxic T cells and macrophages in children who died of acute Kawasaki disease

[17]. Recently, a functional SNP in the inositol 1,4,5-triphosphate 3-kinase (ITPKC) gene was identified which shows a significant association with susceptibility to Kawasaki disease and coronary artery aneurysm [18]. ITPKC acts as a negative regulator of T-cell activation through the Ca^{2+}/NFAT signaling pathway. A polymorphism of the ITPKC gene leads to reduction of the transcript, and seems to cause immune hyper hyper-reactivity [18].

At molecular levels, matrix metalloproteinases (MMPs) are implicated in the pathogenesis of aneurysm development. MMPs are upregulated by acute or chronic inflammation, and promote aneurysm formation through excessive proteolysis of extracellular matrix proteins [19] (Figure 1). According to some reports, imbalance of serum levels of MMPs and TIMPS (tissue inhibitors of metalloproteinase) is observed in patients with coronary artery aneurysm originating from atherosclerosis [20, 21] or Kawasaki disease [22]. In addition, certain MMP-3 allele is associated with a higher level of gene expression, and is more common in patients with coronary artery aneurysm [23]. Recently, it is reported that endothelial MMP-9 acts as a flow-sensitive effector on the basis of an observation that shear stress upregulates MMP-9 via activation of c-Myc [24]. Therefore, hemodynamic wall stress per se, as well as tissue inflammation, may induce imbalance of MMPs/TIMPs and increase susceptibility to the development of coronary artery aneurysm. In addition to MMPs, cathepsins of the cysteine protease family play an important role in ECM remodeling [25] (Figure 1). Pharmacological inhibitiors of MMPs or cathepsins may have therapeutic effects on the prevention of coronary artery aneurysms [25, 26].

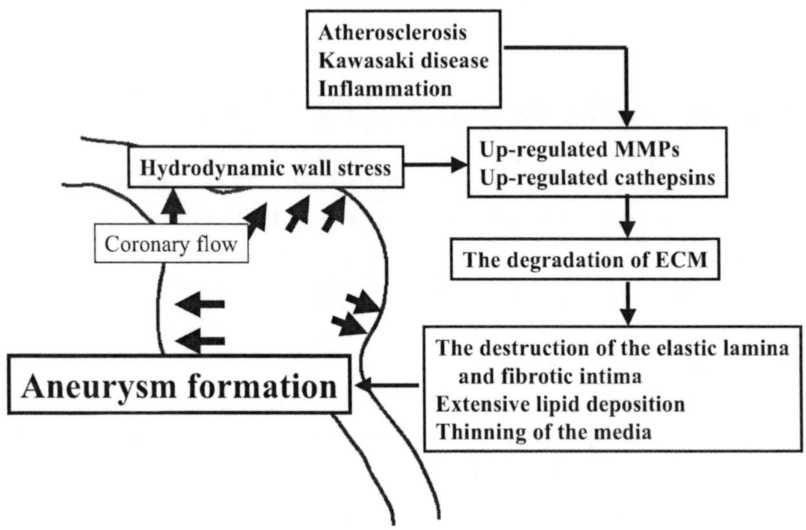

Figure 1. Pathogeneisis of coronary artery aneurysm

Treatment of Coronary Artery Aneurysm

Since there has been no controlled trial due to the rare incidence, the appropriate therapy for coronary artery aneurysm is still unknown. Anti-coagulation with warfarin or anti-platelet therapy are recommended to prevent thromboembolic complications [27]. For patients with coexisting stenotic lesions or ischemic symptoms, percutaneous and/or surgical coronary intervention will be needed. Patients with Kawasaki disease should be treated with aspirin, warfarin and intravenous γ-globulin [28]. For patients with life-threatening compications such as thromboembolism or rupture, prompt surgical procedures should be indicated.

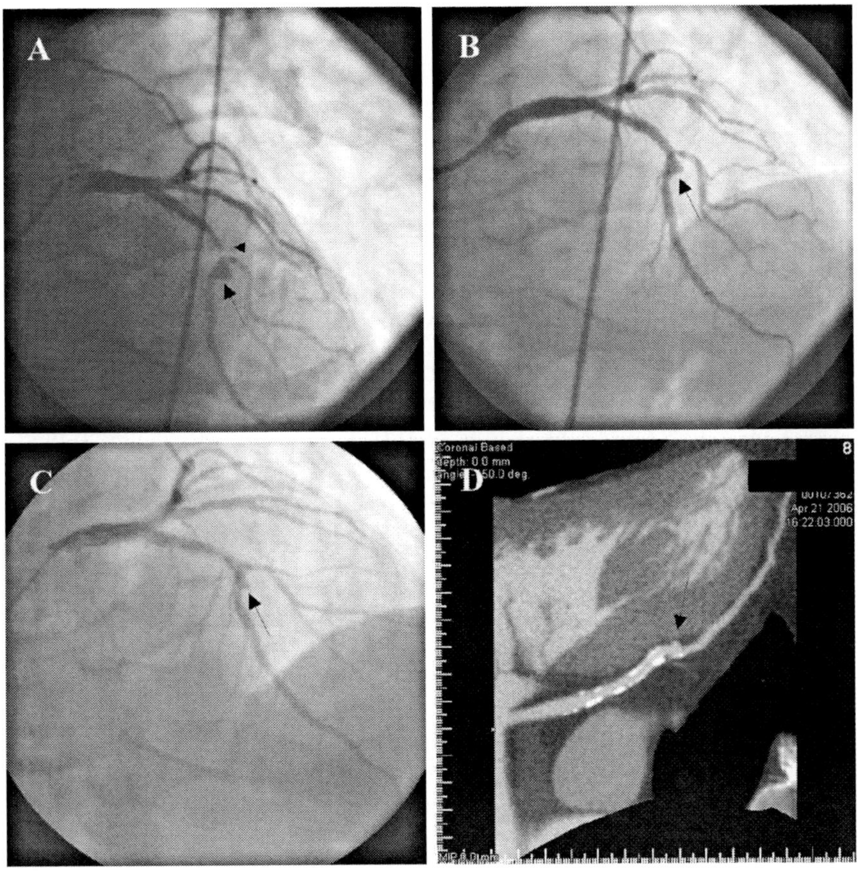

Figure 2. Conventional coronary angiograms from right superior anterior view acquired: (A) before performing percutaneous coronary intervention; (B) immediately after stenting; (C) seven months after stenting; (D) Curved planar reconstruction images of enhanced 64-slice computed tomography acquired six months after stenting

A: Coronary severe stenosis (99% TIMI 1) at the mid-portion of the left anterior descending (LAD) coronary artery (arrowhead), followed by coronary aneurysm (arrow), 5.3mm in diameter, located just distal to the stenotic site, can both be observed.

B: Immediately after stenting, the diameter of the aneurysm was reduced to 4.8 mm (arrow).

C: Seven months after stenting, the diameter of the aneurysm was furthermore reduced to 3.3mm (arrow).

D: there is no evidence of a thrombus or dissection in the coronary aneurysm (arrow).

We recently reported a case of a 70-year-old man who underwent a percutaneous coronary intervention with stenting, for a severe stenosis (99 % TIMI 1, arrowhead Figure 2A) complicated by a coronary aneurysm (arrow Figure 2A) just distal to the stenotic site [29]. Notably, coronary angiograms showed an immediate (arrow Figure 2B) and progressive reduction in the size of coronary aneurysm after stenting (arrow Figure 2C). Curved planar reconstruction images of the enhanced CT showed no thrombus and no dissection of the coronary aneurysm (arrow Figure 2D). We speculate that coronary stenting might decrease the velocity of coronary flow through the stenosis. Consequently, stenting might attenuate the hydrodynamic wall stress on the aneurysm, and, in addition, improve the degradation of the extracellular matrix structure through the regulation of MMPs. Regression of coronary aneurysm after stenting requires further investigations, because stenting may become a potential means for treating post-stenotic aneurysms.

Closing Remarks

Coronary artery aneurysm is not an uncommon form of coronary artery disease, observed in 1.2~4.9 % of patients who undergo coronary angiography. At present, many issues remain unanswered regarding etiology, pathophysiology and prognosis. Especially, an optimal guideline for management is not present. As more reproducible and less invasive imaging apparatus, such as multi-sliced computed tomography, are routinely available in clinical use, a greater number of cases will be discovered incidentally. Under such circumstances, prospective and controlled studies will be feasible that are designed to address these unanswered issues about coronary artery aneurysm.

References

[1] Swaye, PS; Fisher, LD; Litwin, P; Vignola, PA; Judkins, MP; Kemp, HG; Mudd, JG; Gosselin, AJ. Aneurysmal coronary artery disease. *Circulation*, 1983, 67, 134-138.

[2] Pahlavan, PS; Niroomand, F. Coronary artery aneurysm: a review. Clin. *Cardiol*, 2006, 29, 439-443.

[3] Ramappa, P; Kottam, A; Kuivanemi, H; Thatai, D. Coronary artery ectasia-is it time for a reappraisal? Clin. *Cardiol*, 2007, 30, 214-217.

[4] Porter, GF; Gentles, TL. Giant coronary artery aneurysm in Kawasaki's disease. *N Eng J Med.*, 2001, 345, 98.

[5] Syed, M; Lesch, M. Coronary artery aneurysm: A review. *Prog Cardiovasc Dis.*, 1997, 40, 77-84.

[6] Tunick, PA; Slater, J; Kronzon, I; Glassman, E. Discrete atherosclerotic coronary artery aneurysms: a study of 20 patents. *J Am Coll Cardiol,* 1990, 15, 279-282.

[7] Rigatelli, G; Gemelli, M; Franco, GF; Menini, A ; Rigatelli, G. Unusual combination of coronary artery, abdominal aortic and iliac artery inflammatory aneurismal disease. *Int J Cardiol*, 2004, 96, 105-107.

[8] Androulakis, AE; Andrikopoulos, GK; Kartalis, AN; Stougiannos, PN; Katsaros, AA; Syrogiannidis, DN; Tapanlis, EN; Stefanadis, C; Kallikazaros, IE. Relation of coronary artery ectasia to diabetes mellitus. *Am J Cardiol,* 2004, 93, 1165-1167.

[9] Markis, JE; Joffe, CD; Cohn, PF; Feen, DJ; Herman, MV; Gorlin, R. Clinical significance of coronary arterial ectasia. *Am J Cardiol,* 1976, 37, 217-222.

[10] Baman, TS; Cole, JH; Devireddy, CM; Sperling, LS. Risk factors and outcomes in patients with coronary artery aneurysms. *Am J Cardiol,* 2004, 93, 1549-1551.

[11] Tokgozoglu, L; Ergene, O; Kinay, O; Nazli, C; Hascelik, G; Hoscan, Y. Plasma interleukin-6 levels are increased in coronary artery ectasia. *Acta Cardiol*, 2004, 59, 515-519.

[12] Turhan, H; Erbay, AR; Yasar, AS; Aksoy Y; Bicer, A; Yetkin, G; Yetkin, E. Plasma soluble adhesion molecules; intercellular adhesion molecule-1, vascular cell adhesion molecule-1 and E-selectin levels in patients with isolated coronary artery ectasia. *Coron Artery Dis.,* 2005, 16, 45-50.

[13] Burns, JC; Shike, H; Gordon, JB; Malhotra, A; Shoenwetter, M; Kawasaki, T. Sequelae of Kawasaki disease in adolescents and young adults. *J Am Coll Cardiol,* 1996, 28, 253-257.

[14] Kato, H; Ichinose, E; Kawasaki, T. Myocardial infarction in Kawasaki disease: clinical analyses in 195 cases. *J Pediatr,* 1986, 108, 923-927.

[15] Suzuki, A; Kamiya, T; Kuwahara, N; Ono, Y; Kohata, T; Takahashi, O; Kimura, K; Takamiya, M. Coronary arterial lesions of Kawasaki disease: cardiac catheterization findings of 1100 cases. *Pediatr Cardiol,* 1986, 7, 3-9.

[16] Kato, H; Sugimura, T; Akagi, T; Sato, N; Hashino, K; Maeno, Y; Kazue, T; Eto, G, Yamakawa, R. Long-term consequences of Kawasaki disease; A 10-to 21-year follow-up study of 594 patients. *Circulation*, 1996, 94, 1379-1385.

[17] Brown, TJ; Crawford, SE; Cornwall, ML; Garcia, F; Shulman, ST; Rowley, AH. CD8 T lymphocytes and macrophages infiltrate coronary artery aneurysms in acute Kawasaki disease. *J Infect Dis.,* 2001, 184, 940-943.

[18] Onouchi, Y; Gunji, T; Burns, JC; Shimizu, C; Newburger, JW; Yashiro, M; Nakamura, Y; Yanagawa, H; Wakui, K; Fukushima, Y; Kishi, F; Hamamoto, K; Terai, M; Sato, Y, Ouchi, K; Saji, T; Nariai, A; Kaburagi, Y; Yoshikawa, T; Suzuki, K; Tanaka, T; Nagai, T; Cho, H; Fujino, A; Sekine, A; Nakamichi, R; Tsunoda, T; Kawasaki, T; Nakamura, Y; Hata, A. ITPKC functional polymorphism associated with Kawasaki disease susceptibility and formation of coronary artery aneurysms. *Nat Genet*, 2008, 40, 35-42.

[19] Galis, ZS; Khatri, JJ. Matrix metalloproteinases in vascular remodeling and atherogenesis the good, the bad, and the ugly. *Circ Res.,* 2002, 90, 251-262.

[20] Tengiz, I; Ercan, E; Aliyev, E; Sekuri, C; Duman, C; Altuglu, I. Elevated levels of matrix mettaloprotein-3 in patients with coronary aneurysm: A case control study. *Curr Control Trials Cardiovasc Med.*, 2004, 5, 10.

[21] Finkelstein, A; Michowitz, Y; Abashidze, A; Miller, H; Keren, G; George, J. Temporal association between circulating proteolytic, inflammatory and neurohormonal markers in patients with coronary ectasia. *Atherosclerosis*, 2005, 179, 353-359.

[22] Senzaki, H; Matsutani, S; Kobayashi, J; Kobayashi, T; Nakano, H; Nagasawa, H; Sasaki, N; Asano, H; Kyo, S; Yokote, Y. Circulating matrix mettaloproteinases and their inhibitors in patients with Kawasaki disease. *Circulation*, 2001, 104, 860-863.

[23] Lamblin, N; Bauters, C; Hermant, X; Lablanche, JM; Helbecque, N; Amouyel, P. Polymorphisms in the promoter regions of MMP-2, MMP-3, MMP-9 and MMP-12 genes as determinants of aneurysmal coronary artery disease. *J Am Coll Cardiol,* 2002, 40, 43-48.

[24] Magid, R; Murphy, TJ; Galis, ZS. Expression of matrix metalloproteinase-9 in endothelial cells is differentially regulated by shear stress. *J Biol Chem.*, 2003, 278, 32994-32999.

[25] Lutgens, SPM; Cleutjens, KBJM; Daemen, MJAP; Heeneman, S. Cathepsin cysteine proteases in cardiovascular disease. *FASEB J.* 2007, 21, 3029-3041.

[26] Raffetto, JD; Khalil, RA. Matrix metalloproteinases and their inhibitors in vascular remodeling and vascular disease. *Biochem Pharmacol*, 2008, 75, 346-359.

[27] Wang, KY; Ting, CT; St John Sutton, M; Chen, YT. Coronary artery aneurysms: A 25-patient study. *Catheter Cardiovasc Interv.,* 1999, 48, 31-38.

[28] Newburger, JW; Takahashi, M; Gerber, MA; Gewitz, MH; Tani, LY; Burns, JC; Shulman, ST; Bolger, AF; Ferrieri, P; Baltimore, RS; Wilson, WR; Baddour, LM; Levison, ME; Pallasch, TJ; Falace, DA; Taubert, KA. Diagnosis, treatment, and long-term management of Kawasaki disease: a statement for health professionals from the Committee on Rheumatic Fever, Endocarditis and Kawasaki Disease, Council on Cardiovascular Disease in the young, American Heart Association. *Circulation*, 2004, 110, 2747-2771.

[29] Ohtsuka, M; Uchida, E; Yamaguchi, H; Nakajima, T; Akazawa, H; Funabashi, N; Kobayashi, Y; Shiojima, I; Komuro, I. Coronary aneurysm reduced after coronary stenting. *Int J Cardiol,* 2007, 121, 76-77.

In: Aneurysms: Types, Risks, Formation and Treatment
Editors: Alain Laurent and Ethan Morel
ISBN: 978-1-60741-557-2
© 2009 Nova Science Publishers, Inc.

Chapter 11

Treatment Options in Asymptomatic Infrarenal Aortic Aneurysms

Bernd Muehling*[*], *Ludger Sunder-Plassmann and Karl Heinz Orend
Department of Thoracic and Vascular Surgery, University of Ulm, Germany

1. Epidemiology

Each year 15, 000 Americans die due exsanguination following rupture of an abdominal aortic aneurysm (AAA); it is the 13th leading cause of death in the U.S. The prevalence in screening studies is approximately 5% (Scott 1986). Surgical repair in the emergent situation is associated with high mortality rates of about 80%. Elective repair aims at prevention of death from haemorrhage. The UK small aneurysm trial in 1998 and the Aneurysm Detection and Management (ADAM) trial in 2002 have provided evidence that surveillance to an aneurysm diameter of 5.5cm is justified and patients should undergo surgical repair if aneurysms grow beyond this point. Nonetheless once the diagnosis abdominal aortic aneurysm is confirmed patients are at increased risk for cardiovascular death and should therefore be treated like patients with cardiovascular disease (Brady 2001, Norman 2004).

2. Conservative and Medical Treatment

Although the precise mechanisms which lead to aneurysm formation are still unclear the underlying principle of medical treatment is to slow aneurysm growth rates by reducing inflammatory/immune responses in the medial layer of the aorta and inhibition of proteolytic degradation of connective tissue in the aortic wall along with a reduction of the mural stress by management of hypertension (Baxter 2008). As long as AAA diameter is < 5.5cm best medical treatment should be offered.

Smoking Cessation

Smoking is strongly associated to AAA (Alberto 2008, Badger 2008). The mechanisms by which cigarette smoking lead to aneurysm formation are unknown but it is suspected that smoking leads to inflammation in the aortic wall and subsequently influenced by hypertension and genetic predisposition to fragmentation and degradation of collagen mediated by metalloproteinases (MMP´s) (Annambhotla 2008). Hence the first step in conservative treatment of patients presenting with AAA < 5.5cm is to advise active smokers to stop smoking which is likely to be associated with a 20-25% reduction in annual growth rates (Brady 2004).

Antiplatelet Drugs

In addition to smoking cessation AAA patients should be offered best medical treatment according to the currently best known management of cardiovascular disease. This includes medication with antiplatelet drugs, statins and antihypertensives. There is no evidence if prescription of antiplatelet drugs reduces the risk of aneurysm formation or growth rates; however in randomized controlled trials antiplatelet therapy has been shown to significantly reduce the risk of non-fatal myocardial infarction, non-fatal stroke or vascular death in patients with peripheral vascular disease (Robless 2001). Hence antiaggregation is recommended in conservative management of the vascular patient.

Statins

Another cornerstone in the medical treatment of the vascular patient is administration of statins. They exert favourable effects on multiple interrelated aspects of vascular biology important in atherosclerosis. In particular they have positive effects on inflammation, plaque stabilization, endothelial dysfunction, and thrombosis. Statins have also been shown to be useful in acute vascular events (Rice 2006). As for aneurysm growth rates a retrospective study has suggested an almost 50% reduction of AAA growth rates in patients that had been on statin therapy (Shouten 2006). In surgical specimen of aortic aneurismal tissue the activity of MMP9 – a key enzyme in aneurysm formation- was reduced if patients had been on statin therapy (Evans 2007). To provide further evidence of statin therapy on aneurysm growth rates a randomized trial would be attractive though this is regarded to be unethical because of the beneficial effects of statins on cardiovascular events. Therefore medication with statins is

*Corresponding author: Department of Thoracic and Vascular Surgery. University of Ulm Steinhövelstrasse 9, 89075 Ulm, Germany, Tel: +49-731-500-54044, FAX: +49-731-500-26705, e-mail: bernd.muehling@uniklinik-ulm.de

regarded to be fundamental in the conservative management of AAA patients who are at high risk for death from cardiovascular events (Diehm 2007, Golledge 2007).

Beta Blockers

A randomized trial has tested the hypothesis if administration of beta-blockers would slow aneurysm growth rates but failed to show beneficial effects (Propanolol trial investigators 2002). As a smaller trial showed similar results beta-blockers cannot be recommended to slow aneurysm growth rates; on the other hand beta-blockers are part of the armamentarium in the management of the vascular patient and many guidelines recommend the use of beta-blockers in order to reduce the risk of major cardiovascular events.

Antihypertensives

Patients with the diagnosis of AAA have a history of hypertension in up to 70% and lowering blood pressure in these patients appears to be fundamental in order to reduce the tensile strength in the aortic wall and to slow aneurysm growth rates; there are animal data but no human data demonstrating that angiotensin-converting enzyme inhibitors or losartan, an angiotensin receptor blocker, will decrease the rate of AAA expansion (Baxter 2008). Hence administration of ACE inhibitors can not be generally recommended to prevent aneurysm growth rates, but are part of the basic conservative cure of vascular patients.

Inhibitors of Metalloproteinases

A specific feature of infrarenal aortic aneurysm is chronic inflammation in the medial layer of the aortic wall that leads to degradation of collagen and elastic fibres and as a consequence to aneurysm formation. This process is probably mediated by metalloproteinase (MMP´S) – namely MMP 2 and MMP 9 – that degrade collagen layers. For this reason inhibition of theses MMP´s appears attractive in order to stop aneurysm formation. Medication with doxycycline –a non selective MMP inhibitor- has been proposed in the conservative treatment in a phase II trial (Baxter 2002); however, because of the small size of this randomized study and of the potentially confounding effect of pre-treatment risk factors, doxycycline-based management cannot be justified on the basis of the current results (Mosorin 2001).

Surveillance

Once the diagnosis AAA is confirmed patients should undergo regular surveillance to determine annual growth rates. Ultrasound check-up once a year is the most suitable and easiest available method to control AAA diameter and growth rates. As compared to other diagnostic tools (CT/MRI) ultrasound is the most cost effective and ideal technique for monitoring AAA diameter. As to whether ultrasound should be used as screening method in aged patients in order to reduce mortality is still under debate (Cosford 2007).

In conclusion patients presenting with AAA have a large atherosclerotic burden with related high mortality. The major cause of late death in these patients are cerebor-cardiovascular events. As compared to patients with coronary artery disease (CAD) prognosis is significantly worse as vascular patients receive less cardiac medication than CAD patients (Welten 2008). Hence AAA patients with diameter <5.5cm should be offered the same conservative treatment options that are offered to CAD patients in order to reduce the risk of cerebro-cardiovascular events.

In summary as long as no other data exist conservative management and best medical treatment of patients with AAA includes

- Watch and wait to AAA diameter of 5.5cm
- Smoking cessation
- Administration of antiplatelet drugs and statins
- Management of arterial hypertension
- Surveillance by annual ultrasound

3. Preoperative Assessment of AAA Patients

As mentioned above from an AAA diameter of 5.5cm surgical repair is recommended to prevent patients from rupture and exsanguination; at the moment elective repair is performed either by transperitoneal, retroperitoneal or endovascular approach. Open aneurysm repair (transperitoneal or retroperitoneal) represents a complex surgical procedure with aortic cross clamping and ischemia-reperfusion injury which results in morbidity rates up to 30% and mortality rates up to 8% (Heller 2000, Lee 2004, Dardik 1998). Outcome after elective aortic aneurysm repair is dependent on the individual risk factors of each patient and the surgical approach. Preoperative work-up protocols aim at identifying patients unfit for (open) surgery; optimized perioperative management seeks at reducing surgical stress and should by this means reduce morbidity rates. Endovascular aneurysm repair (EVAR) - a minimal invasive procedure - offers clear advantages in terms of perioperative morbidity and mortality but later stentgraft related complications with the need for secondary interventions or even conversion to open repair may occur which counterbalance the advantages in the short term. That's why indication for surgical repair and the approach – transperitoneal, retroperitoneal or endovascular- should be confirmed on the basis of individual risk factors in each patient.

CT Scanning

In the planning of surgical repair the anatomy of the aneurysm has to be elucidated by CT scanning. By this means it has to be decided if endovascular or rather open aneurysm exclusion is reasonable: in particular the anatomy of the aortic neck and the iliac vessels as primary sealing zones for EVAR have to be documented. According to Chuter et al. (2000) we regard the following criteria as inappropriate for an endovascular approach:

Anatomic exclusion criteria for EVAR

• Neck that is < 1.5cm in length or > 3.2cm in diameter
• Lined thrombus
• Conical neck (>4mm at distal end)
• Severely angulated neck (>80° relative to the aneurysm)
• Concomitant iliac aneurysms >2cm involving the internal iliac artery
• Iliac artery diameter < 9mm or severely angulated

By CT scanning a short and angulated neck that may require suprarenal clamping can be identified and additional useful informations (e.g. presence of horseshoe kidney) obtained. Ultrasonography is not sufficient in the planning of aneurysm exclusion.

Risk Scores

Medical complications are an important source of morbidity after surgical AAA repair. After open repair 35%, after EVAR up to 20% of the patients experience myocardial infarction, pneumonia or renal failure. Preoperative evaluation has to estimate the individual risk factors each patient carries. As aneurysm formation is a disease of the aged it may be considered as a surrogate marker for other systemic diseases (Fisher et al in Endovascular therapies – current evidence, 2006). Across a population of patients with AAA significant co-morbidities occur: coronary heart disease in 67%, arterial hypertension in 63%, peripheral vascular disease in 24%, COPD in 22%, diabetes in 10% and renal insufficiency in 7.3% (Zarins 1999, Schermerhorn 2008). Preoperative assessment has to explore the individual physiological reserve by appropriate investigations: these include EKG, testing of the pulmonary function, echocardiography and routine blood tests; in addition duplex ultrasound of the carotid arteries has to disclose relevant cerebrovascular disease. Standard pre-operative work-up protocols aim at identifying patients at risk whose physiological reserve can be enhanced by intensive preoperative therapy, e.g. improvement of renal function and lowering serum creatinine by i.v. fluid administration; apart from that patients that are not suitable – neither for open nor for endovascular repair- should be identified and planned for surveillance rather than for surgical repair with unfavourable outcome. In this context several risk scoring methods have been proposed to decide whether a patient is unfit for surgical repair: The most widespread risk score for surgical procedures is the Classification of the American society of Anaesthesiologist (ASA) which has been established in 1963; it ranges from ASA I to ASA V (healthy to moribund patient). In terms of elective AAA repair this classification can only act as a crude measurement and hardly predicts outcome: most patients are classified ASA III by definition. To more accurately assess the perioperative cardiovascular mortality in noncardiac surgery the revised cardiac risk index (RCRI) was developed from a prospective study of patients aged 50years and older undergoing non cardiac surgery (Lee 1999); factors predicting risk were high risk surgery, e.g. AAA repair, ischemic heart disease, diabetes, heart failure, cerebrovascular disease and renal insufficiency. Adding up age and detailed classification of type of surgery can improve statistic to predict cardiovascular mortality. A significant proportion of patients with AAA presents with coronary artery disease; therefore some investigators recommend standard preoperative coronary angiography (CAG) and revascularization by either coronary artery bypass graft (CABG) or percutaneous coronary intervention (PCI); however the efficacy of this management remains controversial and no studies have provided evidence that any form of coronary artery revascularization prior to AAA exclusion reduces postoperative cardiac complications (Brilakis 2005). In addition PCI with stenting of coronary arteries and subsequent administration of aspirin, clopidogrel or both renders patients nearly inoperable due to high risk of postoperative haemorrhage. Other risk scores that have been suggested with the purpose to further stratify the risk of patients undergoing elective AAA repair are: the Glasgow Aneurysm Score (GAS), the Vascular Biochemistry and Haematology Outcome Models (VHBOM) and the Estimation of Physiologic Ability and Surgical Stress (E-PASS). In addition to age, presence of coronary heart and pulmonary disease and presence of renal disease they use a number of variables that can be easily assessed at the bedside so they are not too complex for practical use. In the population of AAA patients undergoing elective repair all three scoring systems accurately predict the risk of mortality and morbidity (Tang 2007).

Another attempt to categorize patients for their operative risk has been made from the EUROSTAR registry, the largest prospective registry for EVAR patients. One study from this registry has evaluated the risk factors for patients in normal medical condition (category A), unfit for open surgical repair (category B) and unfit for general anaesthesia (category C) (Buth 2002); factors associated with higher surgical risks were for example old age, presence of ischemic heart disease, COPD, chronic renal failure, obesity and previous laparotomy. Unsurprisingly the high surgical risk group (category B and C) had significant higher 30-day mortality.

In summary the precise definition of the unfit patient is impossible and apart from objective comorbidities – cardiac, pulmonary, renal and metabolic- along with patients age the subjective opinion inevitably influences the decision as to whether a patient is unfit for surgery.

4. Perioperative Management of AAA Patients

Open repair of an infrarenal aortic aneurysm represents a complex surgical procedure due to aortic cross-clamping and subsequent ischemia-reperfusion injury. Optimized perioperative management can contribute to lowering the operative risk in these patients and reduce morbidity and mortality rates; although EVAR is a minimal invasive method patients have nonetheless to be regarded high risk and optimized management is inevitable. This includes adjustment of medication and the use of regional anaesthetic techniques in order to reduce the surgical stress response and improve outcome.

Adjustment of Medication

The patients own medication -especially β-blockers- should be continued perioperatively; if patients are not yet on β-blockers starting off this medication is not necessarily related to better outcome: routine use of β-blockers can only be recommended in high risk patients (RCRI ≥ 3) to reduce morbidity and mortality after noncardiac surgery. In low risk patients prophylactic use may even be harmful (Lindenauer 2005).

Statin medication is well established to reduce cardiovascular events in selected patients. Among patients with acute coronary syndrome acute administration of statins improves outcome (Schwartz 2001, Cannon 2004). The question if perioperative statin administration similarly reduces the operative risk has been addressed in several studies and results have been summarized in a systematic review by Biccard and co-workers (Biccard 2005); although mainly based on retrospective data the authors suggest a potential benefit from the perioperative use of statins.

In conclusion patients scheduled for elective AAA repair should be prescribed statins and in high risk patients beta-blockers should be started heart rate adjusted if patients are not yet on regular medication.

In addition to adjustment of medication optimized perioperative management of AAA patients aims at reducing the surgical stress in order to decrease morbidity and mortality rates; in other surgical specialties so called "fast track" programmes have been established which include elements such as no bowel preparation, no preoperative fasting, use of regional anaesthetic techniques, no fluid overload, avoidance of hypothermia and hypoxia, no routine use of nasogatric tubes, short incisions, early enteral feeding and early ambulation. This concept has been introduced by Kehlet and co-workers. As for AAA repair we have adopted the described elements for elective AAA repair and conducted a prospective randomized trial that revealed favourable results for fast track care in terms of morbidity and mortality (Muehling 2008, acc. WJS). Detailed management is outlined in the following paragraphs:

Use of Epdiural Anesthesia(EDA)

The surgical stress of aneurysm repair induced by aortic cross-clamping represents a crucial factor for patients outcome; the administration of epidural anaesthesia aims at reducing surgical stress with extended effect on postoperative analgesia (Kehlet 2002); by this means the surgical stress response can be diminished as has been shown in patients undergoing coronary artery bypass grafting (CABG) where thoracic epidural anaesthesia led to attenuation of epinephrine release and significant reduction of myocardial ischemia as judged by Troponin T measurements (Kirnö 1994, Loick 1999). To date regional anaesthesia is regarded to be the ideal technique available to attenuate endocrine metabolic responses with extended effect on postoperative analgesia (Liu 1995). Our own experience in a series of 125 consecutive patients has shown that supplementation with EDA resulted in a decreased rate of postoperative assisted mechanical ventilation and in lower morbidity rates (Muehling 2008). These findings are in line with other investigators who favour the use of EDA in order to reduce morbidity rates after aortic reconstructive surgery (Nishimori 2006). The data provided so far do strongly support supplementation of general anaesthesia with epidural anaesthesia for both purposes – reduction of the surgical stress response and proper postoperative analgesia that allows early ambulation of surgical patients.

Avoidance of Hypothermia

The importance of intraoperative normothermia has been shown in a prospective randomized trial in three hundred patients undergoing abdominal, thoracic, or vascular surgical procedures (Frank 1997); intraoperative hypothermia of 35.4°C was an independent predictor of adverse cardiac events by multivariate analysis. In a randomized trial of two hundred patients undergoing colorectal resection it has been shown that hypothermia itself may delay healing and predispose patients to wound infections. Maintaining normothermia intraoperatively is likely to decrease the incidence of infectious complications and shorten hospitalization (Kurz 1996). In an animal model normothermia improves survival rates after experimental sepsis by appropriately modulating the early inflammatory response (Xiao 2005). Hence intraoperative normothermia is an essential for the outcome of surgical procedures.

Avoidance of Fluid Overload

As for perioperative fluid management no evidence based guidelines exist. Some clinical trials have suggested that large amounts of fluids may be associated to increased morbidity and hospital stay (Nisanevich 2005). In a double blind study comparing a liberal to a restrictive fluid management 'liberal' fluid regimen led to a transient improvement in pulmonary function and postoperative hypoxaemia but no other differences in all-over physiological recovery compared with a 'restrictive' fluid regimen after fast-track colonic surgery (Holte 2007). As for AAA repair intraoperative fluid restriction is diffcult to realize as declamping may lead to abrupt fall of blood pressure if not stopped with administration of crystalloids and colloids. Nevertheless during the postoperative course administration of i.v. fluids can be cut down to 1000ml/24h as has been shown in our prospective trial of fast track care (Muehling 2008)

No Routine Use of Nasogatric Tube and Early Enteral Feeding

Another condition contributing to postoperative recovery after major surgical procedures is gastrointestinal function; after abdominal surgery up to 20% require reinsertion of nasogastric tube (NGT) and median time to first defecation is three days (Han-Geurts 2007). In the clinical setting of fast track recovery programmes the necessity of re-insertion of NGT and the number of days required to tolerate full oral food intake can be reduced (Gatt 2005). In our own prospective trial of fast track recovery after elective AAA repair patients were able to tolerate full oral food intake after 5 days (Muehling 2008). As a consequence patients should be allowed to drink clear fluids and carbohydrate drinks from the evening of the operation in order to simulate bowel function.

The above mentioned steps in perioperative care and the combination of these elements that have been proven to be of value can lead to decreased risk of perioperative adverse effects and decreased morbidity and mortality rates after elective AAA repair.

In summary preoperative assessment and perioperative management of AAA patients includes

- CT scan for selection of EVAR patients
- Assessment of co-morbidities and preoperative improvement
- Adjustment of medical treatment
- Administration of epidural anesthesia (EDA) to reduce surgical stress
- Avoidance of hypothermia and fluid overload
- Early ambulation and early enteral feeding

5. Surgical Procedure – Transperitoneal, Retroperitoneal and Endovascular

History of AAA Repair

The first successful open repair of an AAA has been described by Dubost in the 1950's when he replaced the diseased segment of the aorta by a homograft. Since then surgical techniques by the introduction of prosthetic grafts and perioperative care by development of intensive care units have improved leading to mortality rates about 6%, in high volume centres about 1% after elective open AAA repair. The first report of successful endovascular aneurysm exclusion has been published by Parodi et al in 1991. This technique uses guide wires to place a stentgraft in the aneurysm via the femoral arteries. At present endovascular repair is an established alternative to open repair but its role has yet to be clearly determined.

Ttrans-, Retroperitoneal and Endovascular Route

Elective repair of infrarenal aortic aneurysms includes the transperitoneal, the retroperitoneal and the endovascular approach through the femoral arteries. The transperitoneal approach to the infrarenal aorta is achieved via a midline incision; it is the preferred approach in patients with concomitant iliac aneurysms that require insertion of a bifurcated prosthesis. In case of retroperitoneal incision we use a curvilinear incision starting at the tip of the 11th rib without routine resection of the rib and continuing obliquely to a point middish above the os pubis. After dissecting the oblique muscles we use a posterolateral approach to the aorta as supposed by Willliams. As for open surgical aneurysmectomy it is assumed that the retroperitoneal approach is associated to fewer pulmonary complications and gastrointestinal disturbances but randomized trials failed to demonstrate the superiority of the retroperitoneal approach over the transperitoneal (Cambria

1990, Sicard 1995). At least it is accepted that the retroperitoneal approach offers advantages in case of hostile abdomen, horseshoe kidney or in case of an anatomically complex neck which may require suprarenal clamping (Shepard 1991). We see the indication for transperitoneal aneurysmectomy in patients with concomitant iliac aneurysms that require insertion of a bifurcated graft, the retroperitoneal approach is preferred in patients with a anatomically complex neck if suprarenal clamping may be necessary or in case of hostile abdomen. In our institution we choose EVAR in older patients estimated to be at high risk for open surgery and if aneurysm anatomy is suitable; we do not apply a rigourous system of preoperative testing and risk quantification: the usual preoperative work-up protocols as outlined above are applied and thereafter the decision is made individually based on the patients individual risk factors. The decision on which approach to use is always an individual one based on the anatomy of the aneurysm and the patients individual risk factors (age, co-morbidities etc.). At present approximately one third of our patients is treated via the EVAR method. .

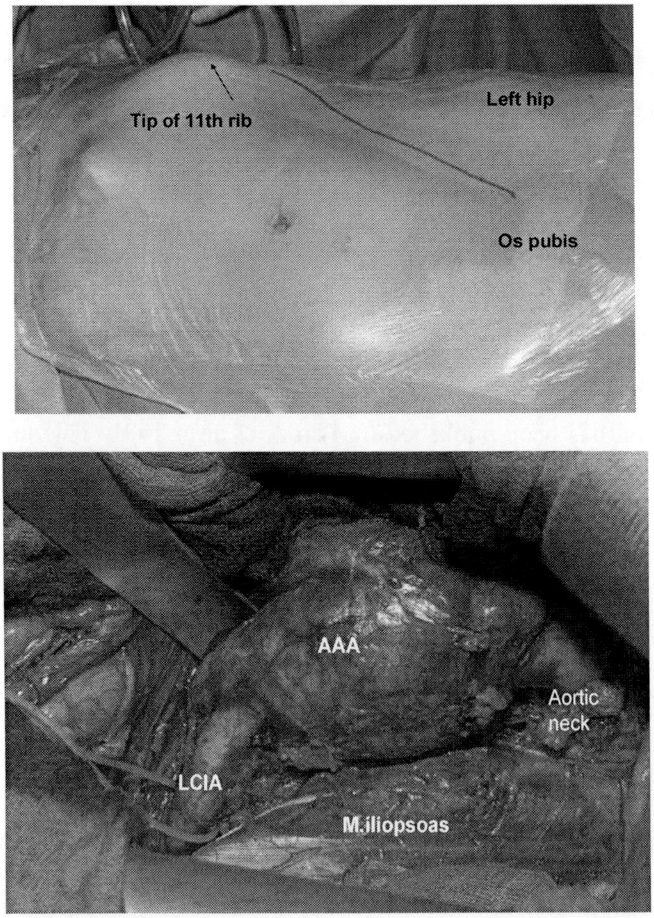

Figure. 1a and b. Positioning of the patient on the operative table and incision for the retroperitoneal approach; intraoperative situs: The center of the picture shows the aortic aneurysm (AAA), the aortic neck being on the right, the common iliac arteries on the left (LCIA: left common iliac artery); the M. iliopsoas serves a landmark for the retroperitoneal route.

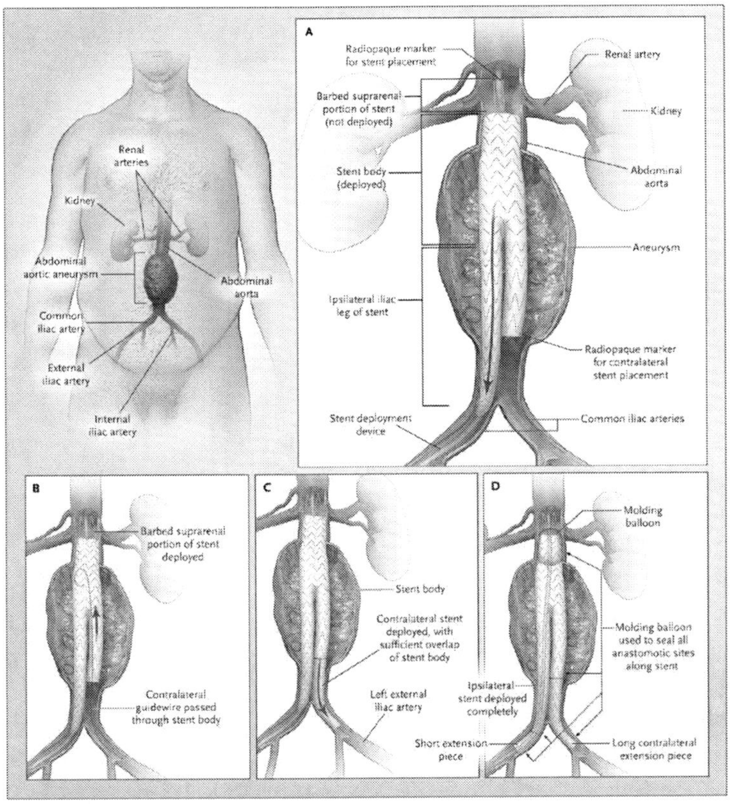

From: Greenhalgh R and Powell J. N Engl J Med 2008;358:494-501

Figure 2. Schematic drawing of the endovascular procedure; the stentgraft consisting of a mainbody and contralateral extension is deployed using guide wires that have been placed via the femoral arteries in the aorta; the procedure is performed under x-ray control.

Perioperative Outcome after Elective Infrarenal Aneurysm Reapir

Large multicentric trials–namely the EVAR1 and the DREAM trial- have demonstrated advantages for endovascular aneurysm repair (EVAR) concerning blood loss, length of stay on intensive care unit and overall morbidity and mortality in patients that were suitable for both approaches: open and endovascular (Greenhalgh 2004, Prinssen 2004). EVAR is by its nature a minimal invasive procedure associated to reduced blood loss, improved postoperative pulmonary function, early ambulation and early consumption of regular diet. These findings have been documented in several studies (Paolini 2008, Prinssen 2004). Furthermore in appropriate cases the minimal access enables the use of local anaesthesia.

The advantages in the short term of EVAR which are attributed to the avoidance of laparotomy and less disturbances in patients haemostasis may be counterbalanced in the long term by the high rate of re-interventions: 2.7% after the first year to 9% in the fourth year which is significantly higher as compared to open repair (Schermerhorn 2008). On the other hand open repair is accompanied by morbidity rates up to 50% and mortality rates up to 8%.

The table summarizes important trials that addressed the value of EVAR compared to open repair in terms of perioperative mortality and our own results.

Table 1. Overview of clinical trials (RCT: randomized controlled trial; NRCT: non-randomized controlled trial) comparing open repair (OR) and endovascular aneurysm repair; our own results have been submitted for publication to the BJS.

Author	Study design	Number of patients	Mortality EVAR vs. OR	In favour of
Prinssen 2004	RCT	345	1.1% vs. 4.5%	EVAR
Greenhalgh 2004	RCT	1,047	1.6% vs. 4.6%	EVAR
Schermerhorn 2008	Cohort Study	45,660	1.2% vs. 4.8%	EVAR
Hansman 2003	NRCT	100	2% vs. 0%	OR
Criado 2003	NRCT	366	0.4% vs. 0%	OR
Becquemin 2000	NRCT	180	2.7% vs. 1.8%	OR
Ulm 2008	NRCT	210	3% vs. 0.6%	Individually adjusted

In the interpretation of the above mentioned trials one has to be aware that trials that favoured EVAR were obtained in patients that were suitable for both: open and endovascular repair; there are also data that are in favour of open repair as in high volume centres mortality rates of open repair are also low. Nonetheless the potential advantages in perioperative outcome deem EVAR as the procedure of choice in patients who appear to be unfit for the surgical stress of open aneurysm exclusion, e.g. patients with severe co-morbidities (Bush 2007). For this reason currently EVAR is regarded the optimal treatment option in older and high risk patients. However a systematic review in older aged patients has described a pooled mortality rate of 4.6% in this high risk group (Henebiens 2007). In this population significant comorbidities reduce life expectancy and the question if EVAR sufficiently will reduce the all-cause mortality to justify its use in these patients is not yet satisfactorily answered. There are only two reports facing this problem: the EUROSTAR registry and the EVAR II trial. In summary these trials showed potential benefits for EVAR in unfit patients if survival is more than 12 months.

In our institution we prospectively collect data from all patients undergoing elective infrarenal aortic aneurysm repair and analysis of this database comparing the surgical approach in 210 patients (trans-, retroperitoneal and endovascular) revealed the following results: Median age in patients undergoing EVAR is significantly higher (78yr) than in patients undergoing transperitoneal (68yr) or retroperitoneal (67yr) repair. ASA classification does not differ between the analyzed groups, the majority is estimated ASA III. Other demographic data (gender, AAA diameter, preoperative haemoglobin and baseline creatinine) are comparable. Datailed overview of our own results are depicted in Table 2.

As expected the endovascular technique exposed clear advantages in terms of need for assisted mechanical ventilation, blood units transfused and total operative time. The in hospital mortality was comparable in all groups and ranged from 0-3%, rates that are in line with the results of other investigators who describe mortality rates of 3.5% for open and 2.7% for EVAR (Chahwan 2007). The reason for the lack of difference between open and endovascular treatment may be the older age of EVAR patients on the one hand and on the other hand the fact that in institutions where endovascular and open techniques are well established, mortality rates of open repair are also low (Ligush 2002, Hertzer 2002, Elkouri 2004).

The frequency of re-operation ranged from 7.5% to 12% in our groups with no significant difference; reasons for re-operation were peripheral embolization, ileus and postoperative bleeding; specific surgical complications in the retroperitoneal group that must be attributed to the technique were spleen rupture and ureter lesion in three patients – complications that have already been described (Shepherd 1991, Dennis1990). Ischemic colitis and mesenteric infarction developed in 2.4% in the RP group and in 4.5% in the EV group. Other reports have documented this complication in 1-6% after open as well as after endovascular aneurysm exclusion (Dadian 2001, Perry 2008). As for medical complications rates of cardio-respiratory and renal failure were similar in all groups; surprisingly overall morbidity showed the highest rate after EV with 39.9%, followed by transperitoneal (30.1%) and retroperitoneal repair (28.3%). This observation may be attributed to two issues: *First* the EV patients had significantly older age: 78 years vs. 68 years and 67years respectively. Age has been demonstrated to be an important predictor of outcome and is even well established in risk scores such as GAS and VBHOM (Patterson 2008). Analysis of population based data in a large number of patients has documented three to four fold higher complication rates in older patients as compared to younger cohorts < 75 years (Schermerhorn 2008). Higher morbidity rates in this high risk group of have been reported (Tefera 2004). *Second*: In high volume centres where both techniques -open and endovascular repair- are well established complication rates for open repair are also low (Ligush 2002, Muehling 2008). As a consequence we recommend referral of patients scheduled for elective AAA repair to high volume centres where all operative facilities are available to face any problems that may arise in elective aneurysm repair. Based on the available literature and on our own experience we feel that advantages and disadvantages of either approach have to be outweighed in the light of the individual risk factors of each patient. By this means in combination with optimized perioperative care elective AAA repair can be performed with low morbidity and mortality rates·

6. Specific Features of EVAR

Endoleaks after EVAR

A specific complication which is unique to EVAR is the occurrence of endoleaks - a phenomenon which implies failure to exclude the aneurysm and which carries the risk of aneurysm growth and eventually secondary rupture. The term has been created in 1996 and a classification scheme has been adopted (White 1996):

Table 2. Perioperative outcome, surgical and medical complications according to the approach: transperitoneal, retroperitoneal and endovascular

	Transperitoneal (n=63)	Retroperitoneal (n=81)	EVAR(n=66)	p-value
Operating time [min]	180 [100-270]	150 [100-270]	120 [45-360]#	#p<0.001
Need for AMV	13/63 (20.6%)	8/81 (9.8%)	2/66 (3%)*	* p= 0.004
Blood units transfused	0 [0-10]	2 [0-28]	0 [0-6]#	# p= 0.001
Duration of ICU [h]	23 [11-336]	22.5 [12-288]	22 [3-336]	p=0.954
Day of discharge [POD]	10 [7-45]	10.5 [6-49]	9 [5-44]	p=0.162
In hospital mortality	0%	1/81 (1.2%)	2/66 (3%)	n.s.
Surgical complications				
Peripheral Ischemia	3	4	2	
Ischemic colitis	0	1	1	
IC req. resection/mesenteric infarction	0	2	3	
Postoperative bleeding	2	0	0	
Wound infection	0	1	2	
Spleen rupture	0	2	0	
Ureter lesion	0	1	0	
Graft occlusion	0	2	0	
Ileus requiring stoma	0	1	0	
Incisional hernia	2	0	0	
Intraoperative graft dislocation	-	-	2	
Re-Operation (patients) Medical complications	8/63 (12%)	9/81 (11%)	5/66 (7.5%)	n.s.
Pneumonia	3/63 (4.7%)	1/81 (1.2%)	2/66 (3%)	
Myocardial ischemia	2/63 (3.1%)	0	2/66 (3%)	
Dysrhythmia	2/63 (2.1%)	5/81 (6.1%)	2/66 (3%)	
ARF	5/63 (7.9%)	9/81 (11%)	/66 (12%)	
ARF req. dialysis	1/63 (1.5%)	1/81 (1.2%)	2/66 (3%)	
Subileus	9/63 (14%)	5/81 (6.1%)	0	
UTI	2/63 (3.1%)	4/81 (4.9%)	7/66 (10%)	
Septicemia	1/63 (1.5%)	4/81 [4.9%)	2/66 (3%)	
Other	0	0	2/66 (3%)	
Total (patients)	19/63 (30.1%)	23/81 (28.3%)	26/66 (39.3%)	n.s.

Classification of endoleaks

Endoleak	Explanation	
Type I	due to incomplete attachement	
	Ia	at the proximal en of endograft
	Ib	at the distal end of endograft
Type II	due to retrograde blood flow from patent arteries (IMA and lumbar arteries)	
Type III	midgraft leak due to graft defect	

The frequency of endoleaks ranges from 24% to 39% (Schurink 1999, Petrik 2001); early reports of endoleaks showed that tube grafts were associated to significant higher rates of endoleaks than bifurcated or aortounilateral (AUI) devices (35% vs. 18%, $p<0.0001$; Shurink 1999). The majority of these endoleaks arose from the distal attachement site (Type Ib); as a consequence at present only bifurcated or aorto-unilateral devices should be deployed. In our own series of bifurcated and AUI devices we had a rate of 38.7% endoleaks, the majority being type II leaks that needed no immediate intervention. Other types of leakage resolved over time without secondary intervention as well. One patient died due to secondary rupture postoperatively, a rare condition in the early postoperative period, but a late complication of endovascular aneurysm repair which must be attributed to incomplete aneurysm exclusion (Lumsden 1995, Torsello 1998). Due to the specific occurrence of endoleakage with incomplete aneurysm exclusion after EV repair lifelong surveillance and careful follow up by either CT scan or MRI is necessary. There is a substantial rate of re-interventions after EVAR -16.2% in a meta-analysis of RCT´s and NRCT´s – with extra surgical or radiological procedures that are of course associated to increased costs and additional morbidity and mortality (Drury 2005). In the rating of EVAR these disadvantages that may cloud the preoperative rewards must be kept in mind.

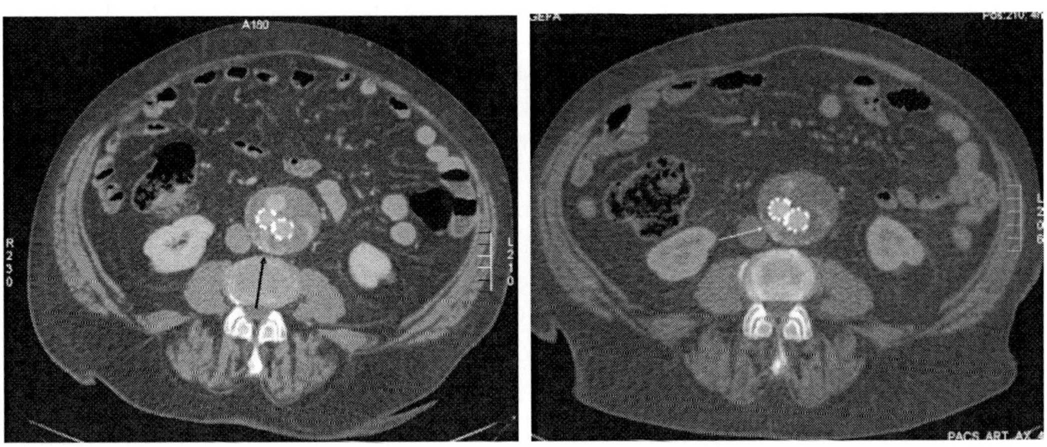

Figures 3a and b. This 72year old patient underwent EVAR due tor severe COPD and ischemic heart disease; the immediate postop CT scan documented a significant endoleak which was suspected to be Typ II. The control 6months later showed the leak regredient without progression of the aneurysm sac. The patient is under close follow up.

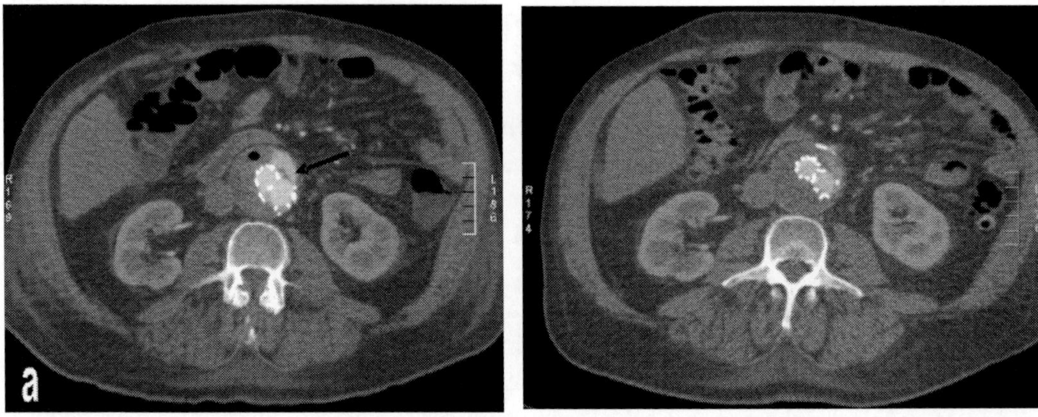

Figures 4a and b. This 69year old patient underwent EVAR due tor severe COPD and ischemic heart disease; the immediate postop CT scan documented a significant endoleak which was suspected to be Typ II or III. The control 3months later showed clear regression of the leak without progression of the aneurysm sac. The patient is under close follow up.

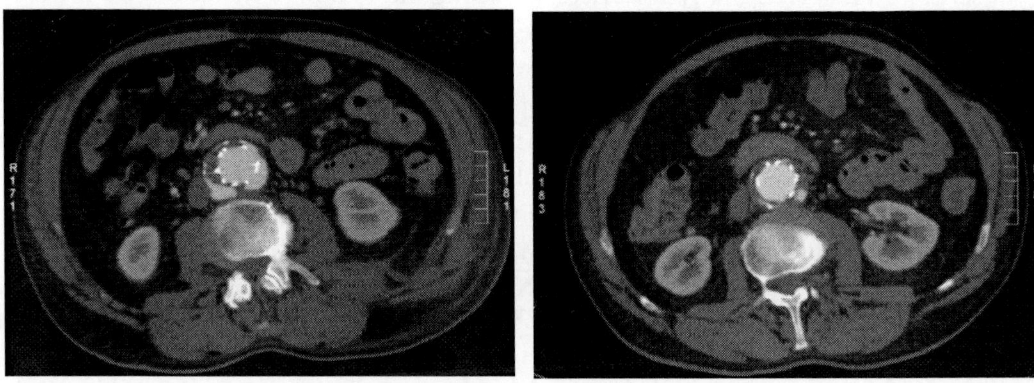

Figures 5a and b. This 69year old patient underwent EVAR because he refused open repair; the immediate postop CT scan documented a significant endoleak which was suspected to be Typ I. The control 3months later showed clear regression of the leak without progression of the aneurysm sac. Herein the leak turned out to be Type II. The patient is under close follow up.

Costs of Elective Aortic Aneurysm Repair

In a period of declining financial resources in all healthcare systems the type of repair has also to be discussed in the light of costs of the procedure. In this context short and long term results must not be considered separately but have to be discussed in the view of short and long term outcomes. From the results of the randomized trials comparing EVAR to open repair it is known that EVAR is associated to higher costs as compared to open repair: higher costs of 3,311£ and 4,293€ respectively over a period of 4 years as compared to open repair (EVAR I trial, Prinssen 2008); the advantages of EVAR in the short term (shorter ICU and in hospital stay) do not compensate the initial costs of the endograft and the subsequent costs of secondary intervention and surveillance.

Requirements of Elective AAA Repair

Elective repair of infrarenal aortic aneurysms – may it be open or endovascular- requires a specialist team where all techniques are well established. Appropriate equipment, facilities, critical care services and follow up management must be provided as after elective repair miscellaneous complications can occur – especially in old and high risk patients.

In summary the decision as to whether patients should undergo transperitoneal, retroperitoneal or endovascular repair has to be outweighed by individual factors

- Individual operative risk: age, co-morbidities
- Life expectancy
- Anatomic suitability for EVAR as judged by CT scan
- Identification of complex aortic neck that may require suprarenal clamping and concomitant iliac aneurysms involving the internal iliac arteries
- Individual anatomic features: obesity, horseshoe kidney, previous laparotomy …
- Is the patient willing for close follow-up by CT scan of MRI
- Cost-effectiveness

References

Alberto, P; Maddalena, G; Giuseppe, G; Ilaria, Q; Franci, B; Campagna, MS; Eugenio, N; Antonio, B; Carlo, S; Ranuccio, N. Prevalence of risk factors, coronary and systemic atherosclerosis in abdominal aortic aneurysm: comparison with high cardiovascular risk population. *Vasc Health Risk Manag*., 2008, 4(4), 877-83.

Alexander, D; Shepard; David, FJ; Tollefson Daniel, J; Reddy, James, R; Evans, Joseph, P; Elliott, Roger, F; Smith, Calvin B. Ernst. Left flank retroperitoneal exposure: A technical aid to complex aortic reconstruction *Journal of Vascular Surgery*, 1991 (Vol. 14, Issue 3, Pages 283-291)

Annambhotla, S; Bourgeois, S; Wang, X; Lin, PH; Yao, Q; Chen, C. Recent advances in molecular mechanisms of abdominal aortic aneurysm formation. *World J Surg*., 2008, Jun., 32(6), 976-86. Review.

Badger, SA; O'Donnell, ME; Sharif, MA; Boyd, CS; Hannon, RJ; Lau, LL; Lee, B; Soong, CV. Risk factors for abdominal aortic aneurysm and the influence of social deprivation. *Angiology*. 2008 Oct-Nov., 59(5), 559-66. Epub 2008 Sep 25.

Baxter, BT; Pearce, WH; Waltke, EA; Littooy, FN; Hallett, JW: Jr, Kent, KC; Upchurch, GR. Jr, Chaikof, EL; Mills, JL; Fleckten, B; Longo, GM; Lee, JK; Thompson, RW. Prolonged administration of doxycycline in patients with small asymptomatic abdominal aortic aneurysms: report of a prospective (Phase II) multicenter study. *J Vasc Surg*., 2002 Jul., 36(1), 1-12.

Baxter, BT; Terrin, MC; Dalman, RL. Medical management of small abdominal aortic aneurysms. *Circulation*, 2008 Apr., 8, 117(14), 1883-9. Review.

Biccard, BM; Sear, JW; Foëx, P. Statin therapy: a potentially useful peri-operative intervention in patients with cardiovascular disease. *Anaesthesia,* 2005 Nov, 60(11), 1106-14. Review.

Brady, AR; Fowkes, FG; Thompson, SG; Powell, JT. Aortic aneurysm diameter and risk of cardiovascular mortality. *Arterioscler Thromb Vasc Biol.,* 2001 Jul., 21(7), 1203-7.

Brady, AR; Thompson, SG; Fowkes, FG; Greenhalgh, RM; Powell, JT; UK. Small Aneurysm Trial Participants. Abdominal aortic aneurysm expansion: risk factors and time intervals for surveillance. *Circulation*, 2004 Jul 6, 110(1), 16-21. Epub 2004 Jun 21.

Brilakis, ES; Orford, JL; Fasseas, P; Wilson, SH; Melby, S; Lennon, RJ; Berger, PB. Outcome of patients undergoing balloon angioplasty in the two months prior to noncardiac surgery. *Am J Cardiol.,* 2005 Aug., 15, 96(4), 512-4.

Bush, RL; Johnson, ML; Hedayati, N; Henderson, WG; Lin, PH; Lumsden, AB. Performance of endovascular aortic aneurysm repair in high-risk patients: results from the Veterans Affairs National Surgical Quality Improvement Program. *J Vasc Surg*., 2007 Feb., 45(2), 227-233; discussion 233-5.

Buth, J; Laheij, RJ Early complications and endoleaks after endovascular abdominal aortic aneurysm repair: report of a multicenter study. *J Vasc Surg*., 2000 Jan., 31(1 Pt 1), 134-46.

Cambria, RP; Brewster, DC; Abbott, WM; Freehan, M; Megerman, J; LaMuraglia, G; Wilson, R; Wilson, D; Teplick, R; Davison, JK. Transperitoneal versus retroperitoneal approach for aortic reconstruction: a randomized prospective study. *J Vasc Surg*., 1990, 11(2), 314-24; discussion 324-5.

Chahwan, S; Comerota, AJ; Pigott, JP; Scheuermann, BW; Burrow, J; Wojnarowski, D. Elective treatment of abdominal aortic aneurysm with endovascular or open repair: the first decade. *J Vasc Surg*., 2007 Feb., 45(2), 258-62; discussion 262.

Chuter, TA; Reilly, LM; Faruqi, RM; Kerlan, RB; Sawhney, R; Canto, CJ; LaBerge, JM; Wilson, MW; Gordon, RL; Wall, SD; Rapp, J; Messina, LM. Endovascular aneurysm repair in high-risk patients. *J Vasc Surg*., 2000 Jan., 31(1 Pt 1), 122-33.

Cosford, PA; Leng, GC. Screening for abdominal aortic aneurysm. *Cochrane Database Syst Rev*., 2007 Apr., 18, (2), CD002945. Review.

Dardik, A: Burleyson, GP; Bowman, H; Gordon, TA; Williams, GM; Webb, TH; Perler, BA. Surgical repair of ruptured abdominal aortic aneurysms in the state of Maryland: factors influencing outcome among 527 recent cases. *J Vasc Surg*., 1998 Sep., 28(3), 413-20, discussion 420-1

Diehm, N; Dick, F; Schaffner, T; Schmidli, J; Kalka, C; Di Santo, S; Voelzmann, J; Baumgartner, I. Novel insight into the pathobiology of abdominal aortic aneurysm and potential future treatment concepts. *Prog Cardiovasc Dis*., 2007 Nov-Dec., 50(3), 209-17. Review.

Elkouri, S; Gloviczki, P; McKusick, MA; Panneton, JM; Andrews, J; Bower, TC; Noel, AA; Harmsen, WS; Hoskin, TL; Cherry, K. Perioperative complications and early outcome after endovascular and open surgical repair of abdominal aortic aneurysms. *J Vasc Surg*., 2004 Mar., 39(3), 497-505.

Evans, J; Powell, JT; Schwalbe, E; Loftus, IM; Thompson, MM. Simvastatin attenuates the activity of matrix metalloprotease-9 in aneurysmal aortic tissue. *Eur J Vasc Endovasc Surg.*, 2007 Sep., 34(3), 302-3. Epub 2007 Jun 18.

Frank, SM; Fleisher, LA; Breslow, MJ; Higgins, MS; Olson, KF; Kelly, S; Beattie, C. Perioperative maintenance of normothermia reduces the incidence of morbid cardiac events. A randomized clinical trial. *JAMA*, 1997 Apr 9, 277(14), 1127-34.

Gatt, M; Anderson, AD; Reddy, BS; Hayward-Sampson, P; Tring, IC; MacFie, J. Randomized clinical trial of multimodal optimization of surgical care in patients undergoing major colonic resection. *Br J Surg.*, 2005 Nov., 92(11), 1354-62.

Greenhalgh, RM; Brown, LC; Kwong, GP; Powell, JT; Thompson, SG. EVAR trial participants. Comparison of endovascular aneurysm repair with open repair in patients with abdominal aortic aneurysm (EVAR trial 1), 30-day operative mortality results: randomised controlled trial. *Lancet*, 2004 Sep., 4-10, 364(9437), 843-8.

Han-Geurts, IJ; Hop, WC; Kok, NF; Lim, A; Brouwer, KJ; Jeekel, J. Randomized clinical trial of the impact of early enteral feeding on postoperative ileus and recovery. *Br J Surg.*, 2007 May, 94(5), 555-61.

Heller, JA; Weinberg, A; Arons, R; Krishnasastry, KV; Lyon, RT; Deitch, JS; Schulick, AH; Bush, HL: Jr, Kent, KC. Two decades of abdominal aortic aneurysm repair: have we made any progress? *J Vasc Surg.*, 2000 Dec., 32(6), 1091-100.

Henebiens, M; Vahl, A; Koelemay, MJ. Elective surgery of abdominal aortic aneurysms in octogenarians: a systematic review. *J Vasc Surg.*, 2008, Mar., 47(3), 676-81. Epub 2008 Jan 22. Review.

Hertzer, NR; Mascha, EJ; Karafa, MT; O'Hara, PJ; Krajewski, LP; Beven, EG. Open infrarenal abdominal aortic aneurysm repair: the Cleveland Clinic experience from 1989 to 1998. *J Vasc Surg.*, 2002 Jun., 35(6), 1145-54.

Holte, K; Kristensen, BB; Valentiner, L; Foss, NB; Husted, H; Kehlet, H. Liberal versus restrictive fluid management in knee arthroplasty: a randomized, double-blind study. *Anesth Analg*, 2007 Aug., 105(2), 465-74.

Immediate repair compared with surveillance of small abdominal aortic aneurysms. Lederle FA; Wilson; SE; Johnson, GR; Reinke, DB; Littooy, FN; Acher, CW; Ballard, DJ; Messina, LM; Gordon, IL; Chute, EP; Krupski, WC; Busuttil, SJ; Barone, GW; Sparks, S; Graham, LM; Rapp, JH; Makaroun, MS; Moneta, GL; Cambria, RA; Makhoul, RG; Eton, D; Ansel, HJ; Freischlag, JA; Bandyk, D. Aneurysm Detection and Management Veterans Affairs Cooperative Study Group. *N Engl J Med.,* 2002 May 9, 346(19), 1437-44.

Kehlet, H; Holte, K. Epidural anaesthesia and analgesia in major surgery. *Lancet*, 2002 Aug 17, 360(9332), 568-9; author reply 569. No abstract available.

Kehlet, H; Mogensen, T. Hospital stay of 2 days after open sigmoidectomy with a multimodal rehabilitation programme. *Br J Surg.*, 1999 Feb., 86(2), 227-30.

Kirnö, K; Friberg, P; Grzegorczyk, A; Milocco, I; Ricksten, SE; Lundin, S. Thoracic epidural anesthesia during coronary artery bypass surgery: effects on cardiac sympathetic activity, myocardial blood flow and metabolism, and central hemodynamics. *Anesth Analg.*, 1994 Dec, 79(6), 1075-81.

Kurz, A; Sessler, DI; Lenhardt, R. Perioperative normothermia to reduce the incidence of surgical-wound infection and shorten hospitalization. Study of Wound Infection and Temperature Group. *N Engl J Med.*, 1996 May 9, 334(19), 1209-15.

Lee, TH; Marcantonio, ER; Mangione, CM; Thomas, EJ; Polanczyk, CA; Cook, EF; Sugarbaker, DJ; Donaldson, MC; Poss, R; Ho, KK; Ludwig, LE; Pedan, A; Goldman, L. Derivation and prospective validation of a simple index for prediction of cardiac risk of major noncardiac surgery. *Circulation*, 1999 Sep., 7, 100(10), 1043-9.

Lee, WA; Carter, JW; Upchurch, G; Seeger, JM; Huber, TS. Perioperative outcomes after open and endovascular repair of intact abdominal aortic aneurysms in the United States during 2001. *J Vasc Surg.*, 2004 Mar., 39(3), 491-6.

Ligush, J; Jr; Pearce, JD; Edwards, MS; Eskridge, MR; Cherr, GS; Plonk, GW; et al. Analysis of medical risk factors and outcomes in patients undergoing open versus endovascular abdominal aortic aneurysm repair. *J Vasc Surg.*, 2002 Sep., 36(3), 492-9.

Lindenauer, PK; Pekow, P; Wang, K; Mamidi, DK; Gutierrez, B; Benjamin, EM. Perioperative beta-blocker therapy and mortality after major noncardiac surgery. *N Engl J Med.*, 2005 Jul 28, 353(4), 349-61.

Liu, S, Carpenter, RL; Neal, JM. Epidural anesthesia and analgesia. Their role in postoperative outcome. *Anesthesiology*, 1995 Jun., 82(6), 1474-506. Review.

Loick, HM; Schmidt, C; Van Aken, H; Junker, R; Erren, M; Berendes, E., et al. High thoracic epidural anesthesia, but not clonidine, attenuates the perioperative stress response via sympatholysis and reduces the release of troponin T in patients undergoing coronary artery bypass grafting. *Anesth Analg.*, 1999 Apr., 88(4), 701-9.

Lumsden, AB; Allen, RC; Chaikof, EL; Resnikoff, M; Moritz, MW; Gerhard, H; Castronuovo, JJ. Jr. Delayed rupture of aortic aneurysms following endovascular stent grafting. *Am J Surg.,* 1995 Aug., 170(2), 174-8.

Medical management of abdominal aortic aneurysm. Golledge, J; Powell, JT. *Eur, J Vasc Endovasc Surg.*, 2007 Sep., 34(3), 267-73. Epub 2007 May 30. Review

Mortality results for randomised controlled trial of early elective surgery or ultrasonographic surveillance for small abdominal aortic aneurysms. The UK Small Aneurysm Trial Participants. *Lancet*, 1998 Nov., 21, 352(9141), 1649-55.

Mosorin, M; Juvonen, J; Biancari, F; Satta, J; Surcel, HM; Leinonen, M; Saikku, P; Juvonen, T. Use of doxycycline to decrease the growth rate of abdominal aortic aneurysms: a randomized, double-blind, placebo-controlled pilot study. *J Vasc Surg.,* 2001 Oct./, 34(4), 606-10.

Muehling, BM; Halter, G; Lang, G; Schelzig, H; Steffen, P; Wagner, F; Meierhenrich, R; Sunder-Plassmann, L; Orend, KH. Prospective randomized controlled trial to evaluate "fast-track" elective open infrarenal aneurysm repair. *Langenbecks Arch Surg.*, 2008 May, 393(3), 281-7. Epub 2008 Feb 14.

Muehling, BM; Meierhenrich, R; Thiere, M; Bischoff, G; Oberhuber, A; Orend, KH; Sunder-Plassmann, L. The retroperitoneal approach combined with epidural anesthesia reduces morbidity in elective infrarenal aortic aneurysm repair. *Interact Cardiovasc Thorac Surg.*, 2008 Sep 30., [Epub ahead of print]

Nisanevich, V; Felsenstein, I; Almogy, G; Weissman, C; Einav, S; Matot, I. Effect of intraoperative fluid management on outcome after intraabdominal surgery. *Anesthesiology*, 2005 Jul., 103(1), 25-32.

Nishimori, M; Ballantyne, JC; Low, JH. Epidural pain relief versus systemic opioid-based pain relief for abdominal aortic surgery. *Cochrane Database Syst Rev.*, 2006, 19, 3, CD005059. Review.

Norman, P; Le, M; Pearce, C; Jamrozik, K. Infrarenal aortic diameter predicts all-cause mortality. *Arterioscler Thromb Vasc Biol.*, 2004 Jul., 24(7), 1278-82. Epub 2004 May 6.

Optimal medical management of peripheral arterial disease. Rice TW, Lumsden AB. *Vasc Endovascular Surg.*, 2006 Aug-Sep., 40(4), 312-27. Review.

Paolini, D; Chahwan, S; Wojnarowski, D; Pigott, JP; LaPorte, F; Comerota, AJ. Elective endovascular and open repair of abdominal aortic aneurysms in octogenarians. *J Vasc Surg.*, 2008 May, 47(5), 924-7. Epub 2008 Mar 21.

Patterson, BO; Holt, PJ; Hinchliffe, R; Loftus, IM; Thompson, MM. Predicting risk in elective abdominal aortic aneurysm repair: a systematic review of current evidence. *Eur J Vasc Endovasc Surg.*, 2008 Dec., 36(6), 637-45. Epub 2008 Oct.

Pfeffer, MA; Skene, AM. Pravastatin or Atorvastatin Evaluation and Infection Therapy-Thrombolysis in Myocardial Infarction 22 Investigators.Intensive versus moderate lipid lowering with statins after acute coronary syndromes. Cannon, CP, Braunwald, E; McCabe, CH; Rader, DJ; Rouleau, JL; Belder, R; Joyal, SV; Hill, KA. *N Engl J Med.*, 2004 Apr 8, 350(15), 1495-504. Epub 2004 Mar 8, Erratum in: *N Engl J Med.*, 2006 Feb 16, 354(7), 778.

Prinssen, M; Verhoeven, EL; Buth, J; Cuypers, PW; Van Sambeek, MR; Balm, R; et al; Dutch Randomized Endovascular Aneurysm Management (DREAM)Trial Group. A randomized trial comparing conventional and endovascular repair of abdominal aortic aneurysms. *N Engl J Med.*, 2004 Oct 14, 351(16), 1607-18.

Propranolol for small abdominal aortic aneurysms: results of a randomized trial. Propanolol Aneurysm Trial Investigators. *J Vasc Surg.,* 2002 Jan., 35(1), 72-9.

Robless, P; Mikhailidis, DP; Stansby, G. Systematic review of antiplatelet therapy for the prevention of myocardial infarction, stroke or vascular death in patients with peripheral vascular disease. *Br J Surg.*, 2001 Jun., 88(6), 787-800. Review.

Schermerhorn, ML; O'Malley, AJ; Jhaveri, A; Cotterill, P; Pomposelli, F; Landon, BE. Endovascular vs. open repair of abdominal aortic aneurysms in the Medicare population. *N Engl J Med.,* 2008 Jan, 31, 358(5), 464-74.

Schermerhorn, ML; O'Malley, AJ; Jhaveri, A; Cotterill, P; Pomposelli, F; Landon, BE. Endovascular vs. open repair of abdominal aortic aneurysms in the Medicare population. *N Engl J Med.*, 2008 Jan 31, 358(5), 464-74.

Schouten, O; Van Laanen, JH; Boersma, E; Vidakovic, R; Feringa, HH; Dunkelgrün, M; Bax JJ, Koning, J; Van Urk, H; Poldermans, D. Statins are associated with a reduced infrarenal abdominal aortic aneurysm growth. *Eur J Vasc Endovasc Surg.*, 2006 Jul., 32(1), 21-6. Epub 2006 Mar 6.

Schwartz, GG; Olsson, AG; Ezekowitz, MD; Ganz, P; Oliver, MF; Waters, D; Zeiher, A; Chaitman, BR; Leslie, S; Stern, T. Myocardial Ischemia Reduction with Aggressive Cholesterol Lowering (MIRACL) Study Investigators. Effects of atorvastatin on early recurrent ischemic events in acute coronary syndromes: the MIRACL study: a randomized controlled trial. *JAMA*, 2001 Apr 4, 285(13), 1711-8. Summary for patients in: *Curr Cardiol Rep*., 2002 Nov., 4(6), 485.

Scott, RA; Ashton, HA; Kay, DN. Routine ultrasound screening in management of abdominal aortic aneurysm. *Br Med J (Clin Res Ed),* 1988 Jun., 18, 296(6638), 1709-10.

Sicard, GA; Reilly, JM; Rubin, BG; Thompson, RW; Allen, BT; Flye, MW; Schechtman, KB, Young-Beyer, P; Weiss, C; Anderson, CB. Transabdominal versus retroperitoneal incision for abdominal aortic surgery: report of a prospective randomized trial. *J Vasc Surg*., 1995, 21(2), 174-81; discussion 181-3.

Tang, TY; Walsh, SR; Fanshawe, TR; Seppi, V; Sadat, U; Hayes, PD; Varty, K; Gaunt, ME; Boyle, JR. Comparison of risk-scoring methods in predicting the immediate outcome after elective open abdominal aortic aneurysm surgery. *Eur J Vasc Endovasc Surg*., 2007 Nov., 34(5), 505-13. Epub 2007 Sep 14.

Tefera, G; Carr, SC; Turnipseed, WD. Endovascular aortic repair or minimal incision aortic surgery: Which procedure to choose for treatment of high-risk aneurysms? *Surgery*, 2004 Oct., 136(4), 748-53.

Torsello, GB; Klenk, E; Kasprzak, B; Umscheid, T. Rupture of abdominal aortic aneurysm previously treated by endovascular stentgraft. *J Vasc Surg*., 1998 Jul., 28(1), 184-7.

Welten, GM; Schouten, O; Hoeks, SE; Chonchol, M; Vidakovic, R; Van Domburg, RT; Bax, JJ; Van Sambeek, MR; Poldermans, D. Long-term prognosis of patients with peripheral arterial disease: a comparison in patients with coronary artery disease. *J Am Coll Cardiol.* 2008 Apr 22, 51(16), 1588-96.

White, RA; Donayre, CE; Walot, I; Kopchok, GE; Wilson, EP; Buwalda, R; De Virgilio, C: Ayres, B; Zalewski, M; Mehringer, CM. Preliminary clinical outcome and imaging criterion for endovascular prosthesis development in high-risk patients who have aortoiliac and traumatic arterial lesions. *J Vasc Surg.,* 1996 Oct., 24(4), 556-69, discussion 569-71.

Williams, GM; Ricotta, J; Zinner, M; Burdick, J. The extended retroperitoneal approach for treatment of extensive atherosclerosis of the aorta and renal vessels. *Surgery*, 1980, 88(6), 846-55.

Xiao, H; Remick, DG. Correction of perioperative hypothermia decreases experimental sepsis mortality by modulating the inflammatory response. *Crit Care Med*., 2005 Jan, 33(1), 161-7.

Zarins, CK; Crabtree, T; Arko, FR; Heikkinen, MA; Bloch, DA; Ouriel, K; White, RA. Endovascular repair or surveillance of patients with small AAA. *Eur J Vasc Endovasc Surg.,* 2005 May, 29(5), 496-503; discussion 504.

In: Aneurysms: Types, Risks, Formation and Treatment ISBN: 978-1-60741-557-2
Editors: Alain Laurent and Ethan Morel © 2009 Nova Science Publishers, Inc.

Chapter 12

Pseudoaneurysm Formation in Severed Arteries

N. G. Gregory
Royal Veterinary College, Hawkshead Lane, Hatfield, AL9 7TA, UK.

Abstract

This paper considers four factors which could predispose an artery to false aneurysm (pseudoaneurysm) formation when it is cut. It then describes recent findings on the frequency of pseudoaneurysm formation during slaughter in livestock for meat consumption. Pseudoaneurysms can develop when carotid arteries are severed in cattle, calves and water buffalo, but not in sheep or goats. Bilateral carotid artery pseudoaneurysms occur in 7% of cattle slaughtered by shechita and 8% of cattle slaughtered by the halal method, and this can delay the onset of unconsciousness during the slaughter process. It is proposed that the main mechanism causing pseudoaneurysm formation in this situation is retraction of the artery within its connective tissue sheath. Blood leaving the severed end impregnates the sheath which swells as it becomes congested with blood. In some cases the swelling covers and occludes the severed end. This could have a protective effect during unintended injuries, but it creates complications during routine slaughter.

Introduction

Pseudoaneurysms can form when there is full depth puncture, rupture, severance or degeneration of an artery wall and blood leaks into the surrounding adventitia. Situations where pseudoaneurysms have been reported include invasive and blunt trauma, bone fractures, intrarterial infusions, biopsy procedures, transplantation surgery, arteritis, periarteritis, atherosclerosis and necrotising pancreatitis (Ahn *et al.* 1997; Cox *et al.* 2007; Ding *et al.* 2008; Flati *et al.* 2003; Hussain *et al.* 2008; Spirito *et al.* 2007).

This paper considers pseudoaneurysm formation when arteries have been completely severed. During the course of the studies reported here it was apparent that a proportion of severed carotid arteries in cattle become occluded by pseudoaneurysms forming at the severed end of the artery, and haemorrhage was arrested. This is of practical importance because it interferes with the slaughter process, either by delaying death of animals in abattoirs or delaying the onset of unconsciousness in animals that are not stunned before slaughter. There are four theoretical mechanisms that could explain artery occlusion during pseudoaneurysm formation. Firstly, a true aneurysm could form at the same time as the pseudoaneurysm if there is shredding of the intima of the artery wall when it is cut. This might enable blood to flow between concentric layers within the artery as well as around the outer perimeter. The resulting swelling might constrict the lumen of the artery and impair blood flow. Secondly, a pseudoaneurysm could form if there is retraction of the severed artery within the surrounding connective tissue sheath when both are cut. This could result in blood flowing around the outer wall of the artery and under or within the connective tissue sheath. The subsequent ballooning might compress the artery or cause folding of congested adventitia over the orifice, limiting blood flow from the severed end. Thirdly, an annular spasm could form if there is a smooth muscle spasm in the artery wall as it is severed. This could create a constriction at the severed end, which might restrict blood flow, creating a jet at the orifice, and make the direction of the flow unpredictable. Coupled with the first two mechanisms, localised misdirected flow at high pressure might contribute to the occlusion. Lastly, there could be white clot formation (platelet clot) at the orifice of the severed artery. This would also restrict blood flow and create a jet at the orifice, which could be directed in an unusual direction. Coupled with one of the previous mechanisms, this might also contribute to occlusion of the severed artery.

A pseudoaneurysm in combination with a dissecting aneurysm may form in other circumstances. For example, it probably occurs in emergency situations when arterial bleeding is prevented by grasping the severed end with artery forceps, rotating the forceps and finally pulling to break and release the artery at the clamped end. In this situation there can be separation of endothelium at the twisted end of the artery.

The aims of this report are to explain the frequency of pseudoaneurysms in severed carotid arteries at slaughter in cattle, sheep and water buffalo, to discuss the likely mechanisms and to consider the value of this situation as a model for pseudoaneurysm formation.

Materials and Methods

Slaughter was examined at 13 slaughter premises in five countries on a total of 1365 animals. There were 231 cattle killed by shechita (jewish method), 116 cattle plus 11 water buffalo killed by halal (islamic method), 387 cattle stunned by captive bolt, 20 cattle stunned electrically followed by an electrical current to induce ventricular fibrillation, 189 calves and 411 sheep stunned electrically. All the animals were bled by severing the carotid arteries, but in a limited number of cases the slaughterman failed to cut both arteries.

In all animals the presence and size of pseudoaneurysms was assessed by palpation at about 30 seconds following the cut whilst the animal was bleeding out. The arteries were located by inserting a hand through the skin wound created by the cut, and following the flow of blood back to the severed end of each artery. The outer diameter of the artery or pseudoaneurysm was assessed by gently palpating the artery with the tips of the fingers and thumb without squeezing the artery. The size of each artery was graded using the 0 to 6-point scale reported by Gregory *et al.* (2006), where increasing score corresponds to increasing diameter. When there was doubt about the assessment, the artery was inspected visually and the diameter measured by ruler. Previous experience showed that palpation was a reliable way of assessing the outer diameter of normal arteries and arteries with pseudoaneurysms. The correlation coefficient between estimation of outer diameter by palpation (y) and measurement by ruler (x) was 0.96 (linear regression coefficient = 0.93; Gregory *et al.* 2006). In some cases, and in particular when there was reduced blood flow, the arteries were located by a combination of palpation and visual inspection.

Arteries were removed from a selection of cattle and promptly fixed in 10 % formol saline. Five arteries with a score of one, and three arteries with a score of 3, were sectioned transversely at their tips and at 1 cm intervals along their length from the severed end. The 2 mm thick specimens were processed routinely for histological examination, and embedded in paraffin wax. A section from each specimen (5 μm thick) was stained with haematoxylin and eosin. Each section was assessed for wall thickness and lumen area, as well as structural relations of the connective tissue, blood clot and artery wall. Total arterial wall thickness and lumen area were measured using a microscope eyepiece graticule (Olympus MIC1156-), which was calibrated using a stage micrometer. From these measurements the change in lumen area was calculated, and this was used as a measure of narrowing or enlargement of the severed end relative to its size in an unaffected region.

The behaviour of partially clamped severed carotid arteries was examined when they were perfused intra-arterially with water in a freshly slaughtered calf. This was done after exposing the arteries, and partially clamping the severed end of each artery with a pair of artery forceps positioned in-line with the long axis of the artery. Sixty ml water was infused from a syringe by hand into the artery at a point caudal to the clamp, and in the direction of the clamp. The clamped end of the artery was examined during the infusion. At the end of the infusion, the clamp was released and the end of the artery plus surrounding tissue massaged by hand.

Results

An example of a pseudoaneurysm in a carotid artery from a slaughtered large bovine is shown in Figure 1. The pseudoaneurysm swelling is at the severed end, and for clarity of presentation adventitia proximal to the enlargement has been removed to expose the outer artery wall.

The histological artery sections showed that swelling at the tip of the artery was associated with blood (fibrin and erythrocytes) trapped within the connective tissue sheath surrounding the artery. There were no signs of infiltration of blood within the artery wall. An example of a section near the severed end of a carotid artery is shown in Figure 2. Mean lumen area of the arteries at 2 cm from the severed end minus lumen area at the severed end was 0.3 cm^2 (± 4.3 se) for the grade 1 arteries and 4.5 cm^2 (± 3.1 se) for the grade 3 arteries ($P > 0.05$). Artery wall thickness did not differ between these two grades.

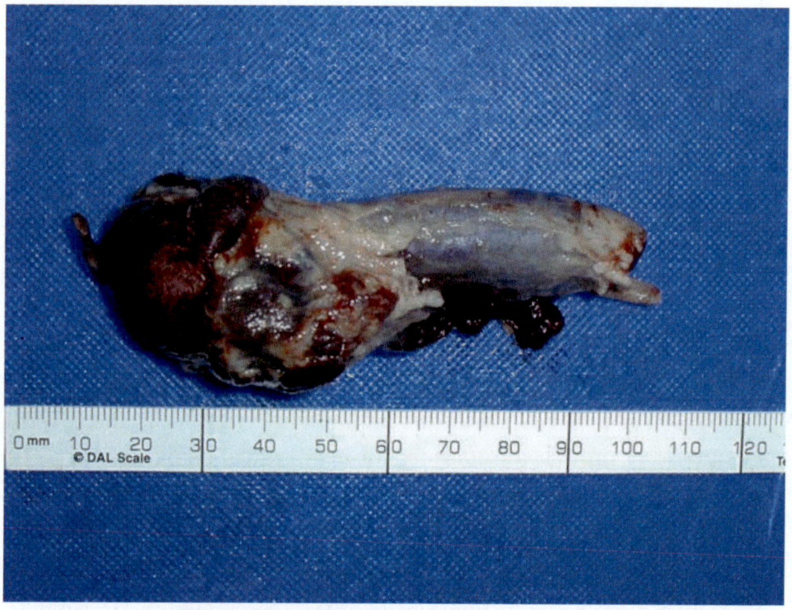

Figure 1. Example of a pseudoaneurysm in a bovine carotid artery.

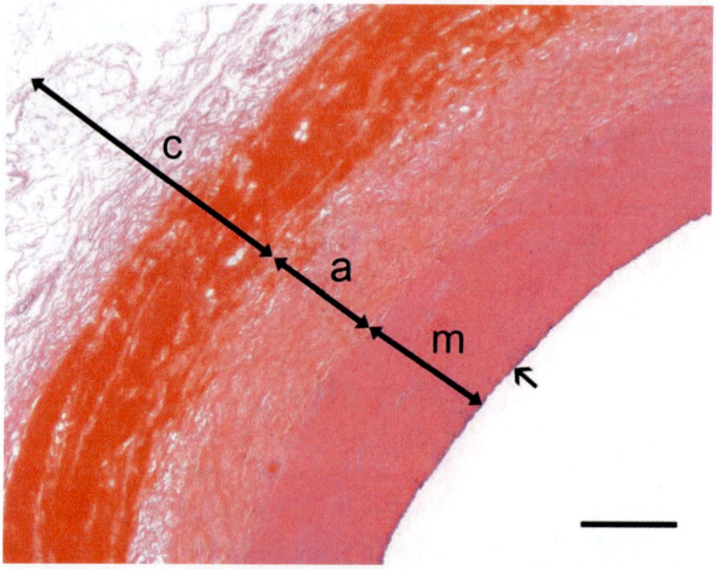

Figure 2. Cross-section of the severed end of a carotid artery. (c) = connective tissue sheath, a = tunica adventitia, m = tunica media. Arrow indicates the endothelial surface. Haematoxylin and eosin. Bar = 0.5 mm.

During infusion of the carotid arteries of the freshly slaughtered calf, the connective tissue sheath welled-up with water at the partially occluded end, and the swelling persisted after the perfusion had stopped, the syringe had been removed and the artery end was massaged. This indicated that enlargement can be a secondary effect of partial occlusion of the severed arteries.

On average, large pseudoaneurysms (outer diameter ≥ 3 cm) were formed in 10 % of arteries during shechita and halal in cattle (Table 1; range 9 to 12 % between countries). The prevalence of animals with one or two pseudoaneurysms larger than 3 cm outer diameter was 18 and 17 % for shechita and halal respectively. In three animals, in which it was noted that arterial blood flow stopped within 20 s after both carotid arteries had been severed, pseudoaneurysm sizes were 2 cm for one artery and at least 3 cm for the other. Using this as an indicator of risk, 8 % of cattle slaughtered by halal and 7 % of cattle slaughtered by shechita were in this category. Three out of the 11 water buffalo had comparable bilateral pseudoaneurysms.

Table 1. Prevalence and size of carotid artery aneurysms following slaughter in stunned and non-stunned cattle and water buffalo

Method	Country	Number of slaughter facilities (slaughter-men)	Number of animals	% carotid arteries according to the size of the severed end, cm diameter					% animals with a carotid artery ≥ 3 cm	% animals with a carotid artery not cut
				≤ 1	2	3	4	5+		
Shechita	Turkey, France and UK	3 (3)	231 cattle	73	12	8	1	<1	18	6
Halal	Bangladesh and France	2 (7)	116 cattle	72	18	9	1	0	17	1
Halal	Bangladesh	1 (1)	11 buffalo	54	14	27	5	0	36	0
Stunning without cardiac arrest †	UK	1 (4)	387 cattle	62	21	10	4	2	25	1
Stunning with cardiac arrest	France	1 (1)	20 cattle	98	0	0	0	0	0	5
Stunning without cardiac arrest	Australia	5 (-)	189 calves	58	17	9	7	9	41	0
Stunning without cardiac arrest	UK	1 (1)	411 sheep	100	0	0	0	0	0	0

The prevalence of pseudoaneurysms with a diameter of 3 or more cm was greater in halal-slaughtered water buffalo than halal-slaughtered cattle (Table 1; $P < 0.01$). The proportion of animals with pseudoaneurysms with a diameter of 3 or more cm was 0 % in sheep.

All the cattle that were electrically stunned and developed ventricular fibrillation before the neck was cut had very little blood flowing from the severed arteries. None of the carotid arteries in those animals had pseudoaneurysms, which indicated that strong arterial pressure was essential for pseudoaneurysm formation.

Discussion

Findings Relevant to Biomedical Sciences

Pseudoaneurysm formation with end occlusion of the severed carotid arteries was sufficiently common to serve as a potential model in biomedical science. The work reported here showed that the condition is seen routinely in bovines in abattoirs. Several questions could be addressed with a bovine model, including what role does an annular spasm at the end of the severed artery play in initiating this type of aneurysm ? Does blade sharpness contribute to arterial wall spasm and pseudoaneurysm formation ? Do co-factors released from platelets play a role in spasm and pseudoaneurysm formation ? When resecting an artery, is it advisable to make the cut near an anchoring point in the connective tissue sheath when wishing to avoid pseudoaneurysm formation ? Understanding the cause of the species differences may direct our thinking about predisposing factors for psuedoaneurysm formation. In addition, a bovine model could be useful in demonstrating the contribution that white (platelet) clot formation can play in arresting a potentially catastrophic haemorrhage.

Platelet clots can form very rapidly at the severed ends of the carotids in calves (Gregory *et al* 1988), but it is not known whether an annular spasm is more important in limiting blood loss. The present work failed to find narrowing of the severed end of cut arteries, and this indicates that annular spasm is not a likely predisposing feature in this type of aneurysm formation. The artery sections showed that blood had infiltrated between the outer artery wall and the inner aspect of the surrounding connective tissue sheath. This supports the view that the enlargement takes the form of a pseudoaneurysm where blood is directed from the cut orifice under the connective tissue sheath. For this to happen the artery probably retracts within the sheath when it is severed, but if there is damage to side branches of the main artery there could also be infiltration within the adventitia. There was no indication of shredding of the artery wall and infiltration of the wall with blood in the sections made in this study, suggesting that true aneurysm formation was unlikely.

The haematoma that was encapsulated in the pseudoaneurysm varied from a uniform concentric layer around the artery to an irregular bulge, which created tortuosity in the artery. It was clear during this study that continued enlargement of the false aneurysm during the early stages of bleeding can lead to obliteration of the vessel. The reasons why some arteries develop pseudoaneurysms and cease to flow whilst others do not were not established, but they could relate to the way blood is directed from the severed end of the artery or from ruptured side branches of the artery into the adventitia. The predisposing factors are also not understood.

This study showed that false aneurysms did not occur when there was an electrically induced ventricular fibrillation. This indicates that the aneurysms do not form when blood pressure is suppressed, and it implies that pseudoaneurysms are more likely to form during the early part of the bleeding period in animals that have a beating heart. There is no reason to suppose that stunning procedures confounded pseudoaneurysm development in the carotid arteries other than through their effect on blood pressure. For example, cattle shot by captive bolt before cutting the vessels in the neck, also developed pseudoaneurysms at the severed ends of the carotids.

Some saccular pseudoaneurysms have a reputation for being friable and tending to rupture when handled (Ding *et al.* 2008), but this was not the experience with bovine carotid artery pseudoaneurysms. This feature could also lend value to their use in model systems.

Implications for Animal Welfare at Slaughter

It has been noted previously that some cattle take a relatively long time to lose brain activity during shechita. For example, in one study the time to loss of somatosensory evoked cortical responses varied between 32 and 126 s (Daly *et al.* 1988). At the time that study was conducted, the reason for this variation was unclear. Similarly, slaughter without stunning in cattle held in an upright position has resulted in long delays (up to 135 s) in some animals before physical collapse (Blackmore 1984). In addition, some cattle have shown a period of recovery, including escape behaviour, following collapse after the shechita cuts (Hoffman, 1900; Klein 1913, 1927; Laux and Bützler, 1927; Levinger 1976). The reason for the variation between individual cattle has not been explained, but the findings in the present study introduce pseudoaneurysm formation, in combination with the collateral supply of blood to the brain through the basi-occipital plexus, as a potential explanation. In the present study, the prevalence of pseudoaneurysm formation during slaughter without stunning was 10% of the arteries and 18% of the cattle.

Pseudoaneurysms can form in calves when their carotid arteries are severed following electrical stunning, and this delays the onset of hypotension and death (Anil *et al.* 1995a). This increases the opportunity for resumption of consciousness following electrical stunning and before the calves die from exsanguination, and the effect may be particularly pronounced in calves because they have a well developed basi-occipital plexus which can serve as a collateral route for blood supply to the brain (Anil *et al.* 1995b).

The primary conclusion from this and related work is that pseudoaneurysm development during shechita and halal slaughter is common (Gregory *et al.* 2008). This could pose a risk of extended consciousness for some of those animals. Since only a proportion of animals are likely to experience the risk, two approaches could be taken when deciding how this situation should be managed. Firstly, the magnitude of the risk of extended consciousness could be determined and then it could be decided whether the hazard warrants further action. Alternatively, the predisposing factors leading to false aneurysm formation could be identified and then ways of overcoming or preventing false aneurysm formation could be considered, to eliminate the risk altogether.

Acknowledgment

This work was partly supported by EU funding under the DIALREL fp6 program.

References

Ahn, J., Trost, D. W., Mitty, H. A. & Sos, T. A. (1997). Pseudoaneurysm formation after catheter dissection of the common hepatic artery: report of two cases. *American Journal of Gastroenterology, 92*, 696-699.

Anil, M. H., McKinstry, J. L., Wotton, S. B. & Gregory, N. G. (1995a). Welfare of calves – 1. investigations into some aspects of calf slaughter. *Meat Science 41*, 101-112.

Anil, M. H., McKinstry, J. L., Gregory, N. G., Wotton, S. B. & Symonds, H. (1995b). Welfare of calves – 2. increase in vertebral artery flow following exsanguinations by neck sticking and evaluation of chest sticking as an alternative slaughter method. *Meat Science 41,* 113-123.

Blackmore, D. K. (1984). Differences in behaviour between sheep and cattle during slaughter. *Research in Veterinary Science, 37*, 223-226.

Cox, M. W., Whittaker, D. R., Martinez, C., Fox, C. J., Feuerstein, I. M. & Gillespie, D. L. (2007). Traumatic pseudoaneurysms of the head and neck: early endovascular intervention. *Journal of Vascular Surgery, 46*, 1227-1233.

Daly, C. C., Kallweit, E. & Ellendorf, F. (1988). Cortical function in cattle during slaughter: conventional captive bolt stunning followed by exsanguination compared with shechita slaughter. *Veterinary Record, 122*, 325-329.

Ding, H., You, C. & Yin, H. (2008). Nontraumatic and nonifectious pseudoaneurysms on the circle of Willis: 2 case reports and review of the literature. *Surgical Neurology, 69*, 4141-417.

Flati, G., Andrén-Sandberg, Å., La Pinta, M., Porowska, B. & Caboni, M. (2003). Potentially fatal bleeding in acute pancreatitis: pathophysiology, prevention, and treatment. *Pancreas, 26*, 8-14.

Gregory, N. G., Shaw, F. D. & Rowe, R. W. (1988). Effect of stunning and slaughter method on brain function and bleeding efficiency in calves. *Proceedings of the 34th International Congress of Meat Science and Technology Workshop on Stunning of Livestock,* 37-38. Brisbane, Australia.

Gregory, N. G., Shaw, F. D., Whitford, J. C. & Patterson-Kane, J. C. (2006). Prevalence of ballooning of the severed carotid arteries at slaughter in cattle, calves and sheep. *Meat Science, 74*, 655-657.

Gregory, N. G., Von Wenzlawowicz, M., Alam, R. M., Anil, H. M., Yeşildere, T. & Silva-Fletcher, A. (2008). False aneurysms in carotid arteries of cattle and water buffalo during shechita and halal slaughter. *Meat Science, 79*, 285-288.

Hoffmann. (1900). Das Schächten; *Archiv für wissenschaftliche und praktische. Tierheilkunde, 26*, 99-121.

Hussain, Q., Maleux, G., Heye, S. & Fourneau, I. (2008). Endovascular repair of an actively haemorrhaging stab wound injury to the abdominal aorta. *Cardiovascular and Interventional Radiology, 31*, 1023-1025.

Klein, C. (1913). Zur Schächtfrage. *Deutsche Schlacht- und Viehhofzeitung, 13*, 81-83

Klein, C. (1927). In: *Sind geschächtete Tiere sofort nach dem Schächtschnitt bewußtlos?* Verlag: Berliner Tierschutzverein, Berlin, Germany. 16 pp.

Laux, H. & Bützler A. (1927). Zur Schächtfrage. *Berliner Tierärztliche Wochenschrift,* 43, 873-875.

Levinger, I. M. (1976). *Physiological and general medical aspects of shechita.* Reprint from: E. Munk & M.L. Munk (Eds.) *Shechita. Religious, historical and scientific aspects,* (214 pp.). Jerusalem: Gur Aryeh Publications.

Spirito, R., Trabattoni, P., Pompilio, G., Zoli, S., Agrifoglio, M. & Biglioli, P. (2007). Endovascular treatment of a post-traumatic tibial pseudoaneurysm and arteriovenous fistula: case report and review of the literature. *Journal of Vascular Surgery, 45*, 1076-1079.

In: Aneurysms: Types, Risks, Formation and Treatment
Editors: Alain Laurent and Ethan Morel
ISBN: 978-1-60741-557-2
© 2009 Nova Science Publishers, Inc.

Chapter 13

May Subclinical Vascular Inflammation Play a Role in the Pathogenesis of Aneurysms?

Ivana Hollan
Lillehammer Hospital for Rheumatic Diseases and Department of Cardiac Surgery, the Feiring Heart Clinic, Norway

Abstract

The pathogenesis of aortic aneurysms is linked to the presence of inflammatory diseases and smoking. In The Feiring Biopsy Study, we found a relatively high occurrence of chronic inflammatory cell infiltrates in deep vascular layers of the ascendant aorta of patients with coronary artery disease. The occurrence and extent of the infiltrates were more pronounced in patients with inflammatory rheumatic diseases (IRD) than non-IRD patients, in current cigarette smokers than non-smokers, and in patients with any history of aortic aneurysms compared to patients without aortic aneurysms. In theory, chronic vascular inflammation may be involved in aneurysm formation and also may contribute to aneurysm instability. Clinicians should be aware of the possibility to detect aortic inflammation using surgical specimens, but also of the pitfalls in the interpretation of the histological criteria of aortitis.

Background

The pathogenesis of aortic aneurysms has not been fully elucidated yet. Several risk factors are known, such as hypertension, smoking or the presence of a chronic inflammatory disease. In addition, inflammation is linked to atheroma formation.

While most research concerns the role of the systemic inflammation for the development of cardiovascular disease, in Feiring Heart Biopsy Study we focused on the local vascular inflammation (1). We hypothesized that vascular inflammation might be common to the disease process in inflammatory rheumatic diseases as well as other conditions associated with a high cardiovascular risk. We further hypothesized thatlocal vascular inflammation might underlie the development of cardiovascular complications.

In this section I will discuss first of all our findings from the aorta (1).

Methods

We analyzed specimens from the aorta of 117 patients with coronary artery disease, included in The Feiring Heart Biopsy Study. Of those, 66 had IRD and 51 had not. The IRD and non-IRD groups were matched for age and sex. The IRD group comprised patients with rheumatoid arthritis (n=23), psoriatic arthritis (n=10), undifferentiated seronegative arthritis (n=1), systemic lupus erythematosus (n=3), ankylosing spondylitis (n=6), reactive arthritis (n=1), giant cell arteritis (n=6), polymyalgia rheumatica (n=14), primary Sjögren's syndrome (n=1), and undifferentiated collagenosis (n=1).

The specimens were obtained during coronary artery bypass surgery (CABG). We collected tissue that was routinely removed for the establishment of aortocoronary anastomoses. Subsequently, part of the adventitia (up to 10x25 mm) was removed from the ventral part of the ascending aorta, and punch holes (4.8 mm in diameter) were made through the vessel wall for proximal aortocoronary anastomoses in the same area. The punch specimens consisted of the intima and media, and sometimes also of a thin layer of the adventitia. To avoid thromboembolic complications, the aortocoronary anastomoses are connected to the aorta in areas with less pronounced gross signs of atherosclerosis. We examined one section from the adventitia, and one from the punch specimens in each patient. In two patients, who underwent repair of an aortic aneurysm during CABG, corresponding specimens were collected from the edge of the aortic incision.

The specimens were stained with haematoxylin and eosin, and scrutinized in a standardized blinded fashion for the presence and extent of inflammatory cell infiltrates in all vascular layers.

Results

Acute inflammatory infiltrate occurred in the adventitia of one non-IRD patient. On the other hand, chronic inflammatory infiltrates were observed relatively frequently in both groups, in all three vascular layers.

Mononuclear cell infiltrates (MCIs) in the intima occurred in the atherosclerotic lesions only, and their occurrences in the IRD and non-IRD groups were similar (5% and 6% respectively, p=0.69). Atherosclerotic lesions were all confined to the intima, and they were present in 21% IRD and 14% non-IRD patients, p=0.35).

MCIs in the adventitia occurred in 30 of 64 (47%) IRD and in 10 of 51 (20%) non-IRD patients (odds ratio=3.6, p=0.002, 95%CI: 1.6-8.5). The number of MCIs and the size of the largest MCI per section were also significantly greater in the IRD group. The MCIs were localized around the vasa vasorum and/or throughout the connective tissue (Figure 1).

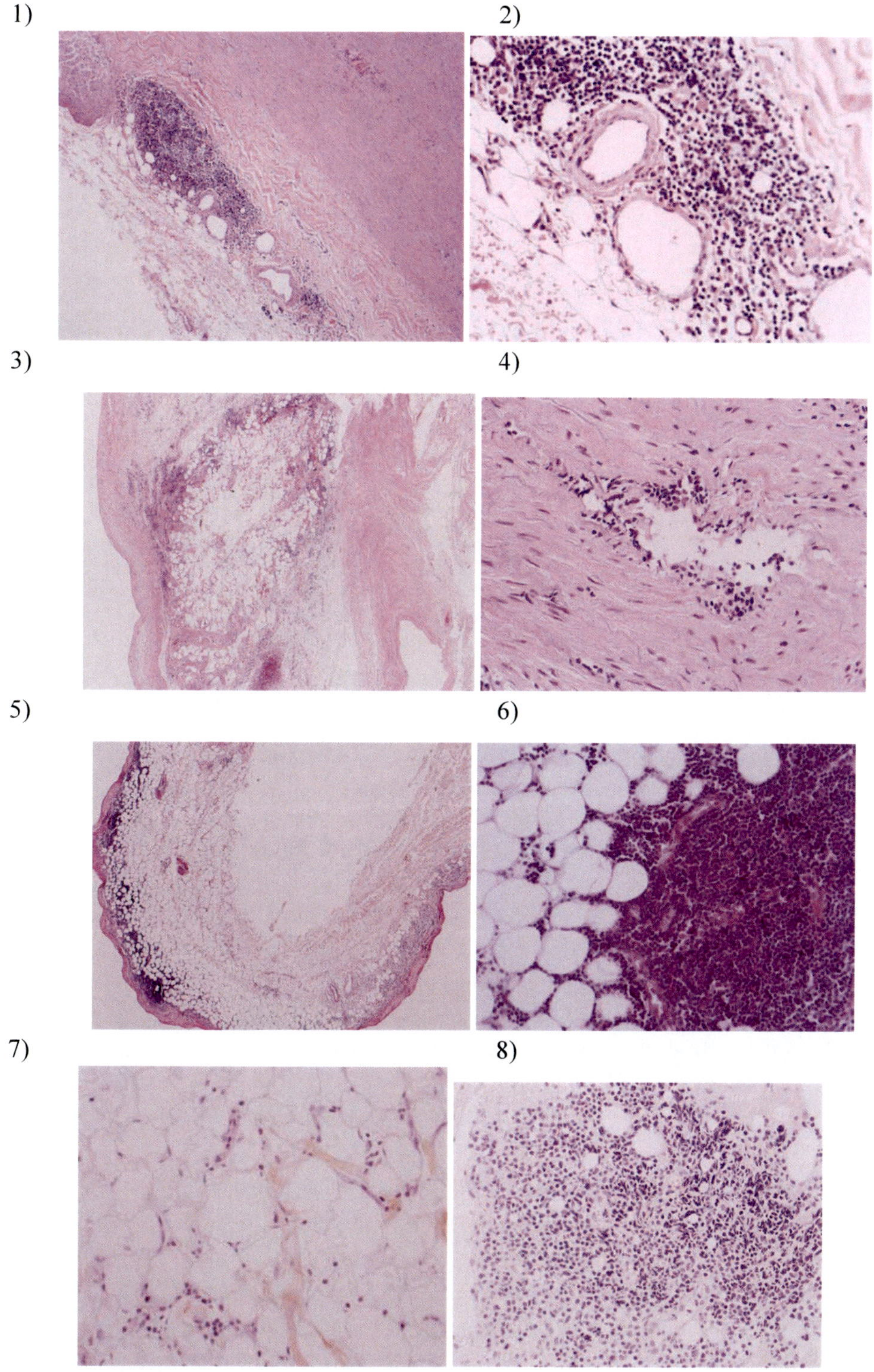

Figure 1. (Continued)

9) 10)

11) 12)

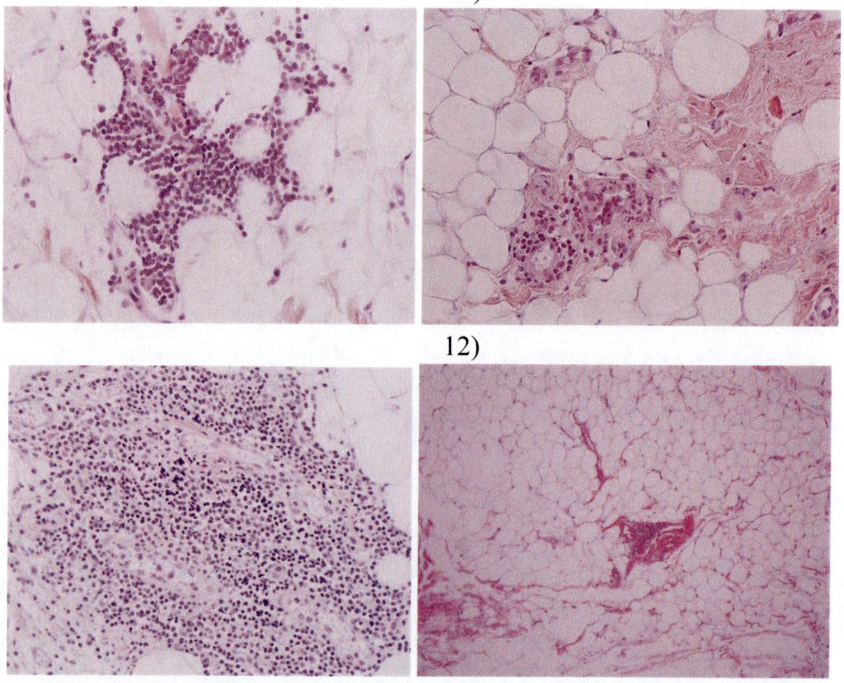

Figure 1. Light microscopy of the aorta: haematoxylin and eosin stain

1) A large MCI in the inner aortic adventitia of a patient with giant cell arteritis (GCA) who underwent repair of ascendant aorta aneurysm during the CABG operation. The patient also had perivascular MCIs in the media, and an atherosclerotic plaque in the intima. The inflammatory changes in the deep vascular layers may be secondary, but also primary to atherosclerosis and/or aneurysm (100×).
2) High-power view of the adventitia from the same specimen as shown in 1 (400×).
3) Pronounced MCI in the aortic adventitia, with fibrosis, of a patient with GCA (40×).
4) MCI in the aortic media of the same patient as in 3 (400×).
5) Pronounced diffuse submesothelial MCIs in the aortic specimen of a patient with RA and thoracic aneurysm. MCIs spread diffusely into the inner adventitia and were also present in the media (40×).
6) High-power view of the adventitia from the same specimen as shown in 5 (400×).
7) Small MCI in the inner aortic adventitia of a control patient (400×).
8) MCI in the inner aortic adventitia of a patient with psoriatic arthritis (400×).
9) MCI in the inner part of the aortic adventitia of a patient with psoriatic arthritis (400×).
10) Perivascular MCI in the inner part of the aortic adventitia of a patient with RA (400×)
11) MCI in the inner part of the aortic adventitia of a patient with ankylosing spondylitis, who had also MCI in the media (400×).
12) MCI in the inner part of the aortic adventitia of a patient with RA, who had also MCI in the media (100×).

Current cigarette smoking was an independent predictor of the adventitial MCIs (OR= 3.93, 95% CI:1.34–11.47, p=0.012 in analyses adjusted for IRD, sex, age and C-reactive protein [CRP]), and was related to the size of the infiltrates.

MCIs in the media were observed only in IRD patients (6 patients):only in those who also had MCIs in the adventitia.

All cases with chronic inflammation in the aorta were subclinical.

Six of 66 patients (9%) with IRD (1 patient with rheumatoid arthritis, 1 patient with polymyalgia rheumatica, 1 patient with systemic lupus, 3 patients with giant cell arteritis) and 1 control patient (2%) had a history of aortic aneurysm. Four of these patients had undergone abdominal aneurysm repair, and 3 patients had a thoracic aneurysm (two underwent aneurysm repair during the actual CABG surgery). The MCIs in the media occurred in 3 of 7 (43%) patients with a history of aortic aneurysm and in 3 of 100 (3%) without such history (p=0.003 by Fisher's exact test). The adventitial MCIs occurred in 6 of 7 (86%) of patients with a history of aortic aneurysm, and in 34 of 108 (32%) of those without (p=0.007 by Fisher's exact test). All patients with thoracic aneurysms had MCIs in the media and pronounced mononuclear cell infiltration in the adventitia, and two (who received an aortic graft during the actual CABG) also had atherosclerotic plaques in the intima. Three of 4 patients with a history of abdominal aneurysm had MCIs in the adventitia of the thoracic aorta (1).

Use of systemic corticosteroids was associated with a lower prevalence and a smaller size of adventitial MCIs in all subgroups, but the effects were not statistically significant. In the RA subgroup, none of 8 patients receiving corticosteroids had inner adventitial MCIs, compared with 6 (43%) of 14 patients who were not receiving corticosteroids; this effect almost reached statistical significance (p=0.051) (1).

Among patients with chronic peripheral arthritis (RA, psoriatic arthritis, or undifferentiated arthritis), inner adventitial MCIs were observed in 2 of 8 patients (25%) treated with methotrexate (MTX), neither of 2 patients (0%) treated with tumor necrosis factor (TNF alpha) inhibitors, 6 of 9 patients (67%) treated with other DMARDs (antimalarial drugs, auranofin, sulfasalazine, CPH82, leflunomide), and 6 of 14 patients (43%) not currently receiving DMARDs (p=0.20).

Among IRD patients, the mean±SD CRP levels in those with and those without adventitial MCIs were 14.4±31.9 mg/liter and 8.5±8.0 mg/liter, respectively (p=0.31). Among control patients, the mean±SD CRP levels in those with and those without adventitial MCIs were 7.4±9.4 mg/liter and 2.9±2.3 mg/liter, respectively (p±0.16).

Discussion

Chronic subclinical inflammatory cell infiltration in the aortic media and adventitia of patients with cardiovascular disease was surprisingly frequent, taking in account that the examined specimens were small and their selection was not based on a suspicion of inflammation.

The occurrence of chronic inflammatory infiltrates in the adventitia of the ascendant aorta was higher in patients with a history of aortic aneurysm (current thoracic aneurysms or surgically repaired abdominal aneurysms) than in patients without such history. Those with thoracic aneurysms had also a high occurrence of MCIs in the media. The medial MCIs may represent a more advanced vascular injury than the adventitial infiltrates.

The clinical significance of the observed chronic inflammation in the vascular media and adventitia is not known. It may be independent of or secondary to aneurysms, but it may also reflect an inflammatory process that induces aneurysm formation or their instability, e.g. by reducing the vessel walls resistance to deformation.

The higher susceptibilities of IRD patients and smokers to the MCIs in the deep aortic vessels may contribute to their increased risk of aortic aneurysms. Smoking is linked to inflammation in lungs and joints as well as trombangiitis obliterans and inflammatory aortic aneurysms. In theory, the high cardiovascular risk in smokers could be, at least partially, related to its proinflammatory effects in the vasculature.

We observed a trend of reduced inflammation in users of certain immunomodulatory drugs. The lower frequency of adventitial MCIs in patients with rheumatoid arthritis treated with systemic glucocorticosteroids compared to the non-users was surprising, because systemic hydrocorticosteroids are usually used in patients with very high disease activity. Therefore, it is possible that the hydrocorticosteroids have a pronounced anti-inflammatory effect on the vessels, which might be protective against development of cardiovascular complications. Thus, their impact on the cardiovascular system might be influenced not only by the negative side effects (such as hypertension), but also the positive anti-inflammatory effects.

The cause of chronic inflammation in deep vascular layers is not known. It may be a result of many various conditions, such as systemic inflammation, pressure, chemical substances, and local infections or auto antigens (such as oxidized low density lipoproteins, heat shock proteins or citrullinated proteins). Or, some of these conditions may play a particular role.

The development of aneurysms may depend both on systemic factors (e.g. traditional risk factors, dysregulation of the immune system or infection), and on local vascular properties (the biochemical composition of the vessel wall, the presence and characteristics of the immunoactive cells in the vessel wall, neurohumoral regulation or microcirculation of the vessel). We note that the adventitial MCIs were often localized around the vasa vasorum, which may be play an important role in the vascular inflammatory process (2).

Both IRD and non-IRD groups had a trend to higher levels of CRP in patients with MCIs in the adventitia compared to those without adventitial MCIs. In theory, the local "subclinical" vascular inflammation might influence the level of circulating inflammatory biomarkers.The opportunities for detecting aortic inflammation are limited. Therefore, it is important to be aware of the possibility to diagnose this condition from surgical specimens. The specimens may be obtained, for example, during aneurysm repair surgery or aortic valve replacement, or from CABG that is a relatively frequent form of surgery.

During our study we became aware of challenges in diagnosing aortitis. Infiltration of the vessel wall by inflammatory cells is one of the criteria for the histological diagnosis of vasculitis. However, there is no defined cut-off for the size or localization of the infiltrates. For example, inflamed atherosclerotic plaques or rare inflammatory cells in the vessel wall are generally not classified as vasculitis. Therefore, additional criteria for distinguishing between vasculitis and atherosclerosis with inflammation are needed. Another possibility is to consider atherosclerosis as a low-grade vasculitis, as some researchers do. Because of the general uncertainty and disparities in the interpretation of the histological criteria, we preferred to present our data in a descriptive form. However, some of our patients had a massive inflammation in their aorta, which would probably be classified as vasculitis in daily clinical practice under a suspicion of vasculitis. It is probablymore important to determine the outcomes of different forms of vascular inflammation than to distinguish between vasculitis vs. nonvasculitis using the presence of inflammatory cells as a criterion.

Additional studies are needed to shed light on the clinical significance of the "subclinical" vascular inflammation. Elucidation of its causes may have implications for the prevention and treatment of aortic aneurysms. In theory, anti-infectious or immunomodulatory treatment such as antirheumatic drugs (e.g. TNF alpha inhibitors, methotrexate or glucocorticosteroids) or statins might be beneficial.

Conclusion

- Chronic subclinical inflammation in the media and adventitia of the ascendant aorta of CAD patients is relatively frequent, especially in those with aortic aneurysms. The vascular inflammation may play a role in the aneurysm formation and/or their instability. The higher occurrence and greater extent of chronic vascular inflammation in IRD patients and smokers may explain why these groups of individuals have a higher susceptibility to aortic aneurysms.
  There is a need for studies that examine the clinical importance of chronic subclinical vascular inflammation, and its treatability.
- Clinicians should be aware of the possibility to detect aortic inflammation using surgical specimens, but also of the pitfalls in the interpretation of the histological criteria of aortitis.

[1] Reference List

[2] Hollan, I; Scott, H; Saatvedt, K; Prayson, R; Mikkelsen, K; Nossent, HC; et al. Inflammatory rheumatic disease and smoking are predictors of aortic inflammation: a controlled study of biopsy specimens obtained at coronary artery surgery. *Arthritis Rheum.*, 2007, 56(6), 2072-9.

[3] Maiellaro, K; Taylor, WR. The role of the adventitia in vascular inflammation. *Cardiovasc Res.*, 2007, 75(4), 640-8.

In: Aneurysms: Types, Risks, Formation and Treatment ISBN: 978-1-60741-557-2
Editors: Alain Laurent and Ethan Morel © 2009 Nova Science Publishers, Inc.

Chapter 14

Reports on Aneurysms in Thailand: A Summary

Viroj Wiwanitkit
Wiwanitkit House, Bangkhae, Bangkok Thailand 10160

Abstract

An aneurysm is an important complication of thromboembolic phenomena. This disorder is considered problematic and requires good medical management. This disorder can be seen in every country with different patterns. Here, the author will review and summarize the previous reports on aneurysms in Thailand. The epidemiology and clinical characteristics (diagnosis and treatment) as well as prevention will be discussed and conclusions will be reached.

Introduction

An aneurysm is an important complication of thromboembolic phenomena. Basically, the thromboembolism occurs when there is a loss in the balance of coagulation and fibrinolysis activity in vivo. This might be due to genetic or acquired etiologies. Three factors— coagulation factor defect, vascular defect and stasis— are the main underlying factors contributing to thromboembolism. When a thrombosis occurs, it can block the physiological flow within the vessel and can cause many problems. The fade of thrombosis is of interest. It can progress in several ways including complete obstruction, induration, elongation, rupture to become an embolism and recanalization. In the case of induration, the thrombus can invade into the media layer of the vessel and might extend further into the externa layer. This invasion brings the destruction of connective tissue in the media layer of the vessel and causes the lost of elasticity. This makes the vessel fragile and if the invasion reaches the externa layer of the vessel, which is a thin layer, the vessel can be deformed into the disorder called aneurysm [1 - 3]. The aneurysm has a very high risk due to its fragility [1 - 3]. Rupture can be seen. Since an aneurysm can be seen in any vessel, the problems can be more severe in specific areas such as the intracranial site and aorta. Rupture of aneuryms in these areas can be fatal. Aneurysm disorder is considered problematic and requires good medical management. This disorder can be seen in every country with different patterns. Here, the author will review and summarize the previous reports on aneurysms in Thailand. The epidemiology and clinical characteristics (diagnosis and treatment) as well as prevention will be discussed and conclusions will be made.

Epidemiology of Aneurysms in Thailand

Similar to other countries, aneurysms can be seen in Thailand. However, knowledge on the epidemiology of aneurysms is limited in Thailand. The first group of reports is on the intracranial aneurysm. In 1998, there was an interesting report from a tertiary hospital on the epidemiology of aneurysms. Phuenpathom et al. retrospectively reviewed the 107 patients on whom direct surgery was done to study the incidence of multiple intracranial aneurysms and found that the incidence was equal to 6.5 % [4]. According to this report, there were 16 aneurysms in 7 cases with multiple aneurysms and there were 2 and 5 patients with 3 and 2 aneurysms, respectively [4]. Phuenpathom et al. reported that the most common site of aneurysm was at the junction of posterior communicating artery and internal carotid artery [4]. Phuenpathom et al. also studied the intraoperative intracranial aneurysm rupture and found that the incidence of intraoperative aneurysm rupture was 7.6 % and its mortality was 33.3 % [5]. Navalitloha et al. performed a similar study in another tertiary hospital in Thailand [6]. Navalitloha et al. found that the incidence of multiple intracranial aneurysms was equal to 8.7 % [6], slightly higher than that reported by Phuenpathom et al. [4]. Navalitloha et al. noted that the patients could be graded according to the scale of Hunt and Hess: 20.1% were classified in Grade I, 33.8% in Grade II, 34.0% in Grade III, 9.6% in Grade IV, and 2.5% in Grade V [7]. Navalitloha et al. found that the mortality and morbidity in all grades were 24.2 % in patients with multiple intracranial aneurysms [6]. Navalitloha et al. concluded that delayed neurological deficit and treatment outcome of poor grade patients significantly contributed to the outcome in patients with multiple intracranial aneurysms [6].

The second group of reports is on intra-abdominal aneurysms. Sriussadaporn et al. reported the epidemiology from a record on surgery of the abdominal aorta at a university hospital in Thailand [8]. They noted that 17.4% of the patients were aged less than 60 years, 77.3% aged 60–80 years, and 5.3% were older than 80 years [8]. They noted that elective abdominal aortic aneurysm repair was the most common indication for abdominal aortic surgery—up to 56.0% [8]. Satdhabudha and Luengtaviboon reported on surgical management for type A aortic dissection from the same setting and indicated very low fatality [9]. Finally, Durongpisitkul et al. reported on an epidemiologic study of Kawasaki disease and noted that abdominal aneurysm was very rare [10].

The last area deals with intracardiac aneurysm. According to the literature search, there is only one report on this topic. Lertsaphacharoen et al. studied infective endocarditis in pediatric patients in a tertiary hospital in Bangkok [11]. Lertsaphacharoen et al. found that mycotic aneurysm is a common complication; other complications included congestive heart failure, cerebral emboli and septic shock [11].

Diagnosis of Aneurysms in Thailand

There are some reports on the advents in diagnosis of aneurysms in Thailand. Most of the reported cases involve the diagnostic feature of imaging technology. Thammaroj et al. reported on predictive CT features in ruptured abdominal aortic aneurysms [12]. They said that a maximum size of aneurysm greater than 5 cm with positive hyperattenuation crescent sign was a sign predicting an aneurysm rupture [12]. Visrutaratna et al. studied the CT findings on mycotic aneurysm of the left subclavian artery and found that CT, particularly multidetector CT, helps in visualisation of mycotic aneurysms [13]. Visrutaratna and Oranratanachai also reported clinics in diagnostic imaging on cerebral aneurysmal arteriopathy [14]. They reported that fusiform dilatation of the segment of the artery was the sign of an aneurysm [14]. Tongprasert et al. reported on prenatal sonographic diagnosis of a congenital ductus arteriosus aneurysm [15]. In this case, Tongprasert et al. found markedly enlarged and tortuous ductus arteriosus with saccular dilation at the distal end, just before joining the descending aorta [15]. They noted that postnatal echocardiography could confirm the prenatal findings [15]. Panchavinnin et al. studied the accuracy of two-dimensional echocardiography in the diagnosis of aortic dissection [16]. Panchavinnin et al. indicated that two-dimensional echocardiography was a reliable non-invasive method for diagnosis of aortic dissection in either the acute or chronic form and proximal or distal aortic dissection [16]. Sahasakul et al. also mentioned that doppler, colour, and cross-sectional echocardiography were useful non-invasive techniques for diagnosing a ruptured aneurysm of the sinus of Valsalva without the need for cardiac catheterisation [17].

Treatment of Aneurysms in Thailand

There are some reports on the advents in treatment of aneursyms in Thailand. Most reports are on the success in treatment by surgical procedures. Some important reports on unusual, difficult, and interesting procedures will be hereby presented. Mutirangura et al. reported on endovascular abdominal aortic aneurysm repair in high risk patients [18]. They reported that this treatment was a safe and effective alternative to open abdominal aorta aneurysm repair, especially in high-risk patients [18]. Wongwanit et al. reported on treatment of iatrogenic pseudoaneurysm of the brachial artery with percutaneous ultrasonographically guided thrombin injection [19]. Wongwanit et al. concluded that percutaneous injection of bovine thrombin under ultrasound guidance is possible as one of the minimally invasive procedures to treat the pseudoaneurysm of the extremity artery [19]. Sriussadaporn et al. reported on successful management of a superior mesenteric artery aneurysm by ligation [20]. They concluded for the success in application of this surgical technique [20]. Chittithavorn et al. reported on repair of extra-cranial internal carotid artery aneurysm with application of modified carotid shunt [21]. Chittithavorn et al. said that they did not expect this shunt to represent the standard commercially available shunt but only an alternative in limited resource setting [21]. Finally, Kamchanapandh et al. reported on obliteration of a ruptured partially thrombosed giant m1 fusiform aneurysm with coil embolization at distal m1 after extracranial-intracranial bypass [22]. Kamchanapandh et al. concluded that combined distal bypass and endovascular obliteration of the aneurysmal sac with coils was a good alternative if vascular reconstruction was difficult [22].

Prevention of Aneurysm in Thailand

Due to the nature of disease, aneurysms usually present to the patient at a late stage, sometimes upon rupture. Therefore, prevention is usually not possible. However, there are some specific prevention measures in some special cases (such as in some specific arterial diseases). In Thailand, preventive medicine is not promoted therefore, only a few reports are available on this topic. Khaosathit et al. reported on treatment of Kawasaki disease with a moderate dose (1 g/kg) of intravenous immunoglobulin and proposed that this was a preventive method for aneurysm development [23]. A similar report was published by Tantiprasit et al. [24].

Conclusion

Although aneurysms are not uncommon in Thailand, the reports on aneurysms are limited. Most reports are only case studies with few further applications in clinical practice. The reports cover a broad area but are very limited in the area of prevention. Promotion of further research on aneurysms is recommended.

References

[1] Aronow, WS. Etiology and pathogenesis of thromboembolism. *Herz.* 1991 Dec., 16(6), 395-404.

[2] Sekhar, LN; Heros, RC. Origin, growth, and rupture of saccular aneurysms: a review. *Neurosurgery*. 1981 Feb., 8(2), 248-60.

[3] Breslin, DJ; Jewell, ER. Peripheral aneurysms. *Cardiol Clin*., 1991 Aug., 9(3); 489-96.

[4] Phuenpathom, N; Ratanalert, S; Sripairojkul, B. Multiple intracranial aneurysms in Songklanagarind Hospital. *J Med Assoc Thai*., 1998 Feb., 81(2), 75-9.

[5] Phuenpathom, N; Ratanalert, S; Saeheng, S; Sripairojkul, B. Intraoperative intracranial aneurysm rupture. *J Med Assoc Thai*., 1999 Apr., 82(4), 332-5.

[6] Navalitloha, Y; Taechoran, C; O'Chareon, S. Multiple intracranial aneurysms: incidence and management outcome in King Chulalongkorn Memorial Hospital. *J Med Assoc Thai*., 2000 Dec., 83(12), 1442-6.

[7] Navalitloha, Y; Taechoran, C; O'Chareon, S. Outcome in treatment of intracranial aneurysm 10 years retrospective study at King Chulalongkorn MemorialHospital. *J Med Assoc Thai.,* 2000 Oct., 83(10), 1150-7.

[8] Sriussadaporn, S; Pak-Art, R; Chiamananthapong, S; Tangchai, W; Nivatvongs, S; Sirichindakul, B; Kitisin, P; Smavatkul, V; Navicharern, P; Tharavej, C; Chatamra, K; Chulakadabba, A; Sangsubhan, C; Tanprayoon, T; Rojanasakul, A; Vajarabukka, T. Surgery of the abdominal aorta: experience of a university hospital in Thailand. *J Med Assoc Thai.,* 2001 Dec., 84(12), 1655-60.

[9] Satdhabudha, O; Luengtaviboon, K. urgical management for type A aortic dissection: 38 cases experience in King Chulalongkorn Memorial Hospital: early result and longterm follow-up. *J Med Assoc Thai.*, 2002 Jun, 85 Suppl 1, S156-62.

[10] Durongpisitkul, K; Sangtawesin, C; Khongphatthanayopthin, A; Panamonta, M; Sopontammarak, S; Sittiwangkul, R; Pongpanich, B. Epidemiologic study of Kawasaki disease and cases resistant to IVIG therapy in Thailand. *Asian Pac J Allergy Immunol.*, 2006 Mar., 24(1), 27-32.

[11] Lertsaphacharoen, P; Khongphatthanayothin, A; Chotivittayatarakorn, P; Thisyakorn, C; Pathmanand, C; Sueblinvong, V. Infective endocarditis in pediatric patients: an eighteen-year experience from King Chulalongkorn Memorial Hospital. *J Med Assoc Thai.*, 2005 Sep., 88 Suppl 4, S12-6.

[12] Thammaroj, J; Vungtal, S; Srinakarin, J. Predictive CT features in ruptured abdominal aortic aneurysm. *J Med Assoc Thai.*, 2006 Apr., 89(4), 434-40.

[13] Visrutaratna, P; Charoenkwan, P; Saeteng, S. Mycotic aneurysm of the left subclavian artery: CT findings. *Singapore Med J.*, 2006 Jan., 47(1), 77-9.

[14] Visrutaratna, P; Oranratanachai, K. Clinics in diagnostic imaging (75). HIV encephalopathy and cerebral aneurysmal arteriopathy. *Singapore Med J.*, 2002 Jul., 43(7), 377-80.

[15] Tongprasert, F; Tongsong, T; Sittiwangkul, R. Prenatal sonographic diagnosis of congenital ductus arteriosus aneurysm: a case report. *J Med Assoc Thai.*, 2005 Apr., 88(4), 541-4.

[16] Panchavinnin, P; Sahasakul, Y; Chaithiraphan, S. Accuracy of two-dimensional echocardiography in diagnosis of aortic dissection. *J Med Assoc Thai.*, 1990 Jun, 73(6), 308-14.

[17] Sahasakul, Y; Panchavinnin, P; Chaithiraphan, S; Sakiyalak, P. Echocardiographic diagnosis of a ruptured aneurysm of the sinus of Valsalva: operation without catheterisation in seven patients. *Br Heart J.*, 1990 Sep., 64(3), 195-8.

[18] Mutirangura, P; Kruatrachue, C; Ophasanond, P; Chaiyasoot, W; Ruangsetakit, C; Wongwanit, C; Siriapisith, T; Sermsathanasawadi, N; Chinsakchai, K; Phongraweewan, O. Endovascular abdominal aortic aneurysm repair in high risk patients: outcomes of management. *J Med Assoc Thai.*, 2007 Oct., 90(10), 2080-9.

[19] Wongwanit, C; Ruangsetakit, C; Sermsathanasawadi, N; Chinsakchai, K; Mutirangura, P. Treatment of iatrogenic pseudoaneurysm of brachial artery withpercutaneous ultrasonographically guided thrombin injection (PUGTI): a case report and a literature review. *J Med Assoc Thai.*, 2007 Aug., 90(8), 1673-9.

[20] Sriussadaporn, S; Prichayudh, S; Sriussadaporn, S; Kritayakirana, K; Pak-art R. Successful management of a superior mesenteric artery aneurysm by ligation: acase report. *J Med Assoc Thai.*, 2006 Nov., 89(11), 1965-9.

[21] Chittithavorn, V; Rergkliang, C; Chetpaophan, A; Vasinanukorn, P; Chowchuvech, V; Chanchayanon, T. Repair of extra-cranial internal carotid artery aneurysmwith application of modified carotid shunt: a case report. *J Med Assoc Thai.*, 2005 Apr., 88(4), 530-3.

[22] Kamchanapandh, K; Imizu, M; Kato, Y; Sano, H; Hayakawa, M; Kanno, T. Successful obliteration of a ruptured partially thrombosed giant m1 fusiform aneurysmwith coil embolization at distal m1 after extracranial-intracranial bypass. *Minim Invasive Neurosurg.* 2002 Dec., 45(4), 245-50.

[23] Khaosathit, P; Hong-Hgam, C; Khositseth, A; Wanitkun, S. Treatment of Kawasaki disease with a moderate dose (1 g/kg) of intravenous immunoglobulin. *J Med Assoc Thai.*, 2002 Nov., 85 Suppl 4, S1121-6.

[24] Tantiprasit, W; Jamjureeruk, V; Sangtaweesin, C; Layangool, T; Kiravittaya, T. Efficacy of IVIG in prevention of giant coronary artery aneurysm in Kawasaki Disease. *Thai J Pediatr.*, 2001 Oct-Dec., 40,4, 279-287.

In: Aneurysms: Types, Risks, Formation and Treatment ISBN: 978-1-60741-557-2
Editors: Alain Laurent and Ethan Morel © 2009 Nova Science Publishers, Inc.

Chapter 15

Parasitic Aneurysm: A Rare but Interesting Form of Aneurysm

Viroj Wiwanitkit
Wiwanitkit House, Bangkhae, Bangkok Thailand 1060

Abstract

Parasitic infestation is a common infectious disease that can be seen around the world. Parasitic infestation can bring several disorders to the host. An interesting complication of parasitic infestation is the formation of an aneurysm. It should be noted that there is a specific group of parasitic infestations that is classified as blood infection. These infections can directly involve the vessel, and an aneurysm can be a complication of these infections. The situation of heartworm infection and Chagas disease will be reviewed and presented.

Introduction

Parasitic infestation, a common infectious disease that can be seen around the world, can cause several disorders in the host. It is a form of living together between two living things in which one wins and the other loses. Some parasitic infestations can result in complications and death of the host. Vascular complications due to parasitic infestation are rare but are documented in the literature. An interesting complication of parasitic infestation is the formation of an aneurysm. This is an extremely rare but significant complication. It should be noted that there is a specific group of parasitic infestations that is classified as blood infection. By definition, blood infection is any infection of the blood within the vessels. Examples of parasitic blood infestations are malaria, filariasis, trypanosomiasis and leishmaniasis. These infections can directly involve the vessel and an aneurysm can be a complication of some of these infections. The situation of heartworm infection and Chagas disease will be reviewed.

Aneurysm in Heartworm Infestation

Heartworm infestation is an important filarial infestation. This is a specific serious disease of dogs that is potentially fatal. Cardiac involvement in heartworm infestation is common and usually severe. Dirofilariasis can be the cause of a fatal aneurysm. A ruptured aneurysm can bring death in the affected host. Miller et al. reported a case of ruptured aortic aneurysm in a wild animal, the coyote, due to heartworm infestation [1]. In this case, necropsy showed an aneurysm within the thoracic cavity as well as severe heartworm infection, with parasites identified in the caudal vena cava. Histologically, inflammatory cell infiltrates could be detected in the aneurysm and consisted of eosinophils, neutrophils, lymphocytes, plasma cells, and macrophages [1]. Thornton et al. noted that this complication is a common problem for the coyote [2]. However, due to the fact that humans are rarely accidentally infested with heartworm, there has never been a case report of an aneurysm due to heartworm infestation in human beings.

Aneurysm in Chagas Disease

Chagas disease, or *Trypanosoma cruzi* infestation, is an important blood infestation. Millions of humans, especially in Latin America, are at risk for this disease. Chagasic myocardiopathy is well described [3]. Elizari reported that the primary infection could be unrecognized and clinically apparent acute chagasic myocarditis might appear in less than 5% of infected individuals, usually children living in endemic areas [3]. Elizari also mentioned that pathological findings were those of dilated cardiomyopathy in the most advanced stages of chronic chagasic myocarditis and the apical aneurysm with thrombus is a frequent and distinctive finding at autopsy [3]. Bittencourt et al. studied chronic Chagas disease and reported that intracardiac thrombi were present in 55.6%, apical left ventricle aneurysms in 44.4% and parasites in the myocardium in 33.3% of all cases [4]. Rassi et al. concluded that cardiac involvement could result in cardiac arrhythmias, ventricular aneurysm, congestive heart failure, thromboembolism, and sudden cardiac death [5].

There have been some studies of Chagas disease in the rat model. According to the study by Factor et al., numerous areas of focal vascular constriction, microaneurysm formation, dilatation, and proliferation of microvessels were specific for infected rats [6]. However, Oliveira et al. found no differences between control and *T. cruzi*-infected rats with respect to mortality, gross heart lesions, and myocardial histopathology after isoproterenol treatment [7].

Aneurysm in Other Parasitic Infestations

Aneurysm can also be seen in other parasitic infestations that are not blood infections. However, those cases are sporadic. Pagnoux et al. said that these cases might be due to the secondary vasculitides [8]. Good examples will be hereby presented. Zhou et al. presented a case of multiple brain hemorrhages and hematomas associated with ectopic fascioliasis in the brain and eye [9]. Fascioliasis, a parasitic infection caused by accidental ingestion of *Fasciola hepatica* metacercariae, is mentioned as the cause of aneurysm in this case report [9]. Ectopic fascioliasis in both the brain and the right eye of a school-aged boy, which was associated with two unruptured intracranial aneurysms, was presented [9]. Zhou et al. indicated that intracranial infection occasionally caused by *F. hepatica* or other parasites could be implied by a fever of unknown origin, eosinophilia, and iterative intracranial hemorrhages [9].

References

[1] Miller, DL; Schrecengost, J; Kilgo J; Ray, HS; Miller, KV. Ruptured aortic aneurysm in a coyote (Canis latrans) from South Carolina. *J Zoo Wildl Med.*, 2007 Sep, 38(3), 492-4.

[2] Thornton, JE; Bell, RR; Reardon, MJ. Internal parasites of coyotes in southern Texas. *J Wildl Dis.*, 1974 Jul., 10(3), 232-6.

[3] Elizari, MV. Chagasic myocardiopathy: historical perspective. *Medicina* (B Aires). 1999, 59 Suppl 2, 25-40.

[4] Bittencourt, AL; Roters, FA; Da Silva, HC. Chronic Chagas cardiopathy in patients aged 12 to 15 years. *Arq Bras Cardiol,* 1990 Nov., 55(5), 301–3.

[5] Rassi, A; Jr. Rassi, A; Little, WC. Chagas' heart disease. *Clin Cardiol*, 2000 Dec., 23(12), 883-9.

[6] Factor, SM; Cho, S; Wittner, M; Tanowitz, H. Abnormalities of the coronary microcirculation in acute murine Chagas' disease. *Am J Trop Med Hyg.*, 1985 Mar., 34(2), 246-53.

[7] Oliveira, JS; Soares, EG; Muccillo, G; Gaspar, PR. Non-potentiation of myocardial lesions by isoproterenol in T. cruzi-infected rats. *Res Exp Med* (Berl). 1984, 184(1), 33-9.

[8] Pagnoux, C; Cohen, P; Guillevin, L. Vasculitides secondary to infections. *Clin Exp Rheumatol.*, 2006 Mar-Apr., 24(2 Suppl 41), S71-81.

[9] Zhou, L; Luo, L; You, C; Wang, B; Xu, J; Liao, L; Hui, X; Cai, B. Multiple brain hemorrhages and hematomas associated with ectopic fascioliasis in brain and eye. *Surg Neurol,* 2008 May, 69(5), 516-21.

Index

B

C

D

E

F

G

H

I

M

N

O

P

Q

R

S

T

U

V

W

X

Y

Z